The Artery and the Process of Arteriosclerosis

Pathogenesis

ADVANCES IN EXPERIMENTAL MEDICINE AND BIOLOGY

The Artery and the
Process of Arteriosclerosis
Pathogenesis

The first half of the Proceedings of an Interdisciplinary Conference
on Fundamental Data on Reactions of Vascular Tissue in Man
April 19-25, 1970, Lindau, West Germany

Edited by

Stewart Wolf

University of Texas System Professor of Medicine
Professor of Medicine and of Physiology
The University of Texas Medical Branch and
Director, The Marine Biomedical Institute
Galveston, Texas

℗ PLENUM PRESS · NEW YORK-LONDON · 1971

The second half of the proceedings will be published as
The Artery and Process of Arteriosclerosis: Measurement and Modification
(Volume 16B of this series).

Library of Congress Catalog Card Number 70-163284

ISBN 978-1-4684-8132-7   ISBN 978-1-4684-8130-3 (eBook)
DOI 10.1007/978-1-4684-8130-3

© *1971 Plenum Press, New York*
Softcover reprint of the hardcover 1st edition *1971*
A Division of Plenum Publishing Corporation
227 West 17th Street, New York, N.Y. 10011

United Kingdom edition published by Plenum Press, London
A Division of Plenum Publishing Company, Ltd.
Davis House (4th Floor), 8 Scrubs Lane, Harlesden, NW10 6SE, England

DEDICATION

        This volume is dedicated to the memory of Dr. John French,
distinguished pathologist and member of the Steering Committee
for the Lindau Conference. University Lecturer at the Sir William
Dunn School of Pathology and Fellow of St. Cross College, Oxford,
Dr. French's research contributed mightily to our knowledge of the
artery in health and disease. The clarity of his thinking, its
penetrating quality and his incisive comments greatly enriched the
Conference. Most of all his superior qualities as a man will be
missed by his many friends who attended this meeting.

PREFACE

The present volume contains the first half of the edited tran-
script of a six-day Conference, "Fundamental Data on Reactions of
Vascular Tissue in Man," held April 19-25, 1970, in Lindau, West
Germany. The remainder of the proceedings, dealing with the epide-
miologic, clinical and preventive aspects of arteriosclerosis, will
be published in a second volume.

The Conference was held under the auspices of the International
Society of Cardiology, the International Cardiology Foundation and
the European Atherosclerosis Group. The aim of the Conference was
to achieve a synthesis of present knowledge concerning arteriosclerosis. Therefore, workers were brought together from several coun-
tries and from various disciplines that do not ordinarily intercom-
municate for free exchange of data and ideas. Six broad subject
areas were introduced by single papers; three of them are included
in this volume. In the discussion which followed each formal presentation, the participants attempted to reconcile disparate data and
interpretations and to reach a clear identification of important areas
of ignorance and of crucial questions for future research.

The format of the proceedings does not follow precisely that of
the Conference itself. The formal papers are included, somewhat ab-
breviated, and excerpts of the discussion have been gathered under
a series of topics arranged in logical sequence. Therefore, the
quoted statements do not necessarily appear in order or in the place
in the program where they were made. Principal issues, syntheses
and unanswered questions are interspersed among the topics as editorial comments.

The Lindau Conference took place less than six months after the
Second International Symposium on Atherosclerosis in Chicago (Atherosclerosis, Proceedings of the Second International Symposium, Edited
by Richard J. Jones, Springer-Verlag, New York, Heidelberg, Berlin
1970). Despite the proximity in time and the substantial overlap in
participants, the Lindau meeting reflected a further step in understanding the pathogenesis of arteriosclerosis. Each presentation of
data was exposed to a more or less leisurely examination and critical

comment by interested participants of varying background and experience. Unfortunately, the remarks of some of the participants did not
come through clearly enough in the tape recording of the Conference
to enable them to be transcribed and included in the Proceedings.
Apologies are therefore offered to these contributors. The full list
of participants follows:

C. W. M. Adams, England
Pierre Alaupovic, USA
Egil Amundsen, Norway
Max Anliker, USA
Felix Anschutz, Germany
Poul Astrup, Denmark
Peter Barth, Germany
Gunnar Biorck, Sweden
A. Bizzi, Italy
Per Bjurulf, Sweden
G. V. R. Born, England
G. Bornebusch, Germany
C. J. F. Bottcher, Holland
David E. Bowyer, England
G. S. Boyd, Scotland
Bernard B. Brodie, USA
Daniel Brunner, Israel
Lars A. Carlson, Sweden
Cesare Cavallero, Italy
Paris Constantinides, Canada
R. C. Cotton, England
Allan J. Day, Australia
F. Delfs, Germany
Ervin G. Erdos, USA
R. Finlayson, England
Frank Fremont-Smith, USA
John French, England
Meyer Friedman, USA
H. Fritsch, Germany
Sven O. Froberg, Sweden
J. Gasser, Switzerland
G. Genthe, Germany
K. F. Gey, Switzerland
Theodore Gillman, England
John L. Gordon, England
Andres Goth, USA
E. Granzer, Germany
Donald E. Gregg, USA
J. C. Gremaud, Switzerland
G. A. Gresham, England
H. Greten, Germany
J. J. Groen, Holland

C. G. Gunn, USA
S. Habersang, Germany
Curtis C. Hames, USA
W. H. Hauss, Germany
M. Daria Haust, Canada
Robert Hess, Switzerland
Siegfried Heyden, USA
Alan N. Howard, England
D. E. Hyams, England
Thomas N. James, USA
Ernst Jokl, USA
Richard J. Jones, USA
G. Junge-Hulsing, Germany
Ancel Keys, USA
F. Kief, Germany
H. Kleinsorge, Germany
G. Klose, Germany
D. Kramm, Germany
W. Krauland, Germany
Franz Kuthan, Switzerland
Robert Laffan, USA
K. Laki, USA
P. D. Lang, Germany
K. T. Lee, USA
Bernard I. Lewis, USA
J. F. Linhart, Czechoslovakia
J. Linzbach, Germany
Hugh B. Lofland, USA
Karl Matthes, Germany
Henry C. McGill, Jr., USA
W. Mehrhof, Germany
W. W. Meyer, Germany
Tatu Miettinen, Finland
Pierre Moret, Switzerland
Esko A. Nikkila, Finland
Herbert Nowak, Germany
Robert M. O'Neal, USA
Robert C. Page, Jamaica, B.W.I.
Frank Parker, USA
Thomas M. Parkinson, USA
Jeremy D. Pearson, England
Th. Pfleiderer, Germany

W. Pollmun, Germany
Lawrence Pottenger, USA
Lina Puglisi, Italy
M. W. Reinheimer, Germany
J. L. Richard, France
Abel L. Robertson, USA
David D. Rutstein, USA
Sigurd Sailer, Austria
R. Sanwald, Germany
Gotthard Schettler, Germany
Gunter Schlierf, Germany
Robert A. Schneider, USA
Hans Schroter, Germany
Colin J. Schwartz, Canada
P. J. Scott, New Zealand
D. Seidel, Germany
D. Sinapius, Germany
Elspeth B. Smith, Scotland
Jeremiah Stamler, USA

Olga Stein, Israel
Yechezkiel Stein, Israel
G. Stork, Germany
C. Bruce Taylor, USA
H. J. Thomasson, Holland
A. Timms, Switzerland
K. Toki, Japan
Marcel Vastesaeger, Belgium
A. J. Vergroesen, Holland
K. von Berlepsch, Switzerland
Mark L. Wahlqvist, Sweden
E. Weber, Germany
A. Weizel, Germany
N. T. Werthessen, USA
Robert W. Wissler, USA
Stewart Wolf, USA
G. Wolfram, Germany
Ernest L. Wynder, USA
Nepomuk Zollner, Germany

The expenses of the Conference and of the preparation of the Proceedings were covered by generous contributions from the following organizations and firms:

Alabama Heart Association
American Heart Association
British Heart Fund
Fannie E. Rippel Foundation
Federal Republic of Germany
City of Lindau
Office of Naval Research
Oklahoma Medical Research Foundation
University of Heidelberg
University of Texas Medical Branch at Galveston
Ayerst Laboratories
Bayer A.G.
Boehringer Mannheim GmbH
CIBA A.G.
CIBA Pharmaceutical Company
Deutsche Maizena Werke GmbH
Farbwerke Hoechst A.G.
Hoffman-LaRoche A.G.
Imperial Chemical Industries
Kali-Chemie
Knoll AG
Margarine-Institut fur Gesunde Ernahrung
Merck, Sharp and Dohme Research Laboratories
Nattermann and Cie. GmbH
Sandoz A.G.

x

Sandoz Pharmaceutical
Schering A.G.
G.D. Searle and Co.
Smith, Kline and French Foundation
Squibb and Sons Pharmaceutical
Unilever Research Laboratories
Upjohn Company
Warner-Lambert Foundation

Arrangements for the meeting were accomplished under the direction of Professor Gotthard Schettler and Dr. Gunter Schlierf. The warm and generous hospitality of our German hosts is gratefully acknowledged. The staff for the Conference was led by Mrs. Cora Gillett, and included Miss Jane Henson, Miss Carol Wehner, Miss Anneke Rieben and Miss Anita Reinartz. The editing of the Proceedings was greatly expedited by the able editorial assistance of Miss Helen Goodell, and by the expert and devoted secretarial work of Miss Jane Henson, who typed the final manuscript, and who, with Mrs. Barbara Altstatt and Mrs. Harriet Ross, also managed the lengthy correspondence preliminary to the Conference. Miss Mary Steichen and Miss Elizabeth Fitzsimmons provided valuable assistance to Miss Henson in organizing and developing the manuscript. Thanks are offered to all of these ladies.

CONTENTS

Chapter 8

Chapter 9

Chapter 1

THE STRUCTURE OF ARTERIES, GROWTH ADAPTATION AND REPAIR:

THE DILEMMA OF NORMAL

Opening Address by Dr. John French

Sir William Dunn School of Pathology, University of Oxford, England
(Dr. French died shortly after the Conference and before he had an
opportunity to edit his remarks for publication and provide illustrations and bibliography. Therefore his words appear here sub-
stantially as he spoke them.)

I shall concentrate on points that appear to me basic to an
understanding of the pathogenesis of atherosclerosis in man. Thus
in the first place, I shall consider only the main arteries, i.e.
the elastic arteries, the aorta, pulmonary, common carotid, sub-
clavian and common iliac, and the larger muscular or distributing
arteries. And secondly, I would like to emphasize the fact that
there are differences depending upon different hemodynamic factors
in the large arteries in large animals, as opposed to the large
arteries in small animals. I hope these points will emerge and
will be kept in mind.

It is usual to consider the arterial wall in terms of three
coats or tunics: the intima, media and adventitia, but in following this systematization it needs to be kept in mind that this
division may, from a functional point of view, be arbitrary and that
in practical terms the whole arterial wall is operating as a single
functional unit adapted to its specific role at that particular site
in the arterial tree.

If we begin at the inner surface of the arteries, we can note
that this interface between circulating blood and the arterial wall
is exposed throughout life to the possibility of deposition of solid
material from the potentially coagulable blood and also subjected to
injury from hemodynamic forces. Looked at this way, the remarkable
thing is perhaps, not so much that the arteries occasionally lose
their patency, but that they do so relatively rarely in relation to
the total number of years at risk. This raises the question, then,

what is the nature of the homeostatic mechanisms which in general ensure that the arterial surface remains smooth and its cellular lining
intact?

It is, of course, fully established that the arteries are lined
by a flattened pavement of endothelial cells. This endothelium is
almost certainly all of the continuous type, i.e. the cells closely
opposed at their junctions without the gaps or fenestrations in the
endothelium that may appear at some sites in the peripheral vascular
bed.

The protection which endothelium provides against deposition
from the lumen may be largely passive, that is to say that it presents a surface that does not normally activate either blood coagulation or the adhesion of platelets, but the physico-chemical basis
for this property of the endothelial surface is not fully understood.
Earlier proposals that the surface properties of endothelium depended on the adsorption of a protective layer of protein from the plasma
or the secretion of a so-called cement substance on to the surface
have not been supported by electron-microscopic observations in which
standard methods of fixation and staining had been used. However,
a thin coating of material which stains with the dye ruthenium red,
and is therefore thought to be rich in polysaccharide material, has
been demonstrated on the luminal surface of the capillary endothelium.
It is also present on the surface of arterial endothelium.

This extraneous coating is probably analogous to the so-called
glycocalyx, to use Stanley Bennett's term, which is well known to occur on the surface of many types of cells and is well developed on the
luminal surface of the blood vessels in some invertebrates (Bennett,
1963). Its precise composition in the mammalian endothelium is not
known but it may well be responsible for the surface properties of
the wall and its maintenance may be one of the important functional
properties of the normal endothelial cell. This work with ruthenium
red suggests in a way a revival in a somewhat modified form of what
I mentioned just a moment ago as the secretory hypothesis of a protective layer on the surface, though Dr. Copley has recently claimed
that this ruthenium red staining material could still represent the
fibrinogen or fibrin which, he previously argued, covered the endothelial surface. This question, I think, is still open.

Evidence that endothelium plays an active role in the prevention
of surface deposit has been gained from studies on the fibrinolytic
mechanism. The presence of a plasminogen activator was first demonstrated in venous endothelium by means of the fibrin plate technique
introduced by Todd (Todd, 1959) and this has been followed up by other
workers, including Warren in Oxford (Warren, 1963). It is now clear
that this activity is present also in, and can be extracted from, the
endothelium lining the aorta, though it is possibly present in lower

concentration in the aortic endothelium than it is in the venous endothelium. This fibrinolytic activity associated with endothelium might
be important in regulating any deposition of fibrin on the surface,
particularly where the experiments of Ashford and Freiman have indicated (Ashford and Freiman, 1968). There may be a local activation
of the coagulation mechanism at the surface of an injured endothelial
cell. The cell is not destroyed, the findings suggest, but the surface membrane is broken, then you can demonstrate fibrin formation at
that site of injury if fibrinolysis is suppressed. Incidentally, the
relatively high activity of fibrinolytic properties in the adventitia
of arteries can probably be related also to the endothelium of the
vasa vasorum. Whether endothelium may play an active role in the prevention of platelet adhesion other than by covering up the collagen
fibers or basement membrane beneath it, is uncertain. Endothelial
cells contain phosphatases which can break down ADP and, since this
substance is involved in platelet aggregation, these endothelial enzymes might possibly be concerned in the dispersal of any small platelet aggregates that form at the surface, but it is not at present, to
my knowledge, known whether ADP is directly involved in adhesion at
the vascular surface, as distinct from aggregation, or whether platelets can indeed adhere tenaciously at all unless underlying collagen
or basement membrane is exposed by endothelial damage.

The next point I should like to take up is how the structural
integrity of the endothelial layer is maintained in spite of the
hemodynamic forces which are continuously acting on it. In the
elastic arteries, which are subjected to stretching of the wall during
systole, the cells presumably have some measure of extensibility and
are sufficiently firmly attached to one another at their periphery to
prevent them being pulled apart with each pulse movement. However,
if the cells are not injured within the normal limits of stretching,
there is evidence from the recent work of Dr. Fry (Fry, 1968) in the
United States, that the endothelial cells may undergo structural damage at sites where there are high rates of shear at the surface or
turbulence of flow. It can therefore be expected that there will be
greater wear and tear of the endothelium at certain sites in the arterial tree and that there must be some way in which potential destruction by wear and tear is compensated for in the vessel that remains
normal.

The ability of endothelium to regenerate has usually been considered in relation to the repair of relatively large defects of the
endothelial surface caused by experimental injury, or in relation to
the organization of the surface of arterial protheses, or the organization of mural thrombi. Endothelium grows in these situations and
it is established that endothelium can indeed regenerate by mitotic
division of cells from the intact edges of the defect. I would just
remind you of some experiments by Poole, Sanders and Florey (Poole
and Sanders et al., 1958) in which they scraped the endothelium off
from a 2 cm. length in the abdominal aorta of a rabbit and within

a day or two noted endothelial cells beginning to spread over that
area. They demonstrated mitotic figures in endothelial cells just
behind the growing edge.

If we think of this as preserving the integrity of the endothelial
surface, this growth in this way is a process which takes time to
complete, depending on the size of the defect. Actually, with that
2 cm. length defect in the rabbit aorta, it took up to a year for it
to be fully completed, but experiments with smaller defects by other
workers - Bjorkerud in Sweden (Bjorkerud, 1969), for example - have
shown that quite small defects of the endothelium will stimulate mitosis around them within a day or two, and they may be completely
covered within a week. But there is still the question of what is
happening during this interval.

During the healing process, cells from the circulating blood
platelets and leukocytes adhere to the surface, but it is not known
clearly whether this serves any temporary protective function. This
adhesion of platelets is usually considered only as a pathological
process which under the appropriate conditions of blood flow will
lead to thrombosis. The proposal has been made that the leukocytes,
presumably monocytes, from the circulating blood can, by colonizing
the surface, give rise to new endothelium. This is a difficult
question which, I feel, still really lacks conclusive proof, whether
endothelium can regenerate from circulating cells.

When experimental injury is less severe, as for example when a
rubber coated clamp is used to compress a vessel, gross destruction
of the endothelium may not occur but individual injured cells, rather
than whole groups of cells, then undergo shrinkage and are gradually
displaced by cell division in the surrounding endothelium. This seems
to be the most likely way in which injured or effete cells could be
replaced in the normal artery without the creation of temporarily
denuded areas. In this regard, recent studies using tritiated thymidine and autoradiography to demonstrate endothelial cells engaged
in DNA synthesis have indicated that the endothelium is undergoing a
continuous slow replacement and that the rate of turnover is higher
near the sites of branching, for example, where it can be anticipated
that the greater hemodynamic stress might lead to shorter cell survival.
Dr. H.P. Wright (Wright, 1971) is doing experiments on this subject
using a guinea pig aorta. The animals had been injected with tritiated
thymidine 24 and 16 hours before sacrifice. The labelling rate of the
endothelial cells was greatest over the arch, and at the bifurcation.
After creating an artificial aortic constriction a higher rate of
labelling appeared in that region than in the control. This work has
yielded the tentative information that normal endothelial cells survive between 100 and 180 days, but that in some regions, subject to
particular hemodynamic stresses, this survival time is shorter, and
in Dr. Wright's experiments ranging there from 60 to 120.

Now turning to the sub-endothelial space, i.e. the space between
the endothelium and the internal elastic lamina, in the main arteries
of small mammals such as the mouse,
Differences in   rat or rabbit, the outer surface
intima between   of the endothelium is very close to
small and large   the internal elastic lamina and
mammals   in most regions only a narrow zone
of ground substance and possibly
a few fibers separate these two structures. This description of the
intimal architecture applies only to the vessels in a small animal.
The intima is much thicker in comparable vessels of large animals.
Thus in man and in many other large mammals, it is only in the fetus
or the new born that this close approximation of the endothelium and
the internal elastic lamina can be seen in the aorta and main distributing arteries, and in the adult the thickness of the sub-endothelial zone varies widely in different regions and possesses a considerable population of cells and fibers.

Since during the development of arteries, the elastic tissue
which extends to form the ultimately continuous internal elastic
lamina appears first as small islands in the position of the endothelial basement membrane, or the shared basement membrane of endothelium and smooth muscle, it seems likely then that the internal
elastic lamina and basement membrane could basically be analogous
structures and have primarily a supporting function for the endothelium.
The interposition of ground substance may allow some slip of endothelium over the lamina when the arterial wall extends or contracts.

The intima of the aorta in adult man
Thickening of intima   forms about 1/6th of the total thickness
in man with growth   of the wall, and it is not a simple structure.
It consists of a network of fibro-elastic
tissue supported in a mucinous ground substance. In its deeper part,
the elastic fibers are coarser and are associated with smooth muscle
cells to give a rather poorly defined edge to the internal elastic
lamina. In the coronary arteries in man, there is an apparent
penetration by smooth muscle cells of the space between endothelium
and internal elastic lamina during childhood to form this so-called
musculo-elastic layer which we see also in the pig. This formation
occurs first in relation to the orifices of proximal branches, but
later extends widely to form a substantial part of the total thickness of the wall. Then, in man, and to some extent in the pig, an
elastic hyperplastic layer composed of circularly directed elastic
fibers with relatively few cells among them, forms on the luminal
side of the muscular elastic layer, so the intima is getting thicker.
And finally in the third decade of life, an additional connective
tissue layer is formed immediately beneath the endothelium.

The functional significance of the thickened intima in large
arteries with its relatively loose texture and longitudinal orien-

Nutritional role of thickened intima vs response to injury -- perforation in internal elastic lamina

tation of cells and fibers, is not obvious to me, at any rate. In part, it may be an adaptation to longitudinal stress and extension in arteries. It has also been proposed that this thickened intima acts as a sponge which imbibes plasma filtrate from the lumen and that the passage of the pulse wave then has a milking effect which serves to squeeze the filtrate outwards through the wall. In this way it might have a role in the nutrition of the thick wall of large arteries, if the thickening provides a little nutrition, pumps so to speak. But on the other hand there are many features of this intimal thickening which are consistent with a response to injury. Thus, where the thickenings first appear, for example in the proximal part of the coronary arteries in growing animals, there are always discontinuities in the internal elastic lamina at the deep edge of the intima, an apparent protrusion of smooth muscle cells from the media into the sub-endothelial space and an increase in these regions in the metachromatic staining of the ground substance. This has been demonstrated to be a standard response to injury in vessels.

It may therefore appear that a simple elastic lamina close to the endothelium may represent the ideal construction for an artery, and in fact is adopted in the small mammals, but that such a construction may not be strong enough to meet the increasing stretching forces which act on the inner part of the wall of an artery as its diameter increases with growth in the large mammals and beyond a certain size evidence of injury and repair will always be found at certain critical points in the arterial tree in the large mammals

Adaptation to stress vs injury and repair. The dilemma of normal

including man. If this is so, then it becomes extremely difficult to draw a line between growth changes and pathological changes in the structure of the intima. A change that always occurs in the artery of the pig, for example, would, if you saw it in the rabbit, be interpreted as a response to some extraneous injury.

The mechanical properties of the arterial wall can largely be accounted for by the structure of the tunica media. The requirements in the media differ as between the elastic and the muscular arteries, but in each situation they are met by the combined action of elastic tissue, collagen and smooth muscle, each with distinctive properties when examined in isolation. The tunica media of the large muscular arteries, which of course are under fine neural control, consists very largely of smooth muscle cells arranged spirally in concentric layers, but as Burton has pointed out, there is a need for the combination of muscle, collagen and elastic fibers to provide stability. A few bundles of collagen fibers are present between the muscle cells of the media of the muscular arteries and some loose

networks of elastic fibrils are arranged circumferentially, but the
main concentration of elastic tissue is in the well defined internal
elastic lamina between media and intima and, less constantly, in an
external elastic lamina between the media and adventitia.

There may be some advantage in having the elastic membranes
of the muscular arteries condensed to a single dominant lamina but
it does appear that a relatively strong internal elastic lamina has
secondary effects that are relevant to some of the problems in
arterial disease. You could say that on the one hand an intact
internal elastic lamina appears to re-
strict the migration of cells from the
media into the sub-endothelial space,
and that the thickening of the intima
by the cellular migration may occur
when that internal elastic lamina be-
comes defective. So we might think of it as having a restraining
influence on any migration of cells from the media into the intima.
Then, on the other hand, it is usually stated that the presence of
fenestrae in the lamina means that it does not present a barrier to
the passage of plasma filtrate through the wall. There are fenestrations in the internal elastic lamina in the rabbit aorta that
range in width from 2 to 7 micra. Nevertheless, in cholesterol-fed
rabbits very little cholesterol is found beyond the internal elastic
lamina. Thus it does seem to provide a pretty sharp limit to the
extension of cells and to the movement of lipid material presumably
coming from the lumen. These properties of the internal elastic
lamina in relation to permeability and restraint certainly warrant
further investigation.

In the elastic arteries as exemplified by the thoracic aorta,
there are different functional demands on the media. By exerting
the so-called Windkessel effect, these vessels maintain the blood
pressure during diastole and ensure that there is a continuous forward
flow of blood. The structural adaptation to this situation is seen
in the preponderance of elastic tissue with muscle playing a relatively minor role in regulating tension in the elastic laminae. And in
contrast with the situation in muscular arteries, there are in the
thoracic aorta multiple concentrically arranged laminae, evenly
spaced throughout the media. These concentric laminae are cross-
connected by elastic fibers and inter-leaved with circumferentially
arranged smooth muscle cells and thin collagen fibers.

According to Wolinsky and Glagov, (Wolinsky and Glagov, 1964)
the construction of these arteries is such that tensile forces are
distributed uniformly throughout the wall so that any focal defects
in one of the laminae could occur without there being any overall
effect on the properties of the wall. These same workers also propose that each of these elastic laminae with its adjacent compartment

containing collagen and smooth muscle can be considered as a functional
unit in the media of the aorta. The number of units required in a
particular vessel would then depend on the total tension in the wall.
Bearing in mind that the tension in the wall depends on the radius
as well as the pressure, it is understandable that while a mouse may
require only five such units in the wall of its aorta, the rabbit
requires 20, and adult man about 60. Since the thickness of the units
is fairly constant, it is obvious that the structures required to
meet the greater tension in the wall of the aorta in large mammals
can only be accommodated in a much thicker wall (say 0.3 mm thickness
of aorta in the mouse, 1.2 mm in man).

The greater thickness of the walls of the main arteries in large
mammals introduces problems in the nutrition of the wall which are not
encountered at all in small mammals. It appears that the nutrition
can be maintained from the lumen if the total thickness of the wall
in the adult animal does not exceed approximately half a millimeter,
so there is no need for vascularization of the media of the aorta,
and indeed it does not occur in such animals as the rat or the rabbit.
Where the wall exceeds this critical thickness, as in man for example,
the wall is partly vascularized by medial vessels. These medial
vessels can only extend as far inwards, apparently, as the pressure
gradient across the wall will allow. Thus, regardless of species,
there is always an avascular zone in the inner part of the wall of
the arteries and in those species requiring vasa vasorum, this zone
appears to have a remarkably constant structure, as Wolinsky and
Glagov have shown (Wolinsky and Glagov, 1964), being made up of
approximately 29 of the structural units already described.

The vasa vasorum and the avascular zone

I expect that later speakers will
discuss the formation of elastin and
collagen in the arterial wall, particularly
this interesting question of the whorl of
smooth muscle cells in histogenesis and the way in which these fibers
are modelled or remodelled during body growth. I have also neglected
to discuss the cells of the adventitia. We have emphasized endothelium
and smooth muscle, made a passing mention of fibroblasts in adventitia,
but of course in pathological lesions the macrophage is a very important
cell and, no doubt, there will be some discussion later as to the
potential origin of phagocytic macrophages in the arterial wall.

But just to conclude, if I may, I would like to return to a very
brief consideration of what Anitchkov described as the lymph stream
through the wall of arteries, implying a continuing flow of plasma
from the lumen to the lymphatics of the vasa vasorum. His was a
physiological concept upon which many theories, particularly the
filtration hypothesis of atherosclerosis have been based, and yet
I can find remarkably little factual data in the physiological lit-

The lymph stream

erature about this point. This seems
to be something that pathologists
investigate, physiologists in general
do not, though there are exceptions. To my knowledge there is at
present no satisfactory way in which lymph, obtained exclusively by
filtration from the lumen through the wall, can be obtained for
quantitative analysis in experimental animals. Concepts about the
composition of the lymph stream have depended largely on an extra-
polation from what is known to occur in the peripheral vascular bed.
Confirmation that this may actually apply in the arterial wall has
been sought by measurement of the concentration gradient of labelled
material across the wall from the lumen to the adventitia.

As far as the permeability characteristics of small vessels,
capillaries and venules in the peripheral vascular bed are concerned,
two structures, endothelium and basement membrane have been studied
in considerable detail. The endothelium of arteries appears to be
structurally similar to the endothelium in capillaries of the continuous type and its permeability characteristics also appear to be
quantitatively the same. While no absolute agreement has yet been
reached, it now seems probable that the intercellular junctions between
endothelial cells transmit water and solutes, including protein molecules
up to about 40,000 molecular weight, and that larger protein molecules,
which escape only slowly from the circulation, do so through the system
of vesicles in the endothelial cytoplasm.

Arterial endothelium is, of course, exposed to a higher pressure
than capillary endothelium, but the actual pressure drop across the
endothelium is not necessarily any greater. The pressure is thought
to fall quite steeply in the inner part of the wall of elastic arteries,
but presumably this occurs across the internal elastic lamina and not
across the endothelium itself. However, it is known that the permeability of endothelium to protein may be greatly increased by separation of endothelial cells or by direct injury. It can be anticipated,
therefore, that arterial endothelium would similarly be more permeable
at sites of hemodynamic stress and this seems to be borne out by the
finding of regional differences in the ability of protein labelled by
dye or radioactivity to enter the inner part of the wall of apparently
normal arteries.

The comparison of the permeability of the arterial wall with
that of the capillary wall becomes very much more difficult, once you
begin to look beyond the endothelium. Normally the endothelium may
regulate the proportion of the plasma constituents which enter the
inner wall, but their subsequent movement now depends on the properties
of the ground substance and, as has already been suggested, on their
ability to pass through the relatively restricted channels in the successive elastic laminae. I am personally not qualified to discuss the
important question of how the compositon of the ground substance may

restrict the movement of fluid and solutes through the arterial wall
and exert a sieving effect with regard to large protein and lipoprotein molecules, but I hope that this subject will not be neglected
in the discussions which follow.

DISCUSSION

PARTICIPANTS: C.W.M. Adams, G.V.R. Born, D.E. Bowyer, P. Constantinides,
F. Fremont-Smith, John French, T. Gillman, M.D. Haust,
G. Junge-Hülsing, A. Keys, H.C. McGill, Jr., W.W. Meyer,
A.L. Robertson, C.J. Schwartz, E.B. Smith, C.B. Taylor,
K. von Berlepsch, R.W. Wissler and S. Wolf

DR. MCGILL: Dr. French quite properly emphasized the difference
in the thickness of the musculo-elastic layer in the human coronary
arteries and pointed out the differences among animals, particularly
between small and large animals. May I ask for Dr. French's interpretation of the significance of this musculo-elastic layer? Is it
a normal anatomic structure in the human, or is it a response to injury, or can you reconcile these conflicting attitudes?

DR. FRENCH: This is a difficult question, because it really
depends on what you mean by normal. If normal means that it is
always there, then it is normal in man, but it isn't always there in
smaller animals, so that it's abnormal for a rabbit. It would require
an injury to produce it. The change may well have functional significance particularly in relation to the longitudinal tensions that
develop in the inner wall of arteries at points of branching and
where they are tethered by side branches so that one could then
understand why development of longitudinal smooth muscle in the intima might compensate for this. I also mentioned the possibility
that has been suggested, I think largely hypothetical, that this
thickened intima may aid in the nutrition of a relatively thick wall
by, as I say, acting as a sponge. But one is left, nevertheless,
with this extreme similarity in morphology between what happens
spontaneously in these large arteries in large mammals and what happens in response to injury to the internal part of the wall in smaller
experimental animals. The sequence of events in a normal and in a
pathological process seems to be exactly the same, the former state
characterizes a large and the latter a small animal following an
injury or other atherogenic stimulus. A single internal elastic
lamina close to the endothelium may be the ideal state, but there's
something about the nature of elastic tissue that won't allow it to
function when the artery gets too big, or when the internal tension
is exceeding the capacity of a single strong internal elastic lamina
to compensate for it. You may call it injury and repair, or what
Dr. Gillman will call remodeling, a tissue change that's necessary

during the development of the animal. So it's really a question of
terminology, whether one calls it physiological or pathological, but
I think that however one looks at it, there's no doubt that this
development of the intima sets the scene for what happens later on
in the development of the atheromatous lesion. I don't see that one
can be more specific than that.

COMMENT

The similarity of changes in the architecture of the arterial
wall associated with growth, those associated with adaptations to
hydrodynamic forces and those concerned with repair of injury, suggested that the distinction between a normal and abnormal tissue
response is largely a matter of degree. This conceptual thread can
be traced throughout the conference, together with the corollary
implication that over-responsiveness or insufficient modulation of
artery wall metabolism leads to excessive cellular proliferation and
undue thickness of the intima with consequent compromise of nutritional supply, and ultimately necrosis.

QUESTION: The final question is whether intimal cellular proliferation is responsive to some environmental stimulus or whether
it is actually a genetically programmed process of remodeling.

DR. FRENCH: Whether genetic or environmental, I think intimal
proliferation is a price that has to be paid, so to speak, for
arteries getting large in large animals.

Development of aortic   DR. M. DARIA HAUST: Studies of the
wall during fetal life   morphogenesis of the aorta during fetal and
and infancy   early neonatal life may throw light on the
                           development of the musculo-elastic layer
of the intima and on the problem of what is normal intima. Our
observations were made on the vessels of man and swine.

It has not been widely realized that the "clues" concerning the
potentials of tissue to react are best provided from studies on the
morphogenesis of tissues or organs in fetal life; it will be seen
that under pathological conditions such as atherosclerosis, the
components of the organ concerned, i.e., of the artery, "remember"
what they were capable of performing in fetal life and simply revert
to such activities.

The "youngest" human aortic tissue available to us for the study
was after ten weeks of gestation. The endothelium appears to rest
immediately upon the internal elastic lamina which already at this   **HUMAN**
time is prominent and almost continuous. The media consists of
aggregates of cells arranged in loose, and not always well defined,
circular layers. The elastic lamellae that separate these layers of

cells in later life also are not fully developed. By light microscopy it is not possible to determine the nature of these medial cells
for several months of gestation. They are of various sizes and configuration ranging from polygonal to oval, and are reminiscent of
mesenchymal cells. The cytoplasm may be abundant or scanty, the
nucleus is usually large, vesicular, oval to round, and occasionally
indented (FIG. 1).* However, by electron microscopy these cells have
some features of definite differentiation toward smooth muscle cells,
even in our "youngest" aortae. Thus, the largely undifferentiated
cells have many pinocytotic vesicles, and already have acquired their
enveloping basement membrane (FIG. 2), a feature not characteristic
of a developing or mature fibroblast. The spatial relation between
units of elastic tissue (Haust and More et al., 1965) and the basement
membrane of these medial cells is apparent in man as well as in the
swine (FIGS. 3 and 4); collagen fibrils often develop between the
plasma membrane and the basement membrane in the porcine aorta (Haust
and More, 1967), whereas no such relation is observed in the human
vessel. Elastic units, consisting of a central amorphous core
surrounded by microfibrils, fuse to form larger elastic elements
(fibers, lamellae) (FIG. 5), and the collagen fibrils align themselves
in bundles in the growing and maturing vessel. The microfibrils (Haust,
1965) have a composition different (Waisman and Carnes, et al., 1969)
from that of a "whole" elastic tissue (Partridge and Elsden, et al.,
1963) and collagen. Once this extracellular framework is established,
the cells responsible for its elaboration change their morphological
features characteristic of secretion (e.g., prominent rough-surfaced
endoplasmic reticulum and Golgi zone, numerous and various vesicles)
to those of more typical smooth muscle cells, including the shape.
They acquire numerous (myo-)filaments that fill the cytoplasm and dis-
play the triangular and oblong "densities"; the mitochondria, diminished
in number, and the few profiles of rough-surfaced endoplasmic reticulum
are arranged largely in the perinuclear region; the nucleus is elongated
and cigar-like in shape, and its chromatin is distributed in a fashion
characteristic of smooth muscle cells (FIG. 6). At the end of gestation the intima is narrow; it consists usually of endothelium which
rests upon its own basement membrane and is separated from the underlying internal elastic lamina only
by a narrow space containing micro-
Beginnings of   fibrils. At times, however, the
intimal   diffuse intimal thickening that
thickening   usually begins to develop after
birth and is a normal feature of all growing aortae is present in some
areas already at birth. Here, the elaboration of elastic and other
connective tissues proceeds in a fashion similar to that of developing media, including the changes of cytological features described
above.

The following are conclusions drawn from the above studies that
in part are relevant to some aspects of the morphogenesis of athero-

---

*Figures for this chapter will be found on page 30ff.

sclerotic lesions:

1. The connective tissue framework (elastica and collagen) of the developing human and porcine aortic wall is elaborated and organized by cells that have morphological characteristics of smooth muscle cells quite early in the process. Thus, contrary to similar investigations in other species on the basis of which it was concluded that cells elaborating connective tissues in the developing aorta are immature and mature fibroblasts (Karrer, 1960) later transforming into smooth muscle cells, our studies show that, at least in man and swine, such "transformation" does neither take place, nor is it necessary.

2. The cells of developing aorta do not "cease" to be smooth muscle cells because they are involved in the formation of connective tissues; if we continue to define given cells by morphological criteria rather than on the basis of function (or potential!) then these ·cells are, indeed, smooth muscle cells in spite of their ability to form connective tissues. In the latter capacity they resemble several other types of cells in addition to fibroblasts.

3. Under the pathological conditions of atherosclerosis, the potential of the arterial smooth muscle cells for elaboration of connective tissues that was manifested in fetal life, is "called-upon," and, for whatever the reason of Nature, these are largely the cells responsible for the fibrous component of the atherosclerotic plaque (Haust and More, et al., 1959; Haust and More, et al., 1960; Haust and More, 1966).

COMMENT

In response to a challenge of her statement that smooth muscle cells produce collagen and elastin, Dr. Haust referred to the evidence provided by the published work of hers and her co-workers and by the unpublished work of Dr. Russel Ross of the University of Washington, Seattle. Her comments, supported by Dr. Wissler, were to the effect that Ross has grown in tissue culture arterial medial cells derived from cloning single cells and using appropriate labeled precursors; has observed the formation of both collagen and elastin bearing the appropriate lables. He has been able to verify by electronmicrography the "smooth muscle" nature of the cells and the presence of the labels in the collagen and elastic fibers. He demonstrated, in addition, hydroxyproline synthesis by these cells.

Dr. Constantinides then cited evidence that endothelial cells might also have the capability to elaborate connective tissue fibrils and of becoming smooth muscle cells. He also suggested that the

smooth muscle cells of the media might transform to replace lost endothelial cells.

Continuing the discussion of embryological development Dr.
Gillman introduced his concept of remodeling.

DR. GILLMAN: Biologists and perhaps especially anatomists and
pathologists have, for centuries now, accepted that, during the growth
of the individual, bones grow simultaneously in girth and length and
that this involves remodeling by endochondrial osteoclasis and bone
resorption closely geared with epiphyseal and periosteal osteoblastic
neogenesis of bone.

It seems strange indeed that if such rigid and hard tissues,
like those found in all the bones of the body, can indeed be remodeled
to achieve a predetermined shape and size, pari passu with their growth,
that the same notions of temporally
and spatially integrated remodeling
have not been studied in the heart,
in the coronary arteries, the aorta

The concept of
remodeling

itself or any of its multiple branches. For it is highly probable
that such remodeling will occur as the individual (or any of his organs,
like the liver, lungs, heart, brain) grows in overall body size. Yet,
to my knowledge, no one has provided any adequate description(s) of
how the aorta, for example, remodels itself as its caliber and length
increase, probably in intermittent spurts, from the small vessel seen
in the newborn to that large trunk found in fullgrown adults. For,
in man, the final pattern of the vascular tree is laid down, in accordance with the "law of biogenesis," by ontogenetically determined
remodeling and growth of arteries finally derived after earlier phylo-
genetically imprinted patterns of vascular growth, fusion and/or ob-
literation are completed.

After the morphogenesis and differentiation of organ and tissue
anlagen there occur, in man, three major periodic spurts of bodily,
and hence of organ, arterial and other tissue growth, namely one in
the last two thirds (particularly the final trimester) of intra-uterine
life and the second during the first 1-2 years after birth. The third
period of rapid growth is characteristic of adolescence i.e. age 9-19
years during which, for the first time, the two sexes start to differ
notably from each other (Tanner and Whitehouse, 1962).

When Dr. Dalith, Israel, takes X-rays of postnatal aorta he finds
areas of medial calcification which are the direct consequence of our
evolutionary development. The whole aorta does not react simultaneously
in development. There are waves of growth and tissue differentiation
and the elastin wave - elastogenic wave - starts at the arch, goes up
and extends down into the terminal arteries. And in fact many smaller
mammals may be born without elastic tissue in their terminal arteries.

If you interfere with or block elastogenesis you get a swing back onto collagen, or reticulum formation. We have no evidence how these are correlated except indirect morphological evidence. The chemistry we do have is in terms of quantitative chemistry, but not local individual artery chemistry. As we grow from infancy right through adulthood we not only thicken our elastic membranes, but, I think, we grow them both in length and in girth simultaneously. This can only be achieved by some form of remodeling. Rather than growing in caliber and length by laying down new membranes on the outside, the artery appears to undergo interstitial growth in the existing membrane. One sees it beautifully in the embryo, where if one produces ruptures or otherwise interferes with the process, abnormalities and disease ultimately become manifest more readily than if one disturbs the membrane later in life. This may be attributable to the high synthetic activity in the vascular tissues at the time of embryonic development (Fyfe and Gillman, et al., 1968). For, tripping a man when he is running is likely to have more serious effects than when he is walking, i.e. vascular injuries may be more likely, more extensive and more severe in rapidly growing and remodeling than in stable arterial walls, and may have an initially more serious action, even though the long term delayed effects may only be detected 20 or 30 years later. Is it not possible then, that arterial injuries may be more frequent and severe during such periods of active vascular growth although the end results become detectable only much later in life? For, unfortunately, we do not have any function tests of vascular integrity. Hence, the existence of such lesions, if they do indeed occur early in life, would become recognizable only by their late end results, such as occlusions and their consequences. Similar susceptibility to pre-occlusive changes may perhaps also occur during involutionary degrowth and associated remodeling, as shown by our studies of the post-partum involution of both human and sows' uterine arteries (Gillman, 1964; Gillman, 1968). May not similar processes supervene in coronary arteries when the heart "de-grows" or involutes ("atrophies") with age or after its growth during periods of prolonged and intense muscular activities, for example, in retired marathon runners?

COMMENT

The possibility of a genetic regulator of the thickness of the intima is suggested by histologic studies in Israel of coronary arteries of full-term fetuses, infants and children (Vlodaver and Kahn, et al., 1969). The intima and musculo-elastic layers of the coronary arteries were found to be more developed among Ashkenazy than among Yemenite and Bedouins males.

DR. MEYER: In connection with the remarks of Dr. Gillman, I would like to point out certain arterial segments which are subject to a high hemo-dynamic "stress" or strain during the fetal development. As a consequence of

The internal elastic lamina, calcification and vitamin D

this strain and/or some peculiarities in the development of the wall
structure, early calcification occurs almost regularly in these arterial
segments. This has been observed in the common and internal iliac
arteries as well as in the siphon of the
internal carotid artery. In the fetus
the common and internal iliac arteries
transport blood to the placenta. For
this reason they have a considerable lumen in comparison with the
arteries of the lower limb, as can be seen in angiograms. (FIG. 7).
The early calcifications can be demonstrated in these arteries macroscopically by the modified Von Kossa reaction. With this reaction
the calcifications appear as roundish or polygonal black dots spread
over the inner surface of the arterial wall in 2-day-old newborns
(FIG. 8). The calcific incrustations are often arranged along side
of calcium-free bands. These bands correspond to the wide gaps in
the internal elastic lamina which are arranged circumferentially and
whose length is up to half of the circumference (FIG. 9). In consecutive autopsy material such calcifications of the internal elastic
membrane have been found macroscopically in half of all newborns and
stillborns. They were demonstrated in all autopsies of cases dying
after the age of nine months.

Calcification in the
normal arterial wall

The siphon of the internal carotid artery is the second site of
early arterial calcifications in children. In this arterial segment
the calcifications are observed from the age of one year and appear
first in the upper part of the siphon just above the origin of the
ophthalmic artery (FIG. 10). With advancing age the entire wall circumference in this arterial segment is densely interspersed with black
stained calcific deposits. They are located, as in the iliac arteries,
in the internal elastic membrane. In the first years of life calcific
plaques are formed which penetrate the inner layer of the media.
These plaques are often overlaid by a thin grayish connective tissue
layer which develops in the intima.

DR. ADAMS: I visualize that other things, including protein,
might react with the Von Kossa stain. I would like to be quite sure
that these deposits really are calcium.

DR. MEYER: The results obtained with this stain were confirmed
by microradiographic techniques. On the microradiographs of the fresh,
unfixed arteries before and after Von Kossa staining the pattern and
extent of mineralization of the internal elastic lamina are identical.
The calcium deposits were also identified by some other reactions, such
as Voigt's technique.

DR. SCHWARTZ: I was very impressed with the beautiful work on
Von Kossa preparations and I have the impression from looking at these
that the spots of calcification were linear and at right angles to the
direction of the vessel. I recall that in looking at healthy young

vessels - the femoral and iliac arteries in particular, with conventional staining, one sees a serrated transverse pattern. Do these Von Kossa-positive spots, shown by you, in fact correspond with these serrated lines?

DR. MEYER: Yes, they do correspond. In the most muscular arteries, the Von Kossa-positive material appears at the proximal and distal borders of circularly arranged folds of the inner surface of the arteries. Dietrich (Dietrich, 1930) called these folds "Spindles." **HUMAN** The spindles develop in the postnatal period during the first year of life. They become more numerous in the first decade. To the end of the body growth the whole inner surface of the muscular arteries is densely interspersed with spindles. At the site of the spindles the internal elastic membrane is completely interrupted. The calcification takes place in the borders of the membrane gaps. The Von Kossa-reaction shows the gaps delineated as paired black "calcific bands." The gaps in the membrane are probably sites of increased permeability of the vessel wall. With aging there is further calcification at the borders of the gaps and new connective tissue growth appears that ultimately covers over and apparently seals off the gaps so that they presumably lose whatever meaning they may have had for nutrition of the artery wall.

DR. GILLMAN: Professor Meyer, when you showed a picture of a histological section taken across those ridges or spindles of Dietrich the elevated portion didn't seem to have a continuous elastic lamina. The elevated portion seemed to have a number of fine elastic-staining fibrillae. Is that correct?

DR. MEYER: Yes, it is only a network; fine network.

DR. SCHWARTZ: Does this process have any bearing on the development of arterial fibromuscular hyperplasia?

DR. MEYER: There seems to be no relation between the fibromuscular hyperplasia and the system of gaps. However, near the branchings of the arteries, where a pronounced fibromuscular hyperplasia often occurs, a peculiar labyrinth-like pattern of gaps and calcific bands can be observed.

DR. VON BERLEPSCH: Is this finding of gaps in the elastic membrane confined to muscular arteries of humans or is it a phenomenon which is very widespread over many species?

DR. MEYER: The gaps are not confined to the muscular arterial segment and are also seen in the (elastic) common and internal iliac arteries. However, the typical and numerous gaps can be seen only in the muscular arteries. I don't know if similar gaps exist in animal vessels.

DR. SCHWARTZ: If you stretch or put weights on the end does the vessel wall "give" or rupture preferentially at the points of the spindle? In other words, are these points inbuilt zones of weakness within the vessel?

DR. MEYER: The spindles are probably spots of weakness of the vessel wall but I have not tried to stretch the vessels to see whether or not the vessel wall can be interrupted at these points. The spindles, i.e., gaps in the internal elastic membrane, appear to be the consequence of a postnatal longitudinal stretch of the arteries which increases with the growth of the body. Probably spindles are more pronounced in the arteries of the lower extremity which grow faster than some other parts of the body. The greater number of the gaps in these arteries is in accord with this assumption.

DR. VON BERLEPSCH: Have you had any chance to investigate vessels of hyperlipidemic patients and are there also other signs that lipids will infiltrate these parts of the vessel wall more easily?

DR. MEYER: I think so, but so far I have only a few observations. Wilens and McCluskey (Wilens and McCluskey, 1954) perfused the arteries of the rabbit with a hyperlipemic serum and found a more pronounced lipid infiltration of the artery's wall corresponding to the gaps in the elastic membrane.

DR. GILLMAN: Have you stained and looked for mucopolysaccharides microscopically in the ridges?

DR. MEYER: No, I have not studied this question.

DR. GILLMAN: I think it may be very worthwhile to do this because we have, in experimentally induced calcification in rat's arteries, regularly found mucopolysaccharides close to or around calcified areas (Gillman, et al., 1957).

DR. MEYER: It has been shown by Dietrich (Dietrich, 1930) that in the area of spindles the smooth musculature is reduced and there is also an apparent increase in ground substance.

DR. GILLMAN: This is important. If I have correctly understood you, Dr. Meyer, you have said that Dietrich showed there was a defect in the muscle in the ridges, and you are assuming from this that there must be ground substance and probably mucopolysaccharides. I think it is very important to show whether it is so or not. But you can probably do it microscopically with toluidine blue (at the right pH), at least to start with, just as you have done Von Kossa for calcium. If you do get a positive reaction with toluidine blue I think it is very important to go further. That is the first point. Can you tell us whether you have been able yet to analyze the incidence of these re-

actions in relation, perhaps, to sex, age or particular arteries?
How many arteries have you looked at in this way and can you tell us
anything about the incidence of the changes you've described in relation to age? I gather from your first pictures that, as the individual gets older, you get more ridges and there are less ridges in
the young. You also said, I think, that by the second or third decade,
they had reached a maximum. Do they decrease after that or do they
stay the same?

DR. MEYER: In the central part of the spindle, i.e., in the media
underneath the gap in the internal elastic membrane the number of the
muscle cells is reduced. The muscle cells are interspersed with a
ground substance which contains fine collagenous and elastic networks
and connective tissue cells. With age, the amount of collagen increases
and dense networks proceed deeper in the media. So far there are no
detailed studies of the histochemical peculiarities of the spindle
area. As the collagen content increases with age, a considerable
amount of ground substance, rich in mucopolysaccharides could be expected underneath the gaps in the internal elastic lamina.

The number of spindles considerably increases with the growth of
the vessels. In the arteries of the lower extremities (external iliac
artery, proximal segment of the femoral artery) the precursors of the
spindles in circularly arranged whitish stripes appear during the first
year of life. They become numerous and slightly elevated in the first
decade (FIG. 11) and spread over the middle and distal segment of the
femoral artery as well as the popliteal artery in the second decade.
At the end of the body growth the spindles achieve their maximal development. In young adults the inner surface of the large and medium
sized arteries of the lower extremities is densely interspersed with
elevated spindles and many finer folds. (The latter do not always
correspond to the gaps in the internal elastic membrane).

The spindles are most numerous and prominent in the arteries of
the lower extremities (FIG. 12), but they develop also in other
arteries. During the postnatal growth the spindles appear in the
brachial artery, upper mesenteric artery (a. mesenterica cranialis),
splenic and renal arteries. Thus, the spindles and the corresponding
gaps in the internal elastic lamina are a common finding in all larger
and medium sized muscular arteries (FIG. 13).

At the end of the body growth (i.e. to the end of the second
decade) and in the third decade longitudinally oriented elastic and
collagenous networks often appear in the intima of large muscular
arteries and cover the original circularly oriented folds. In this
way the spindles become flattened. However, the gaps in the internal
elastic lamina, which are located in the spindles, stay unchanged
during later life and can be easily found microscopically in the
longitudinal sections. The pronounced calcification, the gaps in

the lamella can be demonstrated grossly by modified Von Kossa reaction in spite of marked age-bound fibrous thickening of the intima.

DR. TAYLOR: Chronic mild hypervitaminosis D may be a neglected factor in the pathogenesis of arteriosclerosis. In the U.S. it is likely that many individuals ingest modest excesses of vitamin D daily because of its addition to certain foods such as milk and bread. Another source of excess vitamin D is the common practice of taking daily vitamin tablets which usually contain at least the daily requirement of vitamin D. Vitamin D has produced human vascular damage and calcification (Seelig, 1969); similar disease has also been produced in rabbits (Hass and Truehart, et al., 1960) and monkeys (Kent and Vawter, et al., 1958). A very recent, alarming finding is the synergism of hypercholesteremia, vitamin D and nicotine in the rapid production of calcific arterial disease in rabbits (Hass and Landerholm, et al., 1966) and monkeys (Liu and Taylor, 1970). With this combination of hypercholesterolemia, vitamin D and nicotine, calcific arteriopathy with severe arteritis and thrombosis have been observed in both rabbits and monkeys after relatively brief periods of exposure to modest doses of these vasotoxins.

Possible accentuation of normal calcification process by ingestion of excessive amounts of vitamin D

DR. JUNGE-HULSING: I wonder if Dr. Meyer's children with pronounced calcification of vessels may have been treated with vitamin D.

We did some experiments with vitamin D. The results of these investigations on changes of connective tissue and calcium metabolism are demonstrated in FIG. 14. You can see that immediately after vitamin D administration the metabolism of connective tissue, in this case measured by incorporation of ^{35}S-sulfate into sulfated mucopolysaccharides of arterial connective tissue, markedly increased. When this mesenchymal reaction begins to decrease, there is an increase of ^{45}calcium incorporation and, somewhat later, of total calcium content of the tissue.

Calcification of connective tissue is a secondary consequence of a primary disturbance of connective tissue metabolism, especially of mucopolysaccharide and collagen metabolism. Of course, we isolated the mucopolysaccharides chemically and measured the specific activity of separated sulfated mucopolysaccharides. In the same way we did it with collagen, and we saw that each kind of calcification is combined with a primary disturbance of connective tissue in the different organs.

Metabolic effects of vitamin D in arterial wall

DR. GILLMAN: I would like to describe some of our findings con-
·cerning the changes in the elastic lamina and related tissue in the
coronary arteries of rats injured acutely by calciferol-induced meta-   **RAT**
bolic disturbances (Grant and Gillman, et al., 1963). Now in these
experiments we gave rats, for the first five days of the experiment
only, toxic doses of calciferol and thereafter no treatment was given.
We merely watched biochemically, histologically and histochemically
what happened to the coronary and other arteries. Now the changes in
the aorta, which is primarily an elastic artery in the rat, are different from those in the muscular arteries. I have taken here as a
muscular artery, the coronary because it has such important meaning
for what happens in the rats.

COMMENT

As detailed in Chapter IX, Dr. Werthessen called attention to the
relatively unstable nature of the cholesterol molecule and pointed
out that calciferol is an oxidation product of cholesterol and referred
to work identifying calciferol in commercial cholesterol mixtures used
to feed animals in experimental atherosclerosis research.

QUESTION: What do you mean by toxic?

Effects of vitamin D
on connective tissue
metabolism in artery
wall

DR. GILLMAN: Toxic in the sense that
they were such large doses of calciferol
that many of the rats in a group died. All
the rats stopped eating their food; they
either died or they got better, after
calciferol dosing was stopped at the end
of the first five consecutive days. The ones that died were autopsied
and examined histochemically and chemically; the ones that recovered
were then killed at various times up to 400 days after the last (fifth) ·
dose. We studied a very large number of rats treated in this way.
You can get all the details from one of our articles (Grant and Gillman,
et al., 1963). So I am simply saying "toxic doses" for the moment.
Now the interesting thing is that when you do give these "toxic" doses
of calciferol not all the arteries calcify at the same time. For
example, the coronary arteries start calcifying by day 3 or 4 (FIG. 15).
Calcium then disappears completely from the coronary arteries within
3 or 4 days after discontinuing calciferol. By the 8th day of the
experiment (counting day one as the day you give the first dose of
calciferol), there is no more demonstrable calcium in the coronary
arteries although there may be some excess in the heart muscle itself -
as estimated chemically.

FIG. 16 shows a healthy coronary artery, half way down in a
control rat's left ventricle showing a typical wavy internal elastic
lamina. Within 30 days after only 5 days of exposure to calciferol
the elastic lamina can be seen to swell and appear "coated" with muco-

polysaccharides (FIG. 17). The increase in mucopolysaccharides in the
loose connective tissue is evident between the cells. A heavy round cell
infiltration and inflammatory reaction is present around the injured arter

DR. MEYER: Do you also find the deposition of fibrin?

DR. GILLMAN: Not in the vessel. FIG. 18 shows the changes in
the coronary artery at the same position in the ventricle and at the
same magnification as the last two figures 60 days after discontinuing
calciferol. The damaged elastic membrane is no longer visible. With
toluidine blue the previously injured vessel wall appears to be thickened and very cellular with a considerable amount of metachromatic
polysaccharide (FIG. 18). Between 200 and 300 days later a toluidine
blue stain shows that the mucopolysaccharide (as defined by meta-
chromatically stained material) has now virtually disappeared (FIG. 19).
The artery's lumen has become very eccentric and very narrow and the
previously injured wall is replaced by collagen. It would seem that
the rat cannot replace the internal elastic membrane of a severely
injured coronary artery. There is fibrosis of the entire wall of
such injured coronaries. We found 90 to 95% of rats had developed
advanced coronary sclerosis and stenosis between 200 and 300 days
after 5 days' dosing with calciferol. So it is a very useful experimental technique for producing coronary stenosis in rats, apart from
teaching us something about how such sclerosis and coronary stenosis
may develop.

QUESTION: May I ask if these animals were hypertensive?

Rats' inability
to regenerate
damaged internal
elastica

DR. GILLMAN: We did not measure blood
pressures. The calcium one could demonstrate
was not in the membrane but rather around it,
a fact we have reported on more fully elsewhere (Gillman, et al., 1957; Gillman and
Grant, et al., 1960).

COMMENT

Dr. Gillman showed slides of ruptured internal elastic lamina
in human renal and mesenteric muscular arteries associated with finer
"reduplicated" elastic lamina. Differences in the staining quality
(Gillman and Penn, et al., 1955; Gillman, 1959) led him to postulate
a difference between "true" and "pseudo" elastic lamina in diseased
arteries, a difference similar to that observed in the elastic material
of human dermis injured by ultraviolet irradiation and in the tunica
propria of human cholesterolic gall bladders. He mentioned that in
1896 Unna (Unna, 1896) had described such elastin-like materials, in
senile dematoses in man. For such elastin-like materials resembling a
form of degenerated collagen, Gillman proposed the name "pseudoelastin."
He then quoted confirmatory work of R.A. Grant (Grant, 1965) who pre-

pared an elastin-like material from collagen by cross-linking it by
means of heat, ultraviolet or gamma ray irradiation or treatment by
glutaraldehyde. He found that the altered collagen now failed to be
digested by repeatedly purified collagenase but became susceptible to
digestion by highly purified elastase. Furthermore, he said that it
displayed all the tinctorial reactions described for "pseudoelastin"
produced spontaneously in vivo. Whether "pseudoelastin" derives from
collagen degeneration or is synthesized de novo in aging or injured
human connective tissues due to derangements in synthesis - including
arterial connective tissue cannot be settled on the basis of present
evidence.

DR. SMITH: Collagen and elastin have quite different amino acid
compositions and I don't see how you convert collagen into elastin.

DR. VON BERLEPSCH: It seems surprising that altered collagen
suddenly becomes susceptible to elastase digestion. This means perhaps
that your elastase contains also an unspecific proteolytic enzyme and
we know very well that denatured collagen will then be digested.
Therefore the specificity of this so-called elastase may not be suf-
ficent to characterize the substrate.

DR. GILLMAN: Right, this is what I showed. Now let me go right
back to the beginning. I said that one sees occurring spontaneously
in nature (in arteries and elsewhere) apparently at least three varieties
of connective tissue fibers. We all agree there is the "true" collagen
fiber, and the "true" elastin fiber each with its own specific amino
acid and composition. But there is apparently also another fiber
which I suggested we call "pseudoelastin," until we know more because
it shows only some of the reactions of elastin. Now I am not saying,
nor have I ever said, that we have changed collagen into elastin but
rather that these develop naturally in arteries, skin, etc. with aging
in vivo and from collagen in vitro - an elastin-like material. Hence
the suggested name, "pseudoelastin."

I want to make it very clear to Dr. Smith that I am not suggesting
collagen has been converted into elastin. Collagen has been altered
so as to resemble elastin at least tinctorially and perhaps in other
ways too.

DR. SMITH: Wouldn't it be better to forget the "pseudoelastin"
because I think it is confusing.

DR. VON BERLEPSCH: It is just another protein which now becomes
stainable with elastic stains.

DR. GILLMAN: Correct, and this altered connective tissue fiber -
"pseudoelastin" - seems to come from collagen degradation and the amino
acid sequences which Grant and coworkers are analyzing may permit them

to tell us something new about it. I don't want to present the findings
of Grant and co-workers incorrectly here, but I think they are finding,
with finger printing techniques, similarities and differences between
the amino acid and peptide sequences in elastin and in "pseudoelastin"
and the results with "pseudoelastin" differ from collagen even though
the "pseudoelastin" was not the "naturally formed" in vivo material
but derived in vitro from collagen, originally by cross-linking some
amino acids in collagen (Grant, 1967; Grant and Cox, et al., 1970;
Cox and Grant, 1968; Grant and Beale, et al., personal communication).

DR. VON BERLEPSCH: This is very surprising. I would rather
expect that the amino acid composition still resembles that of collagen.

DR. GILLMAN: As far as I know "pseudoelastin" has features that
lie between collagen and elastin, but Grant, et al. will, I hope, report their findings fully soon.

DR. ROBERTSON: I would like to refer to sites of calcification
in the arterial wall that are not related directly to the internal
elastic lamina and to the finding of altered collagen fibers that may
be Dr. Gillman's "pseudoelastin." We examined specimens from the
carotid and femoral arteries, as well as of segments of coronary
arteries, obtained during reparative vascular surgery. There were
microscopic areas of "early" calcification particularly in the presence
of severe intimal hyperplasia. These intimal lesions seemed to differ
from calcified lesions found in peripheral arteries such as the carotid,
for example, in that they occurred first at sites of fibrous aggregates,
many of which, at least in the periphery of the lesions, showed by
electron microscopy ultrastructural characteristics of mature collagen
fibers. Many of these fiber aggregates, however, had lost the typical
array of collagen bundles, became more electron dense and did not
possess the typical periodicity and regularity of mature collagen
fibers. The center of the lesion often contained an area of high
electron density with loss or fusion of fibers surrounding an amorphous
core. The earliest stages of this deposition seemed to be formation
of an electron dense nodule within the limiting membrane of the collagen
fiber. The more advanced lesions resembled the "rosettes" of apatite
crystals described by Yu and Blumenthal (Yu and Blumenthal, 1963) or
by Serafini-Fracassini (Serafini-Fracassini, 1963) using X-ray crys-
tallography. It is of interest that this type of calcification
(FIG. 20, a and b) may represent, in fact, different stages of a
series of phenomena involving the modification of both physical and
chemical characteristics of the collagen fiber resulting in precipitation of calcium salts. It is also of some interest that following Gillman's suggestion (Gillman, 1959) these modified collagen
fibers may represent "pseudoelastin," in very early intimal calcifications. I believe these observations support Gillman's concept of
the possible relation of this "pseudoelastin" tissue with collagen and
emphasize the role of abnormal collagen deposition in arterial intimal
calcification.

Another point to be mentioned is the fact that many of the very
"early" lesions are often surrounded by large amounts of sudanophilic
deposits corresponding morphologically to the "fibrous lipid" described
by Dr. E. Smith. The interplay between modifications of the intimal
collagen matrix, calcification and extracellular lipid deposition de-
serve, I believe, further investigation.

COMMENT

The appearance of abnormal collagen or "pseudoelastin" in the
presence of a thickening intima may be explained in part by the work
of Stetten (Stetten, 1949) who showed that the synthesis of
hydroxyproline, an essential component of normal collagen, requires
the presence of molecular oxygen. It would appear that during
adaptation to the demands of growth or mechanical strain the requirement for sturdiness may compromise the vessel's supply of oxygen. Although nourishing juices containing glucose, lipids and amino acids
may be absorbed into an avascular area, clearly the only access for
oxygen must be by diffusion either from the vessel lumen or from the
capillaries of the vasa vasorum into the deeper layers of the artery.

DR. ADAMS: With respect to the nourishment of the artery I
should like to offer evidence that progressive thickening of the
intima is, indeed, accompanied by ischemic damage in the middle
zones of the tunica media. (FIG. 21) shows a diagram of the
thickening aorta. In section, stained by histochemical ATPase
method, one can see that the fibers in the middle of the tunica
media have already lost some of their ATPase. In the case of a
man at the age of 59,not only are the middle fibers of the tunica
media lost, as reflected in the enzyme activity, but so are those
in the inner region. It's quite noticeable that the outer media,
which is nourished by the vasa, retains its normal enzyme activity. This means you have a sort of metabolic barrier in the middle
and inner part of the tunica media.

DR. WISSLER: It might be valuable to know in what way these
early changes in the intima and the internal elastic membrane correspond to the forces acting on the media, mechanical stresses for
example.

I should like to point out that in the human aorta, the tension
per medial layer is probably greater in the abdominal than in the
thoracic segment. Despite this increased stress, the human abdominal
aortic media is relatively devoid of vasa vasorum.

This information is derived from the comparative studies of aortic
structure of Drs. Wolinsky and Glagov (Wolinsky and Glagov, 1969).
These investigators took care to study vessels which had been fixed
while distended at physiological pressures so that some sort of stand-
ardization could be achieved for evaluating vessel diameters, wall

thicknesses and the disposition of the medial layers. They concluded
that the mammalian aortic media is composed of uniform concentric
structural layers which they called lamellar units because each seemed
to sustain a tension of about 2000 dynes/cm regardless of species.
They also noted that medial vasa vasorum were present only beyond
the innermost 29 or so lamellar units regardless of species. The
medial thickness of the human abdominal aorta correspond to its
diameter, but it had fewer lamellar units than would be expected
as compared to thoracic and abdominal aortic segments of other mammals.
Thus, the tension per layer was relatively high and approached levels
of tension usually seen in aortas of large animals furnished with
medial vasa vasorum. Actually the human abdominal aorta had about
29 lamellar units at the level they studied and, as could be anticipated from the data on other mammals, had no medial vasa vasorum.
Thus, medial layers under relatively high stress had relatively litle
vascularization.

For those of us who believe that the metabolism of the medial
cell may be very important to the development of atherosclerosis,
these considerations may be very important. When abnormal substances
such as low density lipoproteins are making their way through the
media their accumulation could be favored by the combined disadvan-
tages of increased cellular mechanical stress and relatively decreased
medial vascularization.

DR. BOWYER: I wonder if the elastic property of elastin is very
important in the preservation of the normal so-called elastic properties
of the arterial wall. I should like to present an hypothesis of Dr.
Kelloway's which is as follows: The normal elastic properties of the
arterial wall may be provided by the tone of the smooth muscle. The
elastica only provides a matrix against which the smooth muscle cells
can do work.

DR. FREMONT-SMITH: Thirty years ago I was able to observe that
during each systole the whole arterial tree elongates in accommodating
for the increase in blood volume in the arterial tree produced by
systole (Fremont-Smith, 1969; Fremont-Smith, 1942).

I observed this elongation frequently in the meningeal vessels
of the dog, cat and monkey, as well as in the mesenteric arteries of
the rat and in the arteries in the tongue of the frog. This observation
has been described also by Dr. Samuel Reynolds (Reynolds and Light,
et al., 1952).

Elongation of vessels with the pulse beat — In man the elongation takes place
with each heart beat in excess of 350
million times per year and thus plays
a role, I believe, in the eventual
tortuosity of the arterial tree (due
to gradual fatigue of the elastic elements in the wall of the arteries).

While observing these vessels under the microscope no lateral expansion of the arteries was observable but the elongation was quite evident. This progressive elongation and tortuosity of the arterial tree with increasing longevity may well play a role in the pathogenesis of atherosclerosis.

In the lungs there is also an elongation and shortening of both arteries and veins coincident with inspiration and expiration respectively.

My attention was drawn to the elongation and shortening of blood vessels during an observation I made in 1926 on the human inferior vena cava (Fremont-Smith, 1942). In discussing this observation with Dr. J. Howard Means, Head of the Medical Department of Massachusetts General Hospital, he said that he believed that longitudinal stretching of a rubber tube would increase its volume. I was able to demonstrate the validity of his statement both with a large diameter rubber tube and with a fresh human vena cava obtained at autopsy. In the literature, as mentioned in my article, I found a reference to a German scientist, Braune, 1870, who pointed out that veins increase their volume when they are elongated and that when a joint is bent the veins on the outside of the joint are elongated and on the inside of the joint are shortened and vice versa, and this plays a role in return of blood to the heart.

DR. KEYS: What about coronary and cerebral arteries - do they expand mainly lengthwise?

DR. FREMONT-SMITH: All the vessels in the heart, the arteries, the veins, and the cerebral vessels are inevitably elongated and shortened with each heart beat.

DR. CONSTANTINIDES: In this connection it is interesting that in many mammals and birds and in most vertebrates injury to arteries elicits a sterotypic syndrome. Regardless of the specific nature of the insult, when elastic tissue is destroyed new musculo-elastic tissue grows on top and it is always reoriented in a longitudinal direction, appearing at right angles to the original circularly arranged medial cells. Dr. Peter Harmon, one of my graduate students, measured this process in humans, in the coronaries of children, and found that the amount of new musculo-elastic layer is directly proportional to the amount of elastic injury underneath it. That is the wider the gaps (with a quantitative technique), the thicker the muscular hyperplasia, and this is exactly what we found in injured animal arteries. We found the same correspondence in experimentally injured arteries of animals: the wider the elastic break the thicker the overlying muscular elastic regeneration. Such areas were always found to be abnormally permeable to particles of various dyes, and to chylomicrons.

DR. BORN: I am still puzzled as to what we are to consider the
reactions of normal as opposed to those of diseased tissues. May I
ask Dr. Gillman to restate his definition for remodeling and to draw
the distinction between remodeling and repair.

DR. GILLMAN: There are probably three major changes which may
occur in connective tissue: 1) Regeneration. When a tissue has been
torn or when renewal of cells is required, as a result of "wear and
tear" alterations, it reconstitutes itself without any architectural
distortion. That is regeneration. 2) Reconstruction is a process of
altering the original cellular and fiber composition and arrangements
to achieve a repair beyond that for which cell and fiber renewal will
alone suffice. There is a replacement of the original tissue by a
somewhat different cell population. 3) Remodeling, on the other hand,
occurs as part of normal growth and development without a known previous
injury.

DR. BORN: Following a suggestion of mine, Dr. Helen Payling
Wright observed that the endothelium in guinea pig aorta replaces
itself more rapidly in the neighborhood of branchings than elsewhere.
Is this normal, and if so, what does normal mean? We started with
the idea that it was due to differences in the nature of the blood
flow but it might equally plausibly represent a phylogenetic adaptation acquired in developmental history. Therefore, I agree that
our distinction between normal and abnormal is rather artificial and
that we should be thinking more in terms of adaptation.

DR. HAUST: Dr. Gross and his associates have studied the coronary
arteries of newborn infants and older children, and demonstrated a
proliferation of intimal smooth muscles without rupture of the elastica.
The new smooth muscle cells migrate into the developing intima through
naturally occurring openings in the plate of the internal elastic
lamina. In the intima they run longitudinally rather than circularly.
This, according to these authors, provides means for the longitudinal
stretch. We have repeated and confirmed these studies. We should
not consider this to be a pathological process, and I agree with Dr.
French, that if we define as normal something that occurs in all individuals, then this criterion applies also to the diffuse intimal thickening, as this is the normal development of the coronary artery with
age.

CHAIRMAN WOLF: This is extremely interesting. It has been
taught that something normal had to be entirely different from something pathological. We seem to be working toward the notion that the
difference between normal and abnormal is a matter of degree.

DR. FREMONT-SMITH: I should like to point out in this connection
of normality and pathology, that any infant is born with a great many
dead glomeruli. Now this is normal, because every infant has it,

but the glomerulus which is dead is not a normal glomerulus, and
therefore the difference between normal and pathological is academic.
It may not be appropriate for us to make such a distinction.

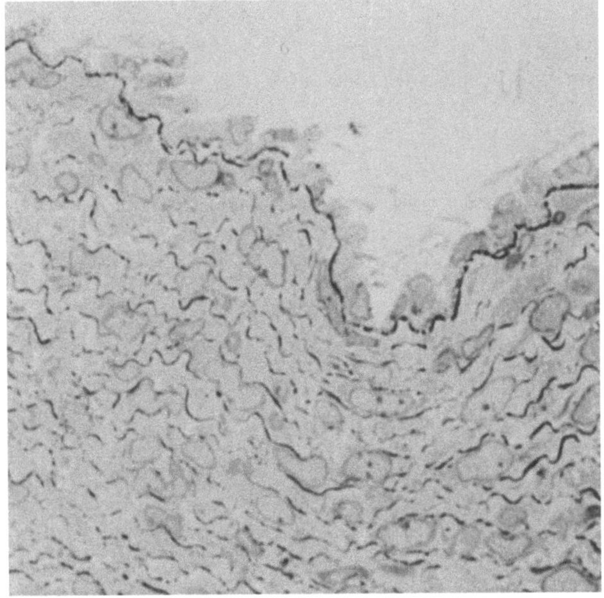

FIGURE 1. Light microscopic appearance of an aorta from a twelve-week-old human fetus. The endothelium rests upon a well-developed, almost continuous internal elastic lamina. The media is composed of circularly arranged cellular layers separated by incomplete elastic lamellae. The medial cells vary moderately in size and shape; their vesicular nuclei are oval to round and occasionally slightly indented. The nature of these cells is not apparent. Epon-embedded tissue; toluidine blue stain; magnification = x 680.

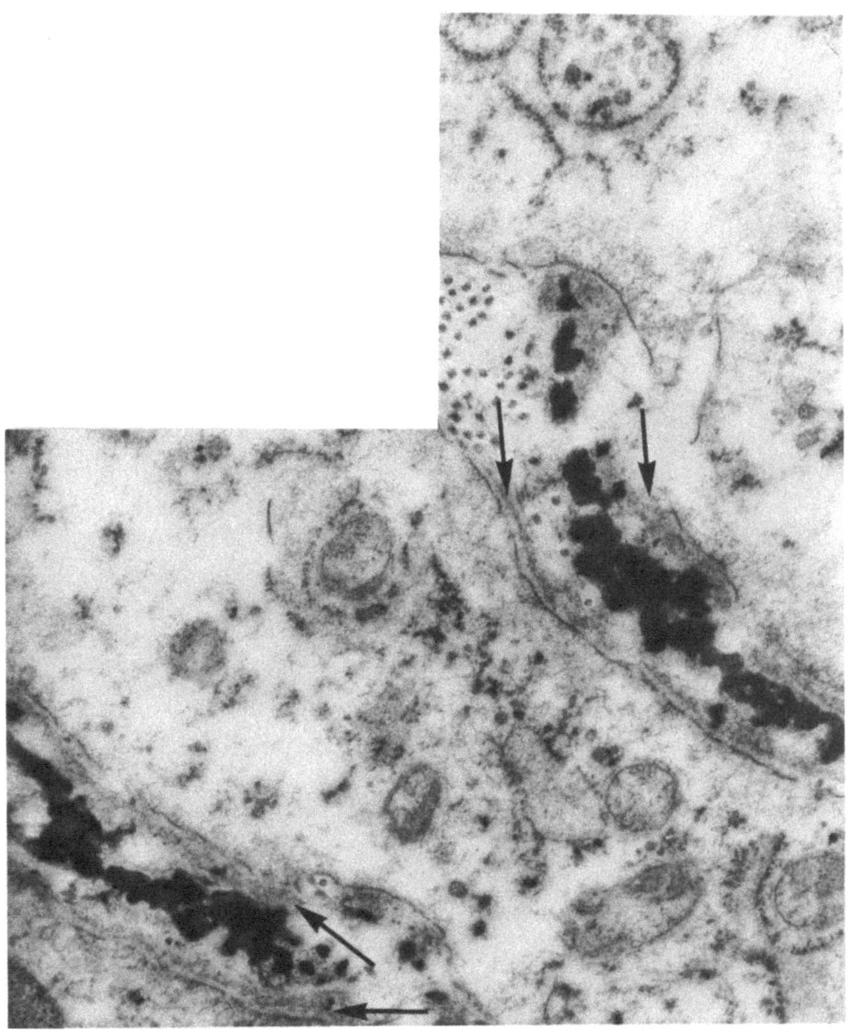

FIGURE 2. Electron micrograph of tissue fixed in glutaraldehyde,
post-fixed in osmium tetroxide, embedded in Epon-812, and stained
with uranyl acetate and lead citrate. Aortic medial cells in a
ten-week-old human fetus. The cells vary in shape and are immature,
but already have partially or entirely enveloping basement membranes
(arrows), and some have numerous pinocytotic vesicles (cell in left
lower corner). Elastic tissue (stained black in this preparation)
develops in close proximity to the basement membranes; magnification =
x 26,000.

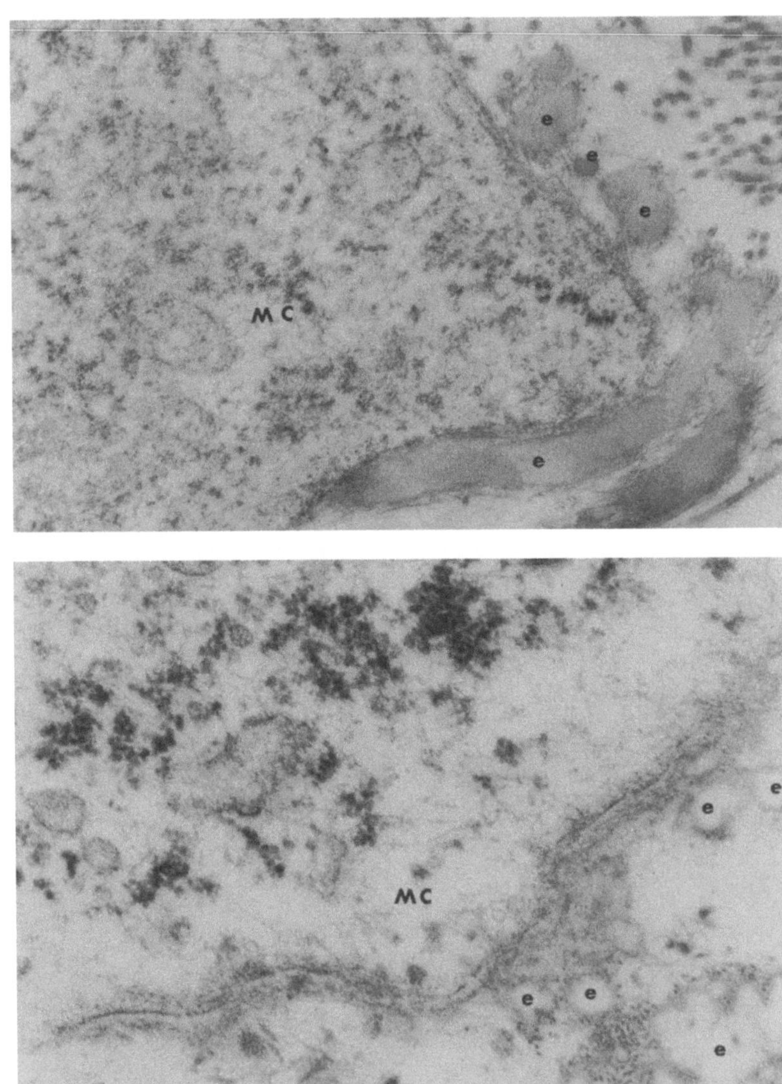

FIGURE 3a and 3b. Electron micrographs of tissues fixed in glutaraldehyde, post-fixed in osmium tetroxide, embedded in Epon-812, and stained
with uranyl acetate and lead citrate. Two examples of an aortic medial
cell (MC) from a ten-week-old human fetus. Units and other elements
of elastic tissue (e) develop in close proximity to the cellular basement membrane; magnficiation: 3a = x 29,000; 3b = x 42,000

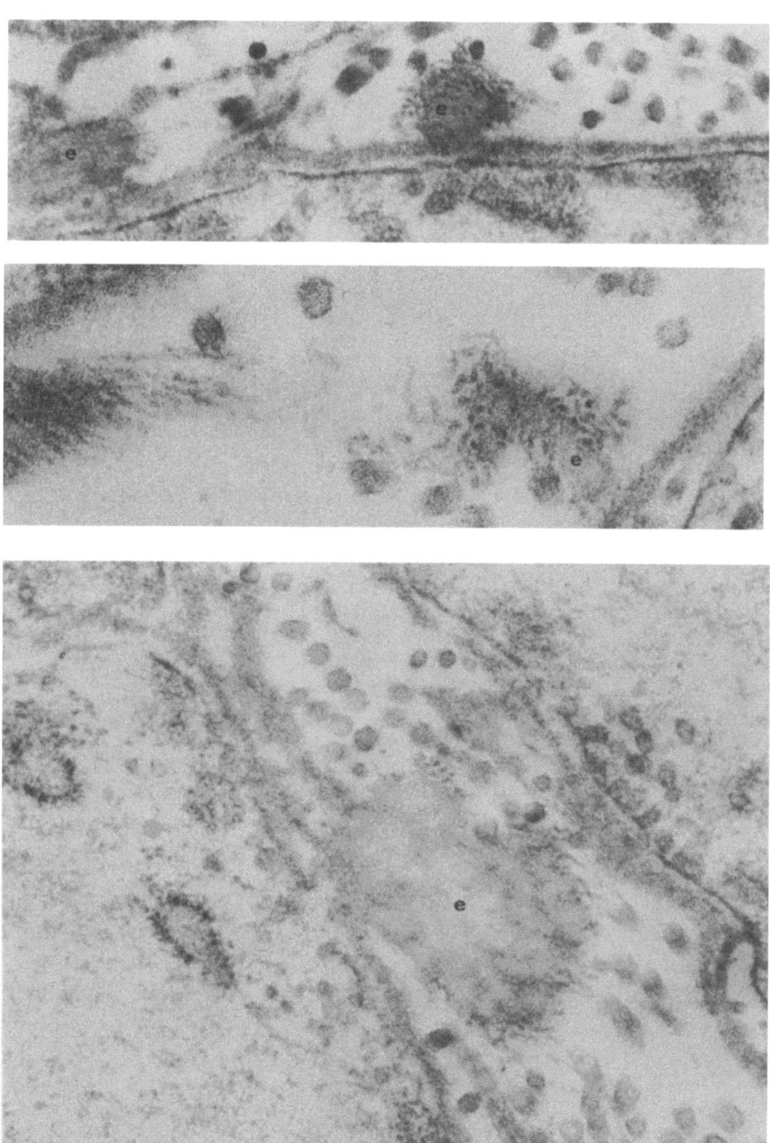

FIGURE 4a, 4b and 4c. Electron micrographs of tissues fixed in
glutaraldehyde, post-fixed in osmium tetroxide, embedded in Epon-812,
and stained with uranyl acetate and lead citrate. Examples of aortic
media from porcine fetus. Elastic tissue units and larger elements (e)
develop in close proximity to the basement membrane of medial cells.
Details of microfibrils surrounding the units are seen on cross (to
right) and longitudinal section (to left) Ø in Figure 4b.
Magnification: 4a = x 72,000; 4b = x 84,000; 4c = x 68,000.

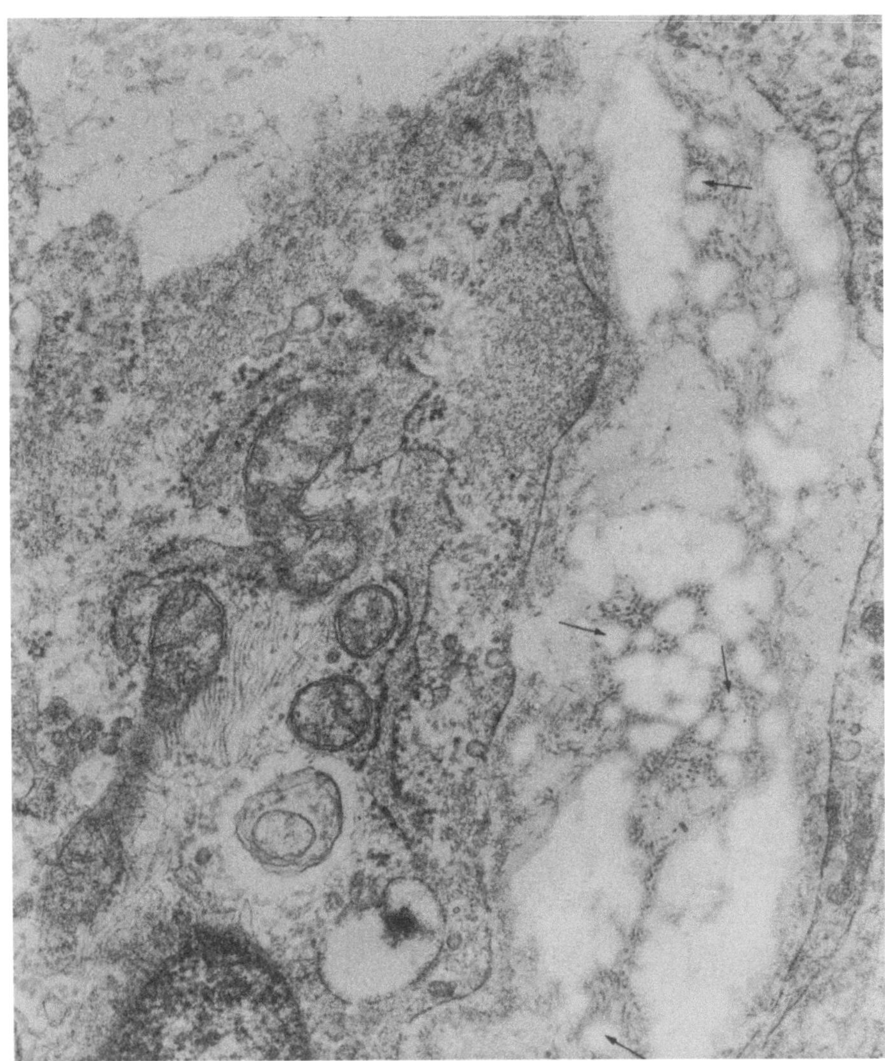

FIGURE 5. Electron micrograph of tissue fixed in glutaraldehyde, post-fixed in osmium tetroxide, embedded in Epon-812, and stained with uranyl acetate and lead citrate. Aortic medial cells in a 15-week-old human fetus. Elastic units (arrows) consisting of a central homogeneous core surrounded by microfibrils fuse to form larger elastic elements. Note that the two smooth muscle cells have many pinocytotic vesicles, prominent mitochondria, and conspicuous, dilated profiles of rough-surfaced endoplasmic reticulum with finely filamentous and granular content; magnficiation = x 42,000.

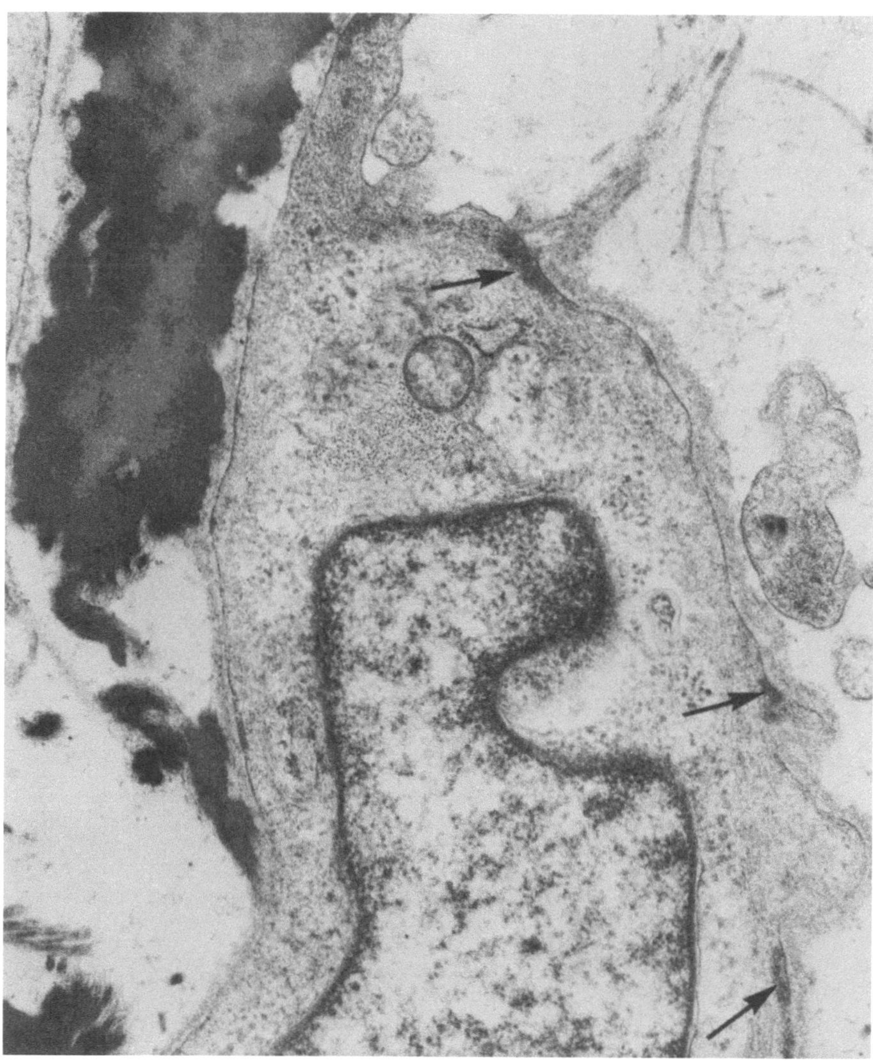

FIGURE 6. Electron micrograph of tissue fixed in glutaraldehyde, post-fixed in glosmium tetroxide, embedded in Epon-812, and stained with uranyl acetate and lead citrate. Aortic medial cell in an 8-month-old human fetus has typical features of a smooth muscle cell: a cigar-like shaped nucleus, numerous myofilaments and triangular densities (arrows), and a prominent basement membrane. Elastic elements of various order (black in this photograph) are in close proximity to the latter; magnification = x 36,000.

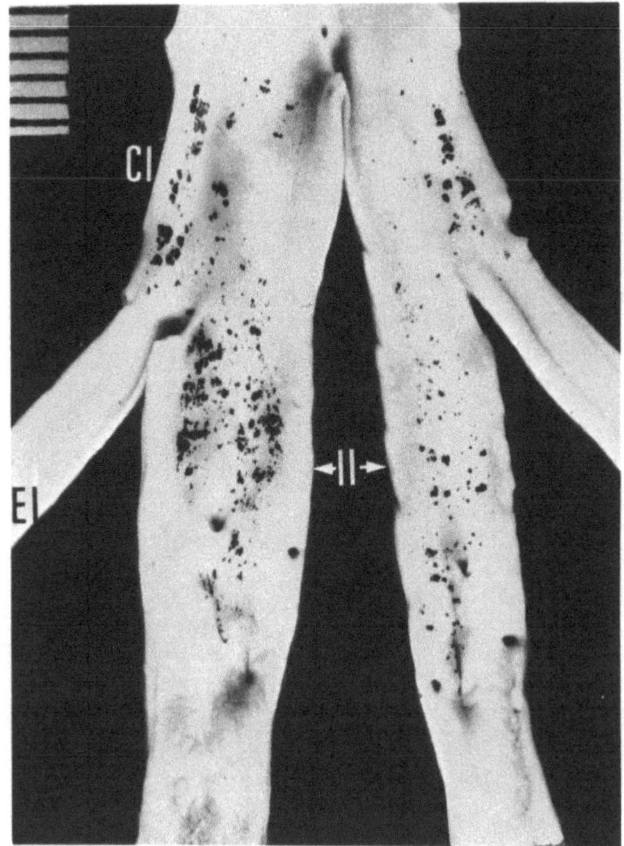

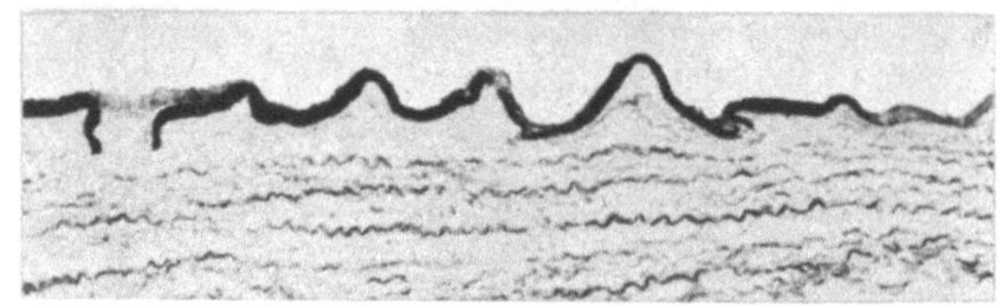

FIGURE 7. Above – Gross demonstration of calcific deposits (black)
in the iliac arteries of a full term stillborn. Von Kossa reaction.
Roundish and polygonal incrustations are scattered throughout the
inner surface of both common (EI) and internal (II) iliac arteries.
No such calcifications are present in the external iliac arteries (EI)
which are much narrower than the internal iliac arteries. Millimeter
scale on the left.
        Below – The microscopic cross section of the right internal
iliac artery. Calcified parts of the membrane are black. x 150.

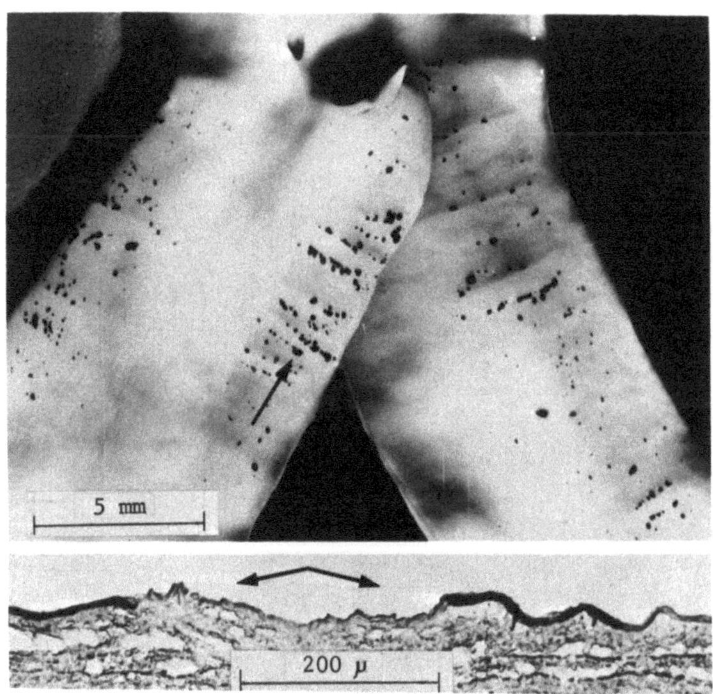

FIGURE 8a, above - Gross demonstration of calcific deposits (black)
in the internal elastic membrane of both common iliac arteries.
2-day-old newborn (internal hydrocephalus, esophageal atresia).
Von Kossa reaction.

FIGURE 8b, below - Longitudinal section of an area indicated by
arrow in FIGURE 8a. Note the gap (arrows) between the calcified
edges (black) of the internal elastic membrane. Such gaps correspond
to the calcium free bands in FIGURE 8a. Near the right border of the
figure a still noncalcified part of the internal elastic membrane is
seen.

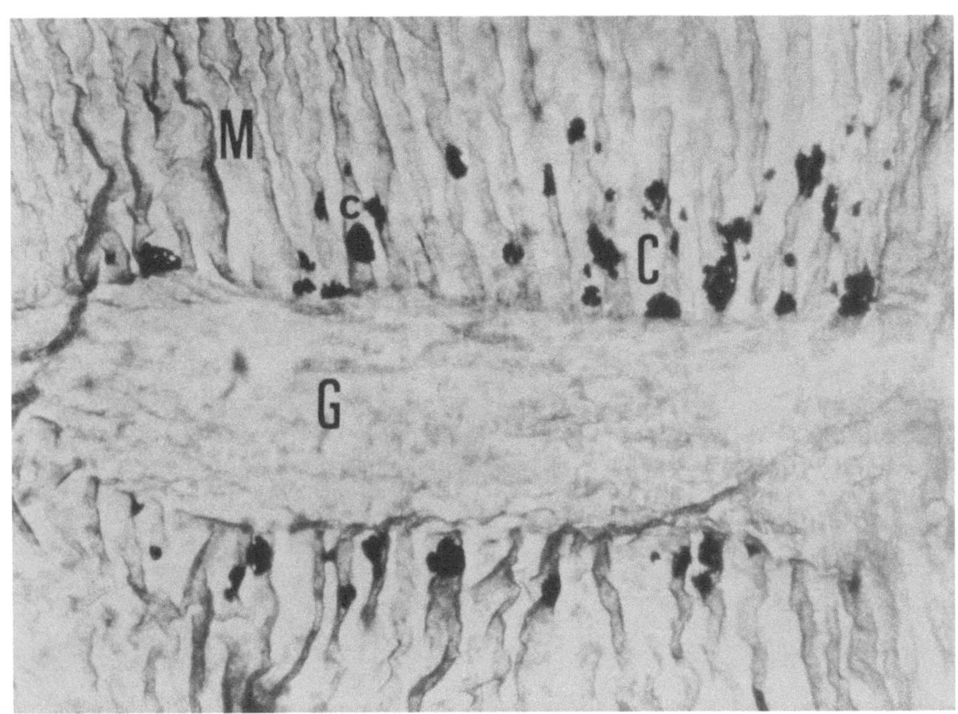

FIGURE 9. Tangential section from the common iliac artery of a newborn (four days old). Von Kossa reaction for calcium and Gomori
elastic stain. The dot-like calcifications (C) are located near a
gap (G) in the internal elastic membrane. Above and below the gap
is seen the typical wavy pattern of the membrane (M). There is no
such pattern in the gap. x 8.

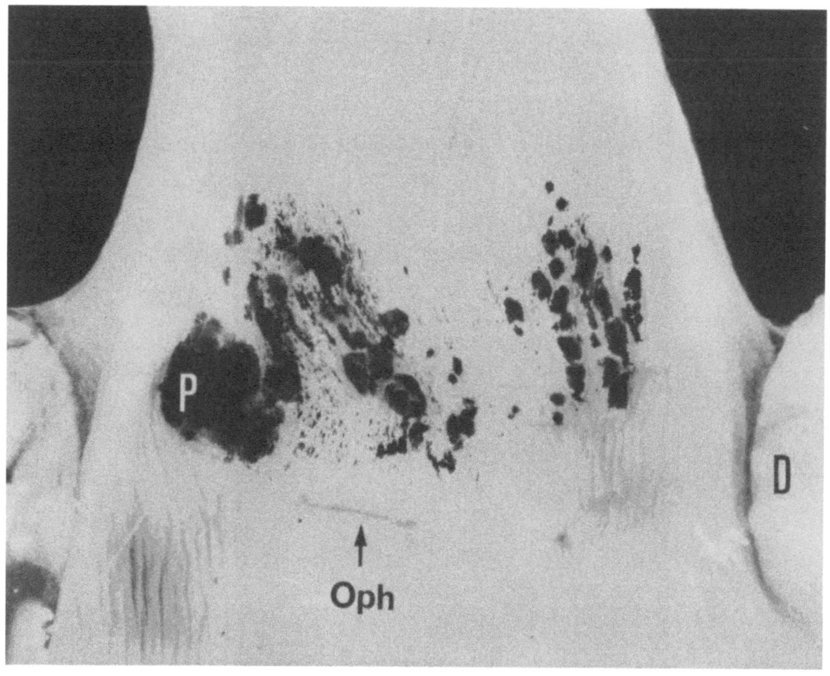

FIGURE 10. Calcifications (black) of the internal elastic membrane
and media in the upper part of the carotid siphon.   Von Kossa reaction.
P: a larger calcific plate, which penetrated in the media. Oph: origin
of the ophthalmic artery. D: Dura mater. 5-year-old girl. Death
after appendectomy. x 12.

(Monatsschr. Kinderheilk., 1971, in print).

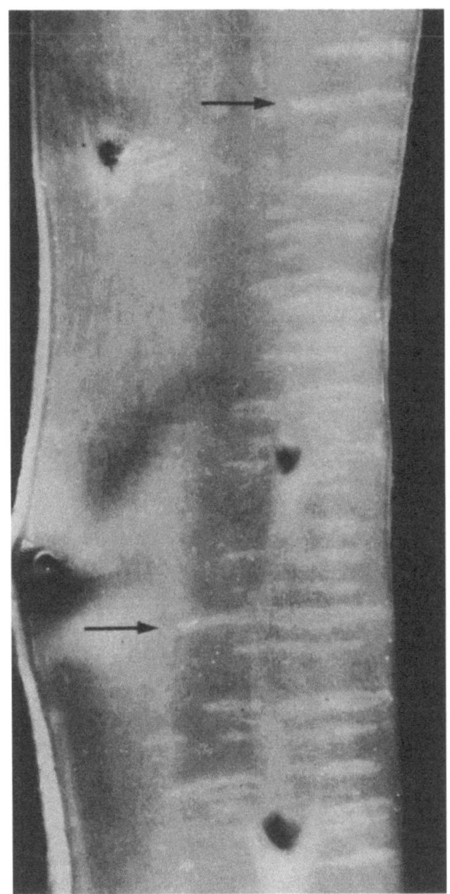

FIGURE 11. Whitish circularly oriented stripes (arrows) on the inner
surface of a femoral artery (two centimeters below the origin of the
deep femoral artery) represent the precursors of the spindles. Five-
year-old girl (56/1968). x 8.

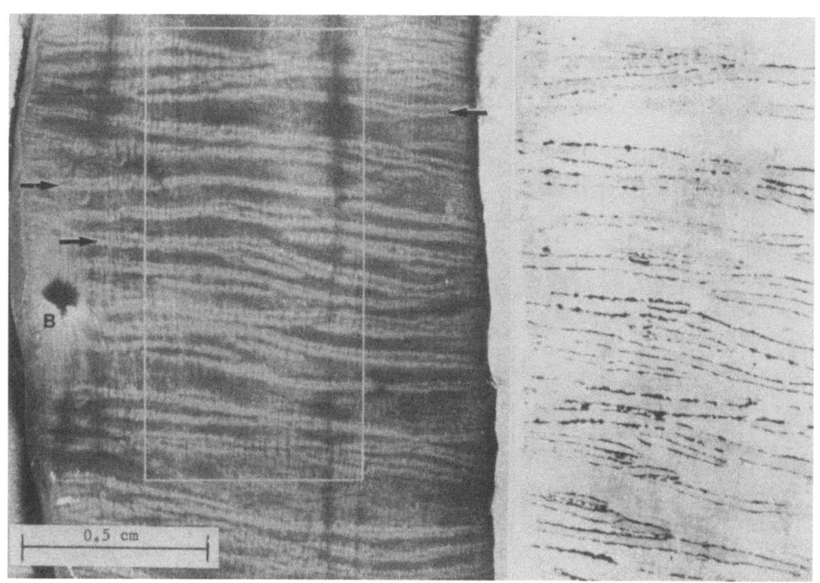

FIGURE 12. Left – Numerous fine circularly oriented spindles
(arrows) at the inner surface of the popliteal artery. B: orifice
of a small branch. The enclosed area is shown in the right figure.

Right – In the tangential section of the enclosed area
(see left) paired calcific bands (black) corresponding to the edges
of spindles are seen after Von Kossa reaction. 19-year-old man.

(Meyer and Stelzig, 1967).

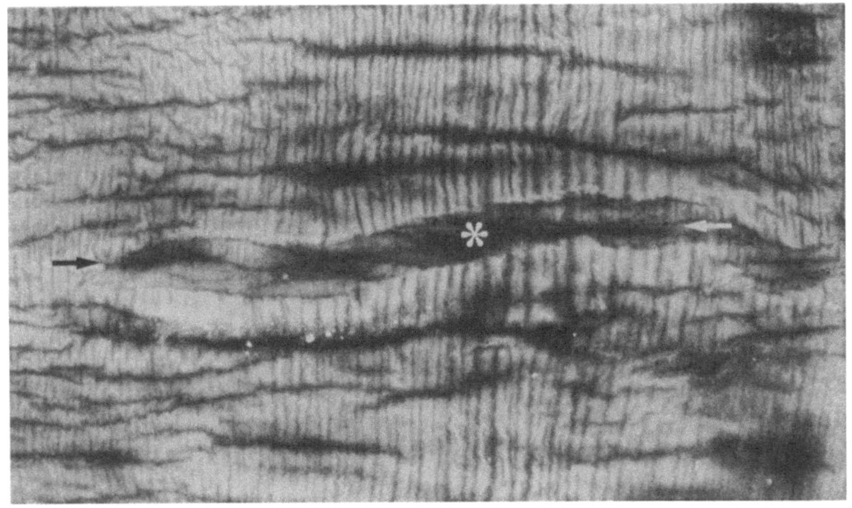

FIGURE 13. The inner surface of the femoral artery of a 20-year-old
man. Magnification 15:1 (millimeter scale below). In the middle
part of the figure a small spindle (arrows) including a gap (*) in
the internal elastic membrane is seen. The wavy appearance of the
membrane (seen everywhere at the inner surface of the artery) is
interrupted at the edges of the spindle. Above and below the spindle
many fine retraction folds of the intima are seen.

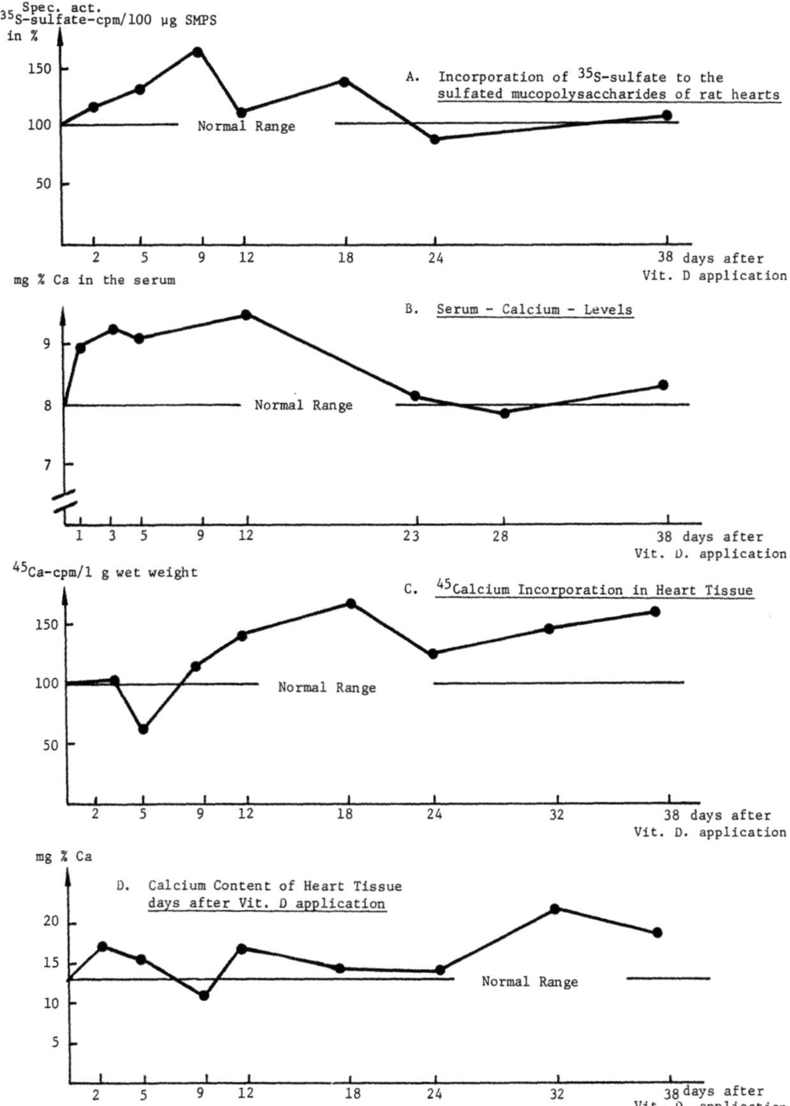

FIGURE 14. Effect of high doses of vitamin D on mesenchyme metabolism, 45calcium-incorporation, calcium concentration in rat-hearts and serum calcium levels.

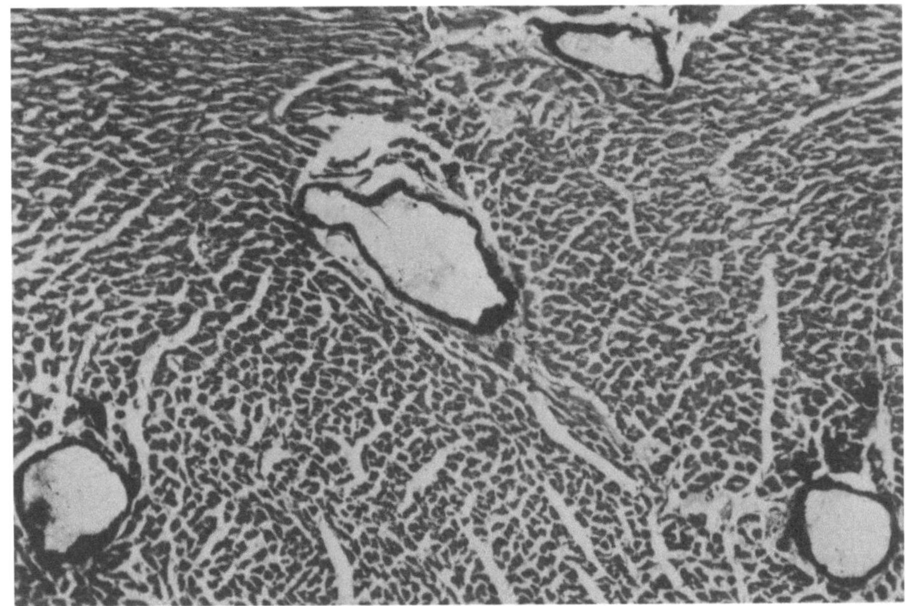

FIGURE 15. Completely calcified walls of 4 quite large, but also
unduly dilated intramyocardial rat's coronary arteries at the fourth
day of the experiments i.e. after receiving 3 daily oral toxic doses
of calciferol. Low power-Von Kossa's method.

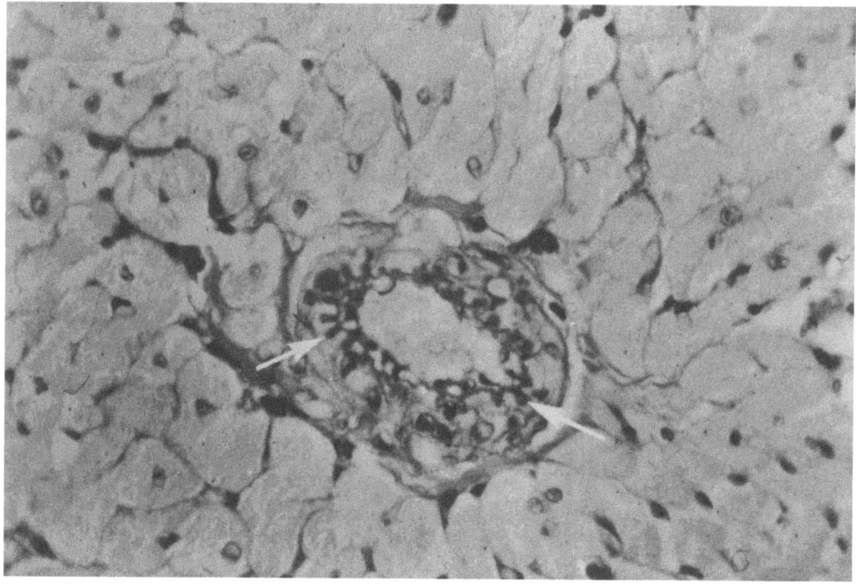

FIGURE 16. Intramyocardial branch of a healthy rat's coronary about
half way down the left ventricle from the A-V valve. Note wave (dark)
PAS-positive internal elastic lamina (arrows) and fairly thin muscular
wall and relatively acellular perivascular connective tissue sleeve.
Stained Periodic Acid Schiff-Haemalum. For comparison with FIGS. 17-
19 all at same magnification and of intramural coronary branches in
about the same position as this vessel.

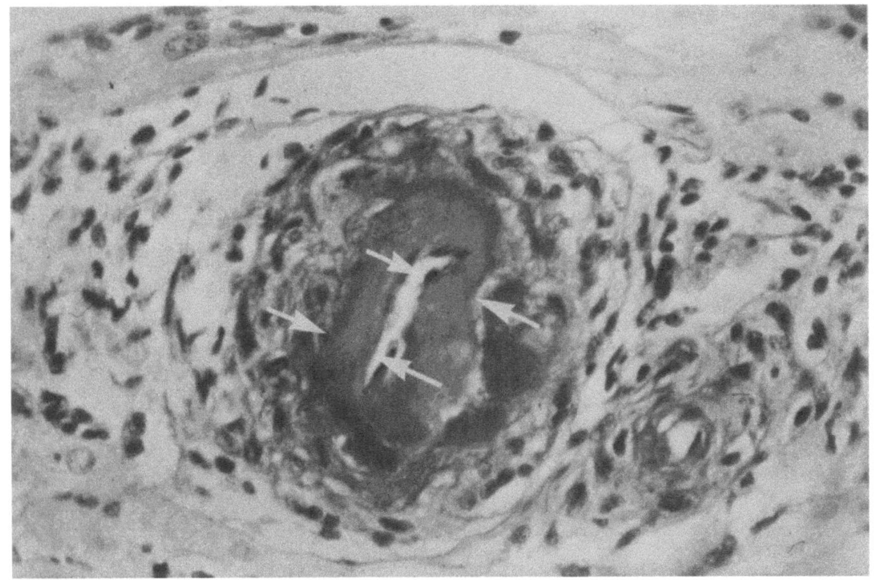

FIGURE 17. Similarly sized and placed intramural coronary artery,
to that in FIG. 16, but 30 days after the last (fifth) daily toxic
dose of calciferol given only up to day 5 of experiments. Note,
narrowed lumen, markedly thicker (swollen) heavily PAS-positive
and now no longer wavy internal elastic lamina (arrows); also swollen
media infiltrated with inflammatory cells and quite heavy round cell
infiltration in perivascular connective tissue. Calcium (histochemically and chemically) has completely disappeared (cf. 15 for
earlier calcified stage) PAS-Haemalum (for comparison with FIG. 16).

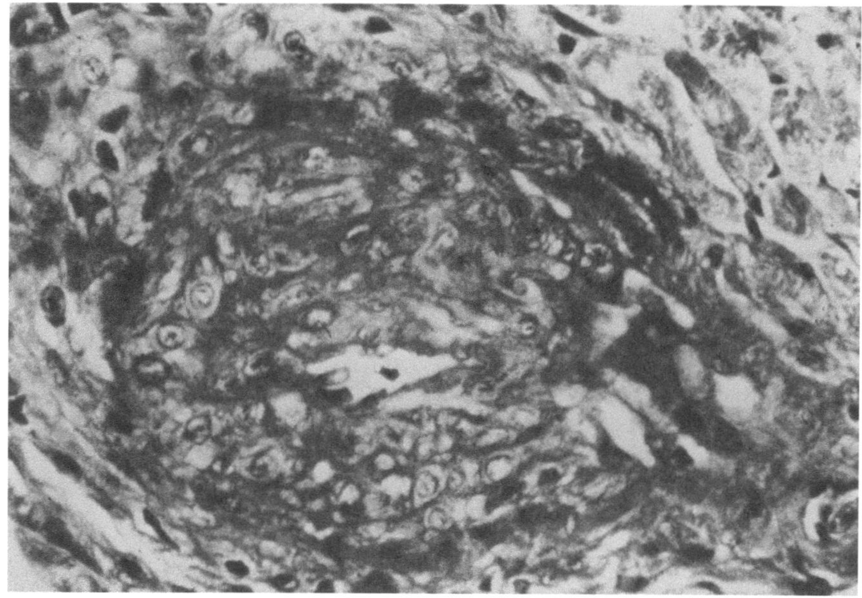

FIGURE 18. Similarly sized and located coronary (to those shown in
FIGS. 16 and 17) but some 60 days after last (fifth) daily toxic dose
of calciferol. The swollen PAS-positive elastic lamina, shown in
FIG. 17, has completely disappeared; the artery's media is much
thickened and comprised entirely of mononuclear cells, many fibro-
blastic-like, between which are pools of metachromatic (darker) polysaccharide. The now much thickened perivascular connective tissue
shows definitive collagen, round cells and fibroblast-like cells.
Stained with Acid Toluidine Blue.

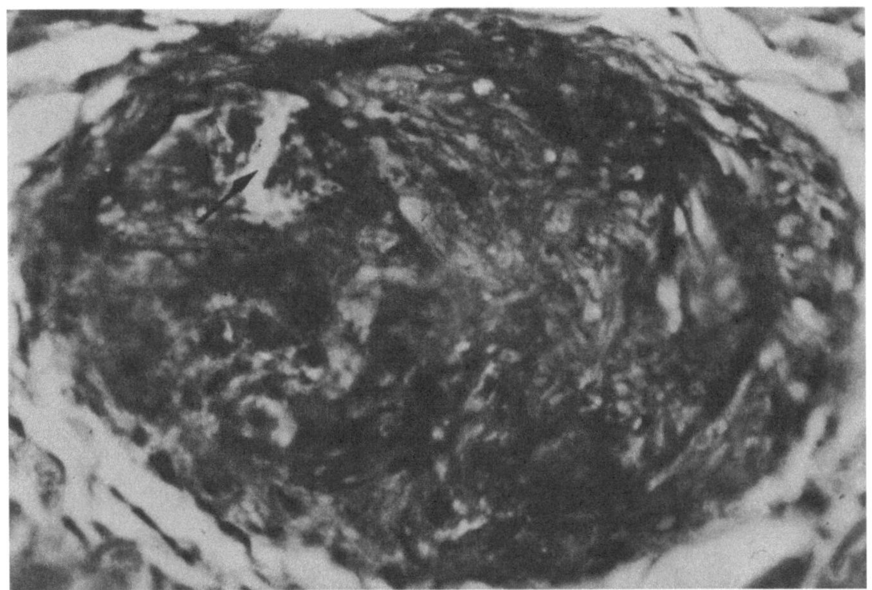

FIGURE 19. Coronary artery (similar to those shown FIGS. 16-18) at
280 days after the last (fifth) daily toxic dose of calciferol. Note
markedly increased thickening of previously totally calcified arterial
wall which, however, is now virtually acellular and comprised almost
entirely of orthochromatic collagen i.e. scar tissue. The perivascular
connective tissue is also acellular, thickened and fibrosed. Metachromatic intercellular material has now disappeared. The lumen (arrow)
is now not only very irregular in outline but quite eccentric. This,
then, is a completely sclerosed and stenosed coronary artery which was
originally severely injured by a single period of insult 275 days
previously. Acid Toluidine Blue (for comparison with FIG. 18).

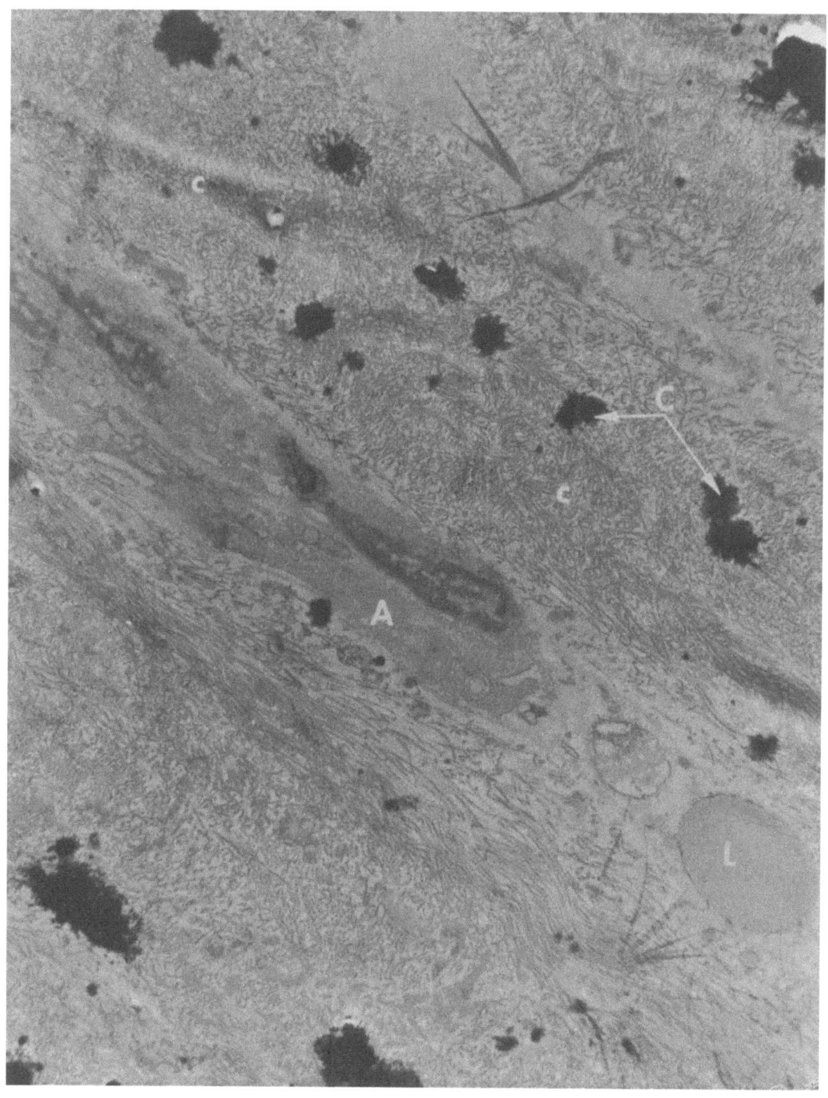

FIGURE 20. A. Electron micrograph of human coronary intimal layer showing early stages of calcification (C) in altered collagen fibers (c) surrounding myointimal cell (atherophil) (A) and an enlarged membrane bound lipid droplet (L).

Uranyl Acetate – Lead Hydroxide Staining   13,100X

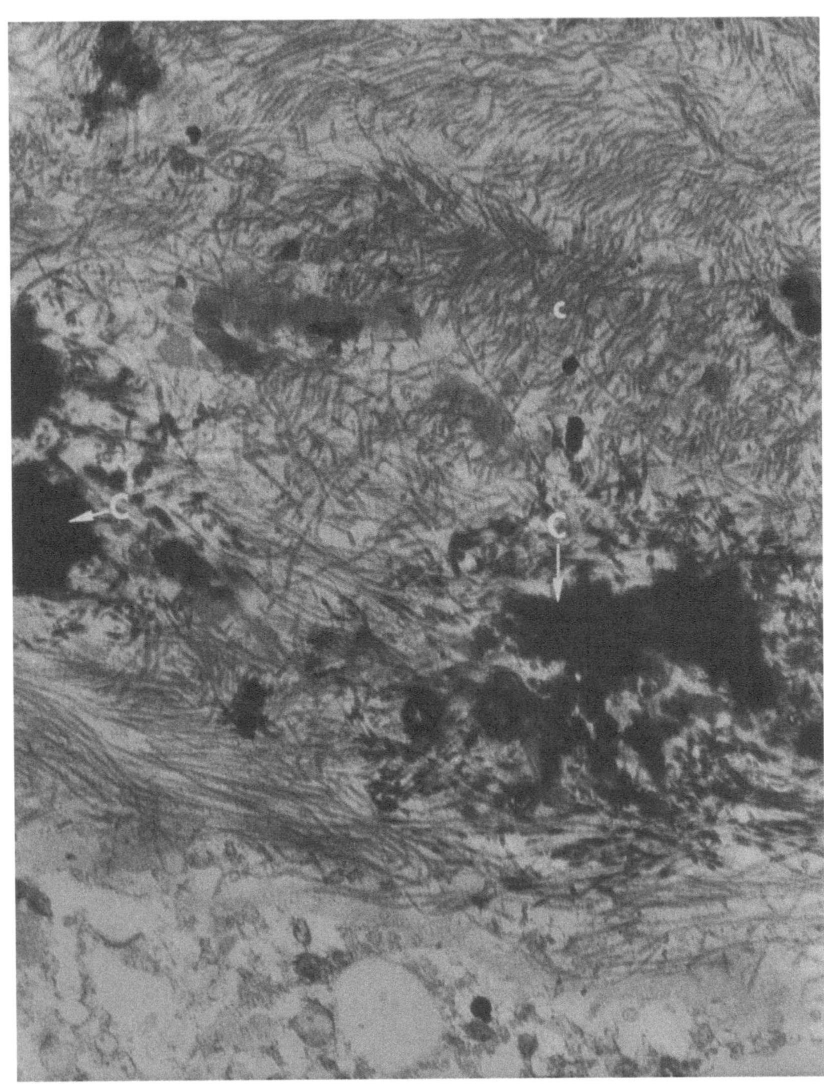

B. Enlargement of similar area as in A showing increased
electron density of pseudoelastin or altered collagen fibers (c)
surrounding amorphous dense deposits that seem to use these fibers
as a matrix for deposition of Ca.
Uranyl Acetate - Lead Hydroxide Staining   36,000X

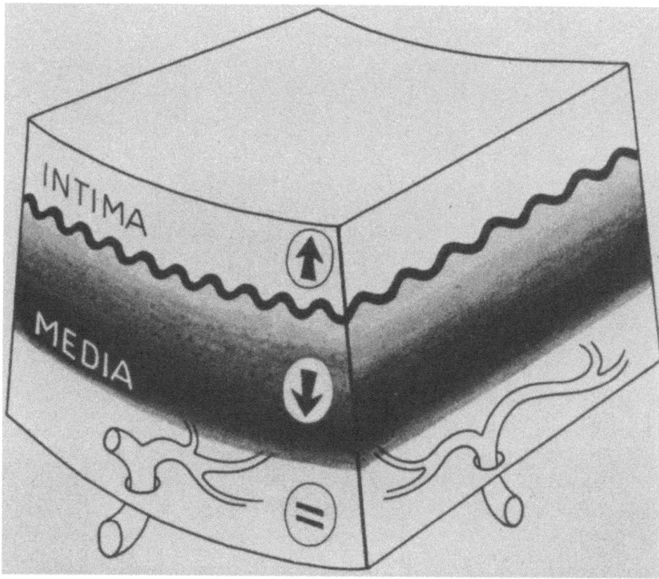

FIGURE 21. Diagrammatic representation of the thickening aorta
of man showing penetration of basa basorum.

Chapter 2

ENDOCRINE, CHEMICAL AND NEURAL REGULATORS AND

THE EFFECTS OF AGING

PARTICIPANTS: Max Anliker, Felix Anschutz, Bernard Brodie,
               Ervin Erdos, Meyer Friedman, Andres Goth, Donald
               Gregg, C.G. Gunn, W.H. Hauss and R.A. Schneider

DR. ERDOS: I believe that a conference on the blood vessel
wall would not be complete without mentioning some of the agents
that act on these tissues. Dr. Brodie will certainly talk about
norepinephrine and epinephrine and Dr. Goth about histamine. I
should like to bring up two peptides, angiotensin and bradykinin,
which have such strong hypertensive and hypotensive effects respectively. The sequence of events which leads to the release and inactivation of kinins in plasma (Erdos, 1970) is more complex than
the one which is responsible for blood coagulation. To state it
simply, the activation of kallikrein leads to the release of bradykinin in plasma. Kallikrein acts as an enzyme on a plasma protein
substrate called kininogen. The active peptide is the product of
the reaction. Kallikreins occur in the blood but also in glandular
tissues and in the urine. Many pathological processes mentioned
in this meeting, such as activation of plasmin or activation of
Factor XII, could lead to the activation of prekallikrein, consequent to the release of a kinin (FIG. 1) which is in turn destroyed
very rapidly in plasma and in tissues. Bradykinin and the related
kallidin are the strongest endogenous hypotensive peptides. They
cause permeability changes, pain, vasodilation and migration of
leukocytes.

The other peptide which should be mentioned here is angiotensin.
As you all know, renin of the kidney acts on a plasma protein, angio-

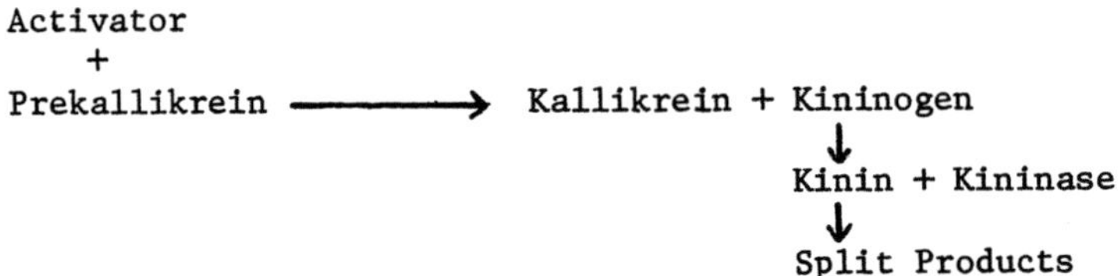

FIGURE 1. Simplified scheme for the relase and inactivation of kinin in plasma

tensinogen, and releases a peptide, angiotensin I. This peptide has to be converted by an enzyme, named converting enzyme, to the active material angiotensin II. The reaction consists of cleaving off a histidyl-leucine dipeptide from the C-terminal end of angiotensin I. Angiontensin II itself is the strongest endogenous vasopressor agent. It is a vasoconstrictor, contracts many isolated smooth muscles and releases aldosterone (FIG. 2). I want to mention only one aspect of our work with these materials. This is the relationship between the metabolism of angiotensin and bradykinin because possibly blood vessels are involved here.

$$\text{Renin + Angiotensinogen}$$
$$\downarrow$$
$$\text{Angiotensin I + Converting Enzyme}$$
$$\downarrow$$
$$\text{Angiotensin II + Angiotensinase}$$
$$\downarrow$$
$$\text{Split Product}$$

FIGURE 2. Simplified scheme for the release and inactivation of angiotensin in plasma.

Human plasma has at least two enzymes which inactivate bradykinin. The first one, called carboxypeptidase N, inactivates it by removing one amino acid, the C-terminal arginine. The second enzyme, which occurs in blood and in tissues such as lung and kidney, acts by removing a dipeptide, the C-terminal phenylalanyl-arginine of bradykinin. It is called kininase II. A C-terminal dipeptide, although a different one, is liberated when angiotensin I is converted to angiotensin II. We showed that in plasma, the same enzyme which inactivates bradykinin can also convert angiotensin I to angiotensin II (Yang and Erdos et al., 1970a; Yang and Erdos et al., 1970b; Yang and Erdos et al., in press); thus, kininase II is identical with an angiotensin I converting enzyme. Very likely, the physiologically important converting enzyme in the lung also functions as a kininase (Yang and Erdos et al., in press). Presumably this enzyme occurs in the lung somewhere on the endothelial surface of the blood vessels. If this assumption is valid, then the blood vessels are involved in the metabolism of both the most potent endogenous hypertensive and hypotensive peptide by inactivating the hypotensive one or releasing the hypertensive peptide.

DR. GOTH: The mast cell is of interest in relation to vascular reactions for a number of reasons. The cell contains such powerful pharmacological agents as histamine, heparin and chymotrypsin-like proteases. Although little is known about the release of these agents under physiologic conditions, there is a great deal of information on their release during anaphylaxis and allergic reactions. Also, many drugs are capable of acting on mast cells without prior sensitization (Goth, 1967).

I should like to summarize some of the current concepts about mast cells and discuss some of our recent experiments which suggest an influence of phospholipids on mast cell function. Although these experiments deal with histamine release and experimental hypersensitivity they may have some relevance to the possible connections between lipid metabolism and the mast cell.

A typical mast cell contains numerous large granules, which in the rat represent packages of heparin bound tightly to a chymotrypsin-like protease. These granules contain also a high concentration of histamine and - in some species - serotonin. It is well established that as a consequence of antigen-antibody reactions, the action of various drugs, basic polypeptides, or certain enzymes, histamine is released from the cell. The release process is not simply a consequence of cell damage. It rather resembles a secretory process consisting of two steps. During the first step, which requires energy, the granules are extruded. Once outside the cell, in a second step, histamine is released from the granule passively by an exchange with cations of the extracellular environment (Uvnäs and Thon, 1966).

The observations on the possible role of phospholipids on mast cell function are an outgrowth of investigations on the anaphylactoid reaction of rats to dextran and ovomucoid. Several years ago we found that this sort of reaction is intimately linked to carbohydrate metabolism (Goth and Nash et al., 1957). In investigating this relationship in vitro, we found as did others (Lagunoff and Benditt, 1960), that despite the susceptibility of rats to dextran and ovomucoid, their mast cells in the test tube failed to react to them. On further investigation we found that dextran and ovomucoid required certain cofactors in order to act on rat mast cells in vitro (Goth, 1966). In recent studies in our laboratory the cofactor present especially in mixed brain lipids, turned out to be phosphatidylserine. This particular phosphatide increases greatly the response of rat mast cells to dextran, ovomucoid, and protein antigens to which the rat has been previously sensitized. It appears that phosphatidylserine is an enhancer of anaphylactic histamine release in the rat. Interestingly, the phosphatide has no effect on the mast cell by itself and it has no enhancing action on histamine release by chemicals, such as compound 48/80.

It is important to point out, that the action of phosphatidylserine is not a simple detergent effect, since a variety of detergents do not show the enhancing action. Furthermore, the ability to promote anaphylactic histamine release is not a general property of phospholipids, since lecithin not only does not enhance histamine release, but actually tends to inhibit it.

It is too early to speculate about the significance of these findings. They may simply represent some curious interactions between phospholipids and mast cells. On the other hand, they may point to a role for phospholipids in mast cell function.

DR. BRODIE: It would be desirable to seek evidence of these processes being controlled by sympathetic nerve endings.

DR. GUNN: In order to understand the role of neural mechanisms potentially regulating arterial wall metabolism, we may gain some insight by looking at arteries that are operating without neural control after denervation.

RABBIT Rabbits fed cholesterol have very little atherosclerosis below the diaphragm. If a bilateral sympathectomy and periaortic stripping are done, the sub-diaphragmatic aorta becomes atherosclerotic (Snyder and Campbell, 1958; Murphy and Haglin et al., 1957).

Recently Marinescu and associates (Mariniscu and Pausescu et al., 1968) have shown some of the arterial wall metabolic consequences of sympathectomy. Decreases in hyaluronic acid, catecholamines, and lactic dehydrogenase activity were seen, while striking increases in adenosine triphosphatase (ATP), alkaline phosphatase, acetylcholinesterase and neutral mucopolysaccharides were noted, especially in the subintimal media. Inability to demonstrate cholesterol by histochemical stains was thought to be due to insensitive techniques.

DOG At the University of Oklahoma, preliminary experiments with Drs. Werthessen, Stout, Stamatis, and Williams (Gunn and Stout et al., in preparation) were designed to investigate possible changes in lipid metabolism in the artery wall when the neural influence was totally removed by denervation similar to that seen in organ transplantation. Using one femoral artery of the dog as a control, a segment of the opposite artery was denervated by removal and immediate replacement autograft or by adventitial and medial stripping and phenol coagulation. Earlier results showed little difference between these techniques except the excision and

Effects of arterial
denervation on
lipid synthesis

replacement technique guarantees complete denervation without risk of rupture and hemorrhage. This autograft technique provided the data shown below.

The animals, eating dry laboratory chow, were sacrificed after either three or six weeks post arterial denervation. Using the exquisitely sensitive chromatographic techniques of Werthessen, Beall and James (Werthessen and Beall et al., 1970), free and esterified cholesterol, phospholipids, triglycerides and free fatty acids were all determined from the same small arterial tissue samples and expressed as micrograms/mg of dry defatted tissue. Lipid synthesis is reflected in C^{14} acetate incorporation in the same lipid fractions as counts/mg of dry defatted tissue. At three weeks, our results (TABLE I) with six dogs suggest that the lipid content is roughly one-third greater in the denervated arteries with the compartmentation as shown. It seems that the greatest differences are in sterol esters, FFA, and phospholipids. There is no significant difference in the triglycerides.

TABLE I

LIPID CONTENT - DOG ARTERIES

(μg./Mg. Dry Wt. - Mean Values)

3 weeks (6 DOGS)	Sterol Esters	Tri- Gl.	Free Sterols	Free F.A.	Phospho- Lipids	Total Lipids
CONTROL -	2.54	2.25	2.45	2.57	22.3	9.84
DENERVATED -	4.64	1.76	3.73	5.41	29.55	15.55
. . . .		. . . . .	. . . . . .	. . . . .	. . . . .	. . . .	
6 weeks (4 DOGS)						
CONTROL -	4.22	7.70	6.00	8.12	-	26.02
DENERVATED -	7.87	9.60	6.17	10.70	-	34.35

When we look at the lipid synthesis data from the C^{14} acetate incorporation into the same lipid fractions from the same arterial samples, (TABLE II) we see evidence of more synthesis in the denervated artery than its contralateral intact control. This difference is greater at three weeks than it is at six weeks. Unfortunately, we can not rule out some reinnervation at this time. There is clearly more denervated artery phospholipid synthesis than the other lipid fractions, but the denervated arteries also show a greater percent increase in triglyceride synthesis than is seen in triglyceride content. Although the numbers are small, the results are consistent in the direction of the differences between denervated arteries and their controls.

TABLE II

LIPID SYNTHESIS - DOG ARTERIES

(C^{14} Incorporation - Counts/Mg. Dry Wt.)

3 weeks (6 DOGS)	Sterol Esters	Tri- Gl.	Free Sterols	Free F.A.	Phospho- Lipids	Total Lipids
CONTROL -	0.92	1.50	3.04	5.31	128.8	10.77
DENERVATED -	13.94	14.19	17.34	26.73	1513.0	72.20
....	....	....	....	....	....	
6 weeks (4 DOGS)						
CONTROL -	0.92	1.27	3.62	13.95	-	19.76
DENERVATED -	2.50	11.95	6.20	22.57	-	43.22

We believe that these preliminary results are consistent with the
concepts that lipid mobilization is suppressed and that lipid synthesis
is increased by denervation. Storage kinetics of exogenous lipids remains to be investigated. It is not too difficult to postulate that
both a suppressed mobilization and an increased synthesis of lipids
within an artery wall may be related to atherogenesis.

Snyder and Campbell (Snyder and Campbell, 1958) showed a number
of years ago as did a researcher named Murphy (Murphy and Haglin et
al., 1957) that sympathectomy will enhance the atheromatous process
in the aorta of a rabbit fed a cholesterol diet. Dr. Friedman and
I also had a series of sympathetically denervated animals that had
markedly sclerotic coronary arteries compared to a non-denervated
but centrally stimulated group, but we let them go too long and they
had regeneration of the sympathetics so we never published this.

In any event, these data strongly suggest that the artery wall
needs the trophic influence of neural stimulation to maintain morphological and functional integrity. Later on I will present evidence
that too much as well as too little adrenergic innervation may be
atherogenic, through what appears to be a different peripheral mechanism. We hope to have more information about cholinergic mechanisms
and also specific adrenergic influences on lipid and protein metabolism soon.

COMMENT

The possible relevance of denervation to the advanced atherosclerosis observed in the coronary arteries of transplanted hearts
is considered in Chapter 8.

DR. BRODIE: It is not generally recognized how necessary the
hormones of the adrenal cortex are to the action of catecholamines.
It is well known that the Addisonian patient is poorly responsive
to sympathetic stimulation and that adrenalectomized rats, especially
when deprived of salt, have almost no response to catecholamines.
Later on in the meeting I shall discuss this aspect in more length.
Meanwhile, I would like to mention some studies carried out by Dr.
Jerome Fleisch in my laboratory (Fleisch and Maling et al., 1970).
It is generally assumed that the smooth muscle of arterial wall contains mainly alpha adrenergic sites. These sites mediate constriction
with epinephrine or norepinephrine. Dr. Fleisch became interested
in the beta adrenergic sites which are also present in arterial smooth
muscle. These beta adrenergic sites mediate relaxation by norepinephrine or epinephrine and thus produce effects antagonistic to those
on the alpha sites. They are thus functionally the equivalent of
the cholinergic nervous system.

To show whether beta sites exist, aortic strips are stimulated **RAT**
by agents such as norepinephrine or histamine, thus producing a con- **RABBIT**
traction of the smooth muscle. The presence of beta sites may now
be shown by the ability of isoproterenol to elicit muscle relaxation. **GUINEA PIG**
Using this technique, he showed that thoracic aortic strips from rats,
rabbits and guinea pigs, but not cats, contained beta adrenergic sites. **CAT**
The dilatation produced by isoproterenol could be prevented by beta
blocking agents. These experiments were carried out in young animals.
However, aortic strips from older rats and rabbits no longer contained
beta adrenergic sites but were capable of relaxation by other agents
such as sodium nitrate.

Loss of beta vaso-   These results indicate that in
dilator sites in arter-   young rats and rabbits the arterial
ies with aging   smooth muscle contained beta sites
                                      which counteracted the constricting
effects elicited by the alpha sites, but that these beta sites disappeared in older rats and rabbits.

It is tempting to consider the possibility that the disappearance
of the beta sites in vascular smooth muscle is part of the aging process. In the absence of the balancing action of the beta sites, the
alpha sites may produce overreaction of the smooth muscle in response
to catecholamines and thus encourage those diseases of the vascular
system that are associated with age. These studies are still in progress and their pertinence to the problem in which this program is
concerned is not yet evident.

COMMENT

Dr. Donald Gregg focused attention on the regulation of the
smooth muscle in the walls of arterioles and small arteries that
regulate the coronary blood flow. He carried the discussion to

studies on the ability of the coronary vessels to dilate and the
permeability characteristics of certain vessels. He pointed out in
dogs that dilatability is the ability of the vascular bed to dilate
after a temporary occlusion of 10-12 seconds and he presented evidence
that flow following brief occlusion increases 35-350 times. Loss of
such ability to increase flow results in collateral vessel development. This dilation is not dependent on coronary innervation (since
totally denervated hearts can dilate their vasculature) but rather on
various substances such as metabolites of the cardiac musculature.
It is not clear what substance or substances are dominant in this
regard. Dr. Gregg suggested two substances, adenosine and potassium
which might be important substances to consider since both are potent
vasodilators of arterioles but it is not clear if these are the crucial metabolites. In addition, Dr. Gregg pointed out that it is not
clear if such substances are released from cardiac muscle cells to
diffuse into arterioles to bring about their effect or if these substances accumulate within the arterioles themselves. Dr. Gregg then
presented evidence to show that as arterial pO_2 decreased, vascular
(arteriolar or small vessel) conductance increased or, to put it
another way, as pO_2 decreased vascular resistance decreased (vessels
dilate). That is, anoxia per se also causes dilatation.

As regards vessel permeability, Dr. Gregg presented data from Dr.
Robert Burns' laboratory where periarteriolar pO_2 measurements were
made in hamster cheek pouch. They could follow a decrease in perivascular pO_2 as they sampled from large artery out to 20μ arterioles. pO_2
was 67 around large vessels and decreased to 20 in areas were 20μ arterioles were present. Since nitroglycerine will dilate 80μ arterioles
in the heart, it might speak for beneficial effects of nitroglycerin.

Lastly, Dr. Gregg commented on studies in dogs with chronically
implanted flow meters (6 months) in the coronary sinus and coronary arteries, who when given isoproterenol or epinephrine got increased coronary blood flow (even before cardiac output increased). Beta-block-
ers prevented this increased flow so that there is some evidence that
even in the intact animal receptors are present in the coronary vasculature. This finding corroborates the in vitro findings reported by
Dr. Brodie earlier in this session. However, Dr. Gregg is unable to
find any relationship between the activity of these receptors and aging
in the dog, as Dr. Brodie has seen in the rat, rabbit and guinea pig.

DR. GREGG: To study the mechanisms controlling coronary vascular
tone, one must have a reference test for dilatability of the normal
coronary vascular bed responding to natural stresses and for dilatability of the coronary insufficient bed. The test generally used is
the maximum increase in flow that follows release of a 10-15 second
occlusion of a coronary artery branch. The magnitude of such dilatability or reactive hyperemia (which may be reduced or disappear in
the diseased coronary bed) is very large in the normal coronary bed,

being 5 to 10 times the control flow and it occurs without change in
systemic dynamics (Khouri and Gregg et al., 1968).

At least two major theories have been advanced to account for
the dilatability of the coronary vascular bed. According to classic
physiology, hypoxic tissue releases a metabolite, as yet unidentified,
which diffuses to small vessels and causes them to dilate. This
mechanism lacks specificity for precapillary sphincters and involves
the assumptions that vascular muscle is a passive oxygen-insensitive
effector, and that oxygen-linked vasodilatation depends on the surrounding tissue. From a number of possible metabolites, Berne (Berne,
1963) has proposed that adenosine may be the transmitter between oxygen
supply and vasomotor tone. The findings of Dr. Olsson, et al., from
our laboratory (Olsson, 1970) using a high resolution biochemical
method heretofore not available, lend some support to this view.

A second view, Guyton, et al., (Guyton and Ross et al., 1964),
and Honig (Honig, 1968) suggests that instead of a diffusible substance, the coupling between tissue metabolism and the circulation
is accomplished through an oxygen-linked metabolite within the vascular
smooth muscle cells. This vascular smooth muscle would "sample" oxygen
availability and adjust vasomotor tone to oxygen demand. Support for
this view is that active vascular smooth muscle apparently has a high
oxygen consumption and that when a whole limb or an isolated small
artery from it is perfused with blood of progressively decreasing
pO_2, the percentage increase in conductance (flow) is as large in
the artery as in the whole limb. The active metabolite has not been
identified.

These views, although lacking experimental proof, are attractive
and provide at least a starting point for our thinking regarding basic
controls of coronary blood flow. In closing, I would refer to some
recent interesting experiments from Dr. Berne's laboratory (Duling
and Berne, 1970). The oxygen tension on the external surfaces of
arterioles and arteries between 8 and 100μ in diameter was measured
with micro oxygen electrodes (2-6μ diameter) in the suffused cheek
pouch of the hamster, the pO_2 of the suffusion fluid being widely
varied. Significant longitudinal gradients were found in periarterial
pO_2. This finding is consistent with the view that significant amounts
of oxygen diffuse from the precapillary vessels and that intravascular
pO_2 falls progressively along the resistance vessels. If this finding
has application in the heart (and at present there is no evidence that
it does), it would provide yet another mechanism for involvement of
oxygen in local regulation of coronary blood flow.

DR. ANLIKER: A difficult situation presents itself when we face
the problem of recognizing the gradual development of a deconditioning
of astronauts as a result of prolonged exposure to weightlessness.
(Known to be associated with decreased adrenergic discharges (Goodall,

1971.) The cardiovascular system of astronauts was shown to undergo
a space adaptation which has been observed in the form of a reduced
tilt-table tolerance even after space flights of only a few days' duration. Without effective countermeasures we are uncertain whether
the cardiovascular system will retain its ability to supply adequate
blood flow to the brain and muscle during reentry from space flights
of longer duration. To establish the effectiveness of proposed countermeasures we have to establish transcutaneous, noninvasive experimental procedures to acquire precise information on the cardiovascular
system parameters without significantly disturbing the subject. For
example, we think of measuring the local distensibility of blood vessels, their geometry and the blood flow pattern without penetrating
the skin by using ultrasound echo ranging devices (Arndt, 1969) and
pulsed ultrasound flow meters (Baker and Watkins, 1967; Peronneau and
Leger, 1969). The data obtained in this manner are obviously only as
reliable and accurate as are the mathematical models introduced for
the transmission, scatter and reflection of ultrasound in biological
tissues and blood and as are the models for the mechanical behavior of
the vessels and the blood they contain. Systematic theoretical and
experimental studies are therefore being supported to develop sufficiently accurate mathematical models and the instruments which would
permit us to evaluate the changes in blood flow and in the mechanical
properties of arteries and veins caused by aging, diseases and exposure
to weightlessness.

     Whereas most theoretical investigations of blood flow and of the
mechanical behavior of blood vessels are based on a linearized analysis, we infer from the literature that practically all earlier experimental in vivo studies are associated with large pressure changes and
as such must be expected to exhibit nonlinear phenomena. A series of
experiments have therefore been performed on anesthetized dogs in which
small sinusoidal perturbations were induced in the aorta, carotid
artery and vena cava in the form of pressure waves and also in the
carotid artery in the form of waves involving primarily axial and
torsion type vessel wall displacements. The experimental setup used
for the aorta is shown in FIGURE 3 (Anliker and Histand et al., 1968),
and those for the carotid artery (Moritz, 1969) and inferior vena cava
(Yates, 1969) are given in FIGURES 4 and 5. Representative tracings
of recordings of the natural pulse wave in the thoracic aorta with
the superimposed trains of sinusoidal pressure waves are illustrated
in FIGURE 6 together with the corresponding diameter changes recorded
with the help of a Pieper diameter gage. The results from the aortic
studies corroborate theoretical predictions that pressure waves with
frequencies between 20 and 200 hertz are essentially nondispersive.
The waves are strongly attenuated, though, primarily due to the visco-
elastic nature of the vessel wall. Relatively strong nonlinear effects
were observed through a marked increase in wave speed with pressure
(see FIG. 7) and the convection of the pressure perturbations by the
mean flow associated with the natural pressure pulse (Histand, 1969).
The findings from the carotid artery verify mathematical analyses

SCHEMATIC OF EXPERIMENTAL ARRANGEMENT

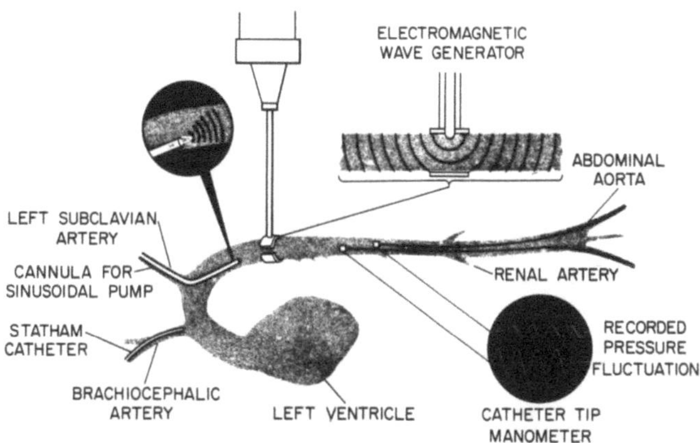

FIGURE 3. Experimental setup for generating small sinusoidal pressure waves in the canine aorta by a sinusoidal pump or an electromagnetic wave generator. The transient signals are sensed by wind
tunnel pressure gages which were adapted for use as catheter-tip
manometers in blood vessels.

(Klip and von Loon et al., 1967; Anliker and Maxwell, 1966) insofar
as torsion and axial waves are being propagated, but their speeds are
much below what would be expected on the basis of the propagation
characteristics of pressure waves in the same vessel. This discrepancy between theory and experiment suggests that the wall of the carotid is anisotropically elastic and has a Young's modulus which is
considerably lower in the axial direction than it is for the circumferential direction. When we want to identify and interpret local
variations of certain cardiovascular parameters like flow velocity,
pressure and wall displacements we may have to take into account the
nonlinear wall elasticity and anisotropy as well as the nonlinear
hemodynamic phenomena documented in these experiments.

The most intriguing feature of blood vessels and perhaps also
the most difficult one to account for in studying the local and regional changes of cardiovascular parameters is that of the active response of the smooth muscle in the vessel wall caused by neural or
humoral stimuli. By measuring simultaneously the internal diameter
and the wave transmission characteristics of the inferior vena cava,
as illustrated in FIGURE 5, it can be demonstrated that the stimulation
of the smooth muscle in the vena cava wall causes the vessel to con-
strict and generally lowers the effective Young's modulus for a given
wall stress. The stimulation elicits an active response of the vessel
which can manifest itself by a paradox situation where we have a decreasing diameter in the presence of an increasing pressure. FIGURE 8

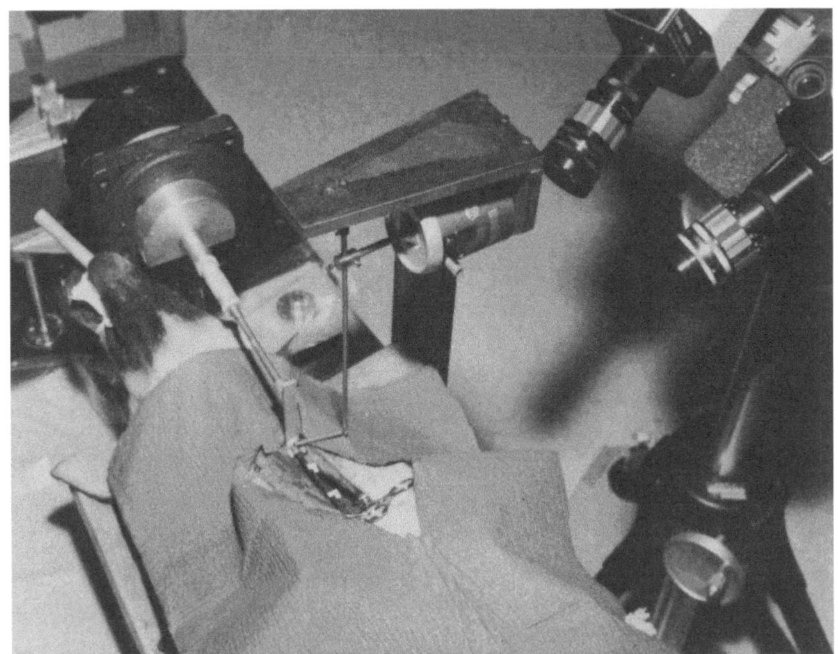

FIGURE 4. Experimental arrangement to determine the dispersion and attenuation of axial, torsion and pressure waves in the exposed external carotid artery of an anesthetized dog. A collar device at the cephalic end of the exposed carotid can be displaced sinusoidally in the axial direction and simultaneously rotated about the axis of the carotid. The small constriction of the vessel caused by the collar device induces not only axial but also pressure waves as it is displaced in the axial direction. Axial and torsion waves are monitored with a pair of PhysiTech electro-optical trackers which detect the axial and circumferential wall displacements of the wall at two locations along the artery. Since the optical tracking system is designed to measure the motion of a line of contrast in two directions perpendicular to the optical axis, special paper targets were attached to the artery. The pressure waves are sensed by miniature catheter-tip transducers located at the sites of the paper targets.

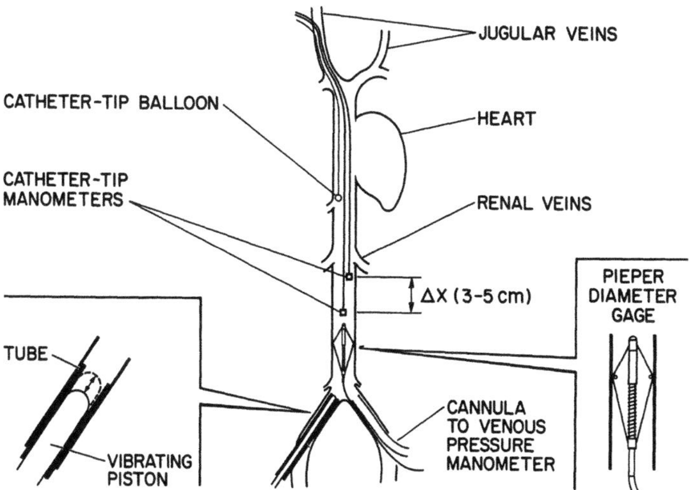

FIGURE 5. General experimental preparation for the study of the
transmission characteristics of small artifically-induced pressure
waves in the abdominal vena cavae of anesthetized dogs. Sinusoidal
pressure signals are generated by the volumetric displacements of a
vibrating piston in the right common iliac vein. To assess the changes
of the mechanical behavior of the vessel with pressure a catheter-tip
balloon is positioned between the heart and the hepatic veins. Its
inflation produces changes in venous pressure from control values of
about 100 mm H_2O within 10 to 20 seconds. The internal diameter of
the vena cava is monitored with a modified Pieper diameter gage.

illustrates such a situation and clearly shows that the stimulated
vessel can be expected to be more distensible than the relaxed vessel.
Knowing the diameter, wall thickness and the speed of pressure waves
at any instant, we can determine the active changes of the effective
Young's modulus E with stimulation. Active changes in E observed for
example in the experiment described in FIGURE 8 are shown in FIGURE 9.
For smaller veins we can anticipate considerably larger changes in E
as a result of stimulation, since smaller veins usually exhibit much
more pronounced relative constrictions. If we wish to delineate and
analyze the control systems which are responsible for maintaining and
regulating circulation or any other physiological processes, it is
essential that we be able to quantify the changes of the controlling
parameters and of the controlled variables.

With the continued progress in ultrasound instrumentation we may
soon be performing the measurements described above on a nontraumatic
basis and with man as the subject. The feasibility of quantifying
quasi-instantaneous velocity profiles and diameter changes with pulsed
ultrasound flow meters has been demonstrated (McLeod, 1970). Profiles
obtained by McLeod at low and high steady flow rates are given in

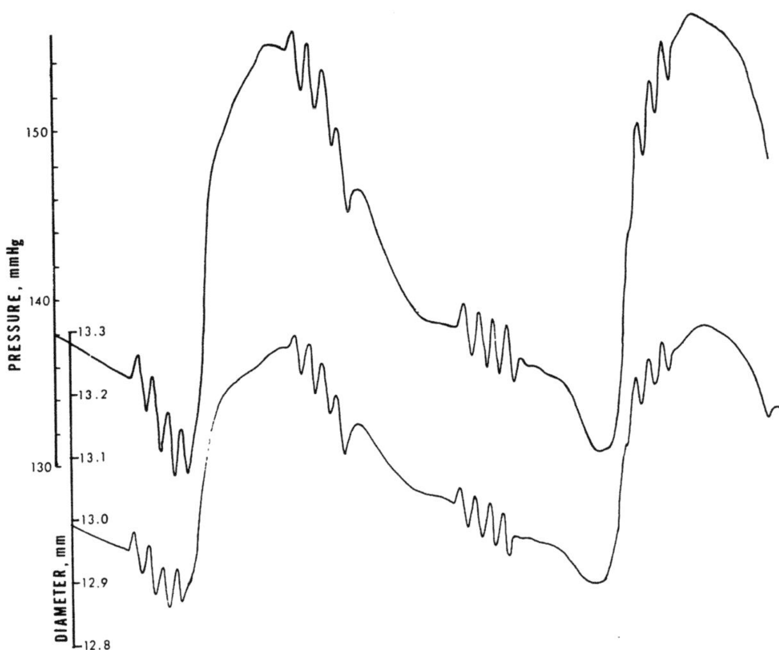

FIGURE 6. Example of actual recording of natural pulse waves prop-
agating downstream in the canine thoracic aorta. The upper tracing
represents the pressure, the lower is the diameter. Transient signals
in the form of finite trains of sinusoidal waves were superimposed on
the natural pressure pulse at various instances of the cardiac cycle.
During transmission in the aorta over distances between 4 and 14 cm
the sinusoidal perturbations retain their sinusoidal wave form, but
they are highly damped.

FIGURE 10. It will be a challenge to examine the possible relationship
between hemodynamic phenomena and the preferred sites of early atheroma
with tools of this kind.

DR. ANSCHUTZ: I should like to comment on the effects of aging
and aortic sclerosis on the elasticity of the aorta. There occurs
an increase in length, width, and weight of the aorta, as the elasticity of the aortic wall decreases (Anschutz, 1970).

FIGURE 11 shows that, with increasing calcification of the
aorta, pulse wave velocity is accelerated. At the same time the
volume of the aorta becomes greater, while the residual volume in
the aorta decreases. Planimetrically measured calcium deposits increase from 5% to a total of 20%.

The significance of aortic rigidity and of the concomitant re-
duction in the ability of the vessel to store blood lies in the fact

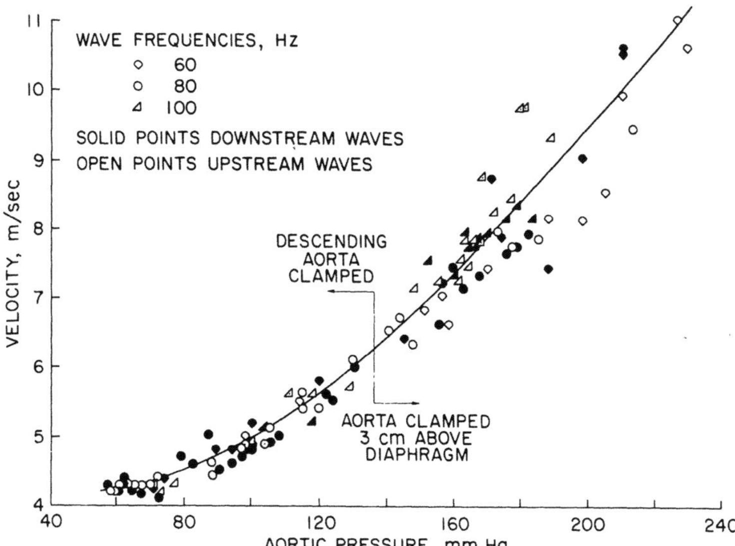

FIGURE 7. Wave speed–pressure variation for a segment of the thoracic aorta in an anesthetized dog. The pressure was varied beyond its normal range by occluding the aorta above and below the segment of interest. The solid points represent waves recorded as they propagate in the downstream direction (away from the heart), while the open points were obtained from waves traveling in the upstream direction (towards the heart). To record simultaneously up- and downstream waves two electromagnetic signal generators were used, one being placed below and one above the aortic segment studied. The sharp rise of the wave speed with pressure suggests that the peak of a large-amplitude pressure pulse travels at a higher speed than does the foot of the pulse. Accordingly such pulses change their shape with propagation.

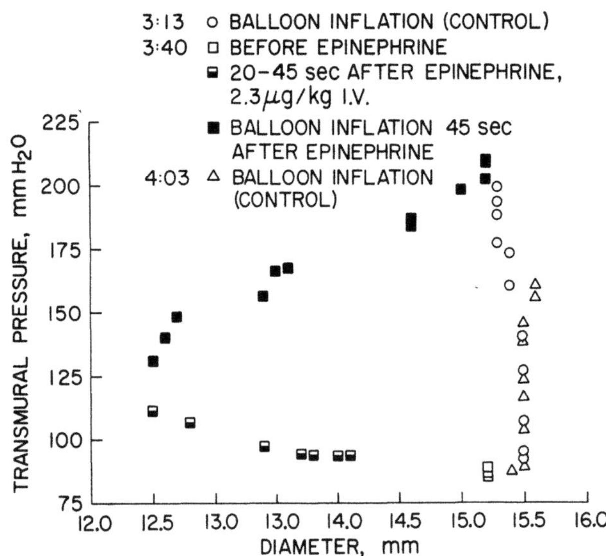

FIGURE 8. Control balloon inflations (see FIG. 5 for experimental
arrangement) before the injection of epinephrine show that the vessel
is "relaxed" but also stiff since it essentially does not change its
diameter with pressure. In response to the epinephrine the vessel
constricts markedly while the pressure increases by about 50%. A
subsequent balloon inflation shows that with rising pressure the diameter of the "stimulated" vessel increases again to its control
value, indicating that the constricted vessel is more distensible
than the "relaxed" vessel.

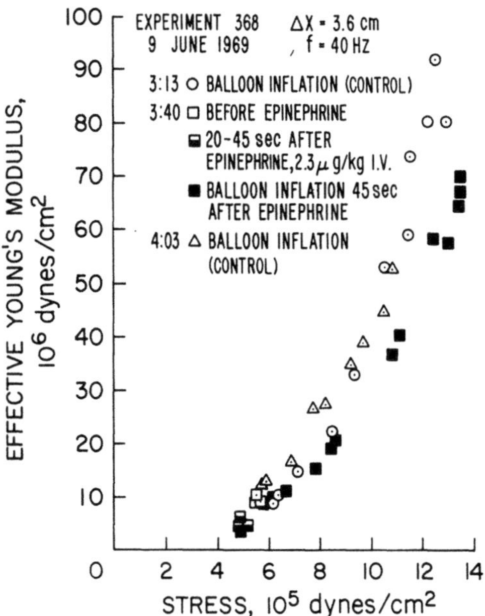

FIGURE 9. Measurements of the wave speed in the vena cava and its
diameter, together with the transmural pressure, during the epinephrine response study illustrated in FIG. 8 can be used to determine
the "instantaneous" effective Young's modulus as a function of the
circumferential wall stress. E is determined from the so-called
Moens-Korteweg equation, according to which:

$$E = 2\rho\frac{a}{h}\,c^2 = 2\rho\frac{a^2}{a_o h_o}\,c^2$$

where ρ is the density of the blood, a and h the instantaneous diameter
and wall thickness respectively. For an incompressible vessel wall
material $ah = a_o h_o$ where a_o and h_o are the radius and wall thickness
at a given reference pressure.

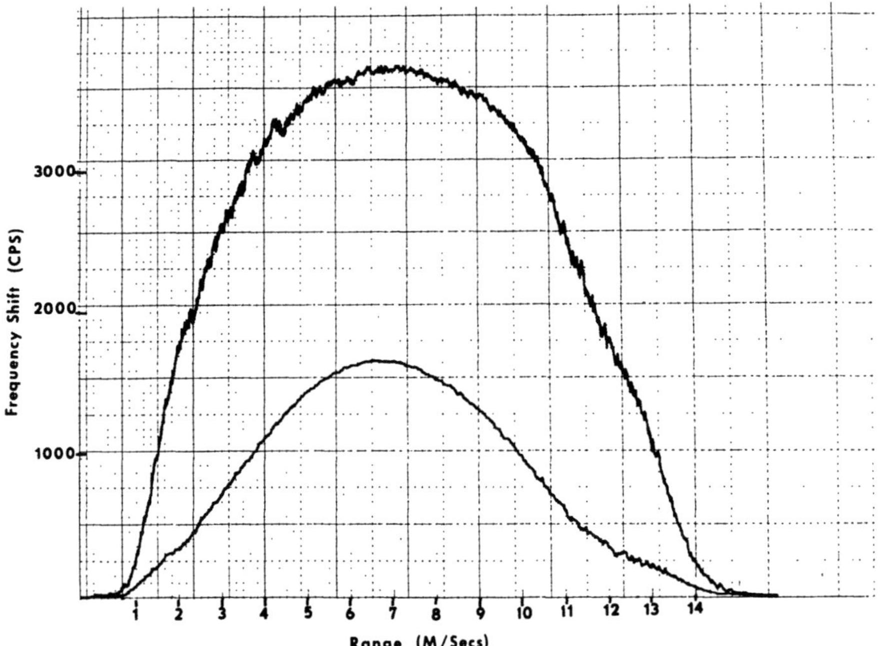

FIGURE 10. Doppler frequency shift distribution representing the velocity profile in dialysis tubing for high (top curve) and low (bottom curve) steady flow with Reynolds numbers of 2650 and 755 respectively.

that the arteries' elastic recoil function is diminished or abolished.
Under normal conditions the purpose of the recoil function is to
transform the aortic pulsations into a uniform flow of arterial blood
in the periphery. An intact recoil function is of relevance in respect to the economy of cardiac work. It also facilitates uniform
circulation in capillaries, and in the vicinity of the heart itself.
Though valid objections have been raised against certain mathematical
analyses of the nature of the 'Windkesselfunktion' of the aorta (Deppe,
1940; Peterson and Lessen et al., 1956; Remington, 1952), there is no
doubt that under physiological conditions the aorta transforms a pul-
sating blood flow into a continuous stream.

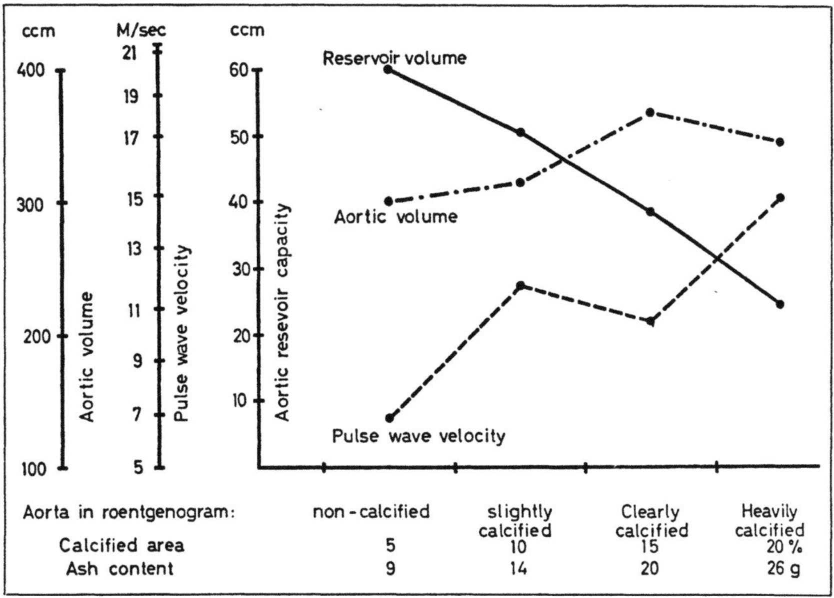

FIGURE 11.   Reservoir and total volume of aorta; pulse wave velocity;
and roentgenographically assessed calcification of aorta.
(Anschutz, 1970)

If the elasticity of the vascular wall is reduced, as much as half
of the cardiac stroke volume can no longer be stored in the aorta during systole. The blood thrown into the aorta with each ventricular
contraction must then be forwarded mainly during systole. This can
be shown if one compares peripheral arterial flow in patients with
heavily calcified aortic sclerosis and in subjects with normal vessels.
In the former, blood flow occurs entirely during systole. The normal
diastolic component of flow has practically disappeared (FIG. 12).

Among the factors which determine the work of the heart (Wiggers,
1932; Evans, 1918; Fahr, 1927; Frank, 1928) the following two are the
most important: The tensile pressure necessary to overcome aortic

pressure, and the force required to accelerate the blood flow in the
aorta. According to Evans and Matsuoka (Evans and Matsuoka, 1915),
the latter factor plays a negligible role. The first factor is the
product of stroke volume and integrated mean systolic pressure of the
aorta. The product represents the main portion of the work load of
the heart.

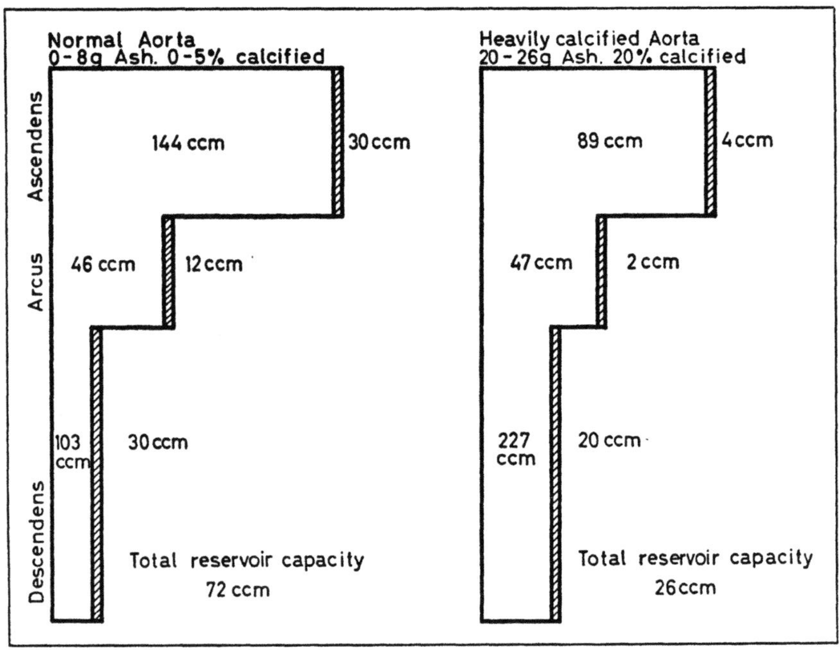

FIGURE 12. Diagrammatic summary of results of measurements of normal and heavily calcified aortae.
(Anschutz, 1970)

The differences between the hemodynamic parameters mentioned
thus far are of relevance in respect to the second factor whose magnitude is expressed as product of accelerated mass and velocity of
a given amount of blood expelled from the left ventricle during systole
divided by two. As shown in FIG. 13, systolic flow velocity is increased in subjects with aortic sclerosis. The factor under analysis
enters the equation from which the work of the heart is calculated
as square potentiator.

What about the factor 'accelerated mass'? If the storage capacity of the ascending aorta and arcus aorta becomes inadequate the
heart must increase during systole not only its ventricular stroke volume but also the contents of the aorta. If one estimates the load thus
imposed upon the heart, using data obtained by anatomical and kymographic analyses, one arrives at increased blood volumes of approx-

imately 370 ml as against normal values of 70 ml. Views that correspond with those detailed above have been derived by Wiggers (Wiggers,
1932) and Rein (Rein, 1937-40) from studies of heart-lung preparations.

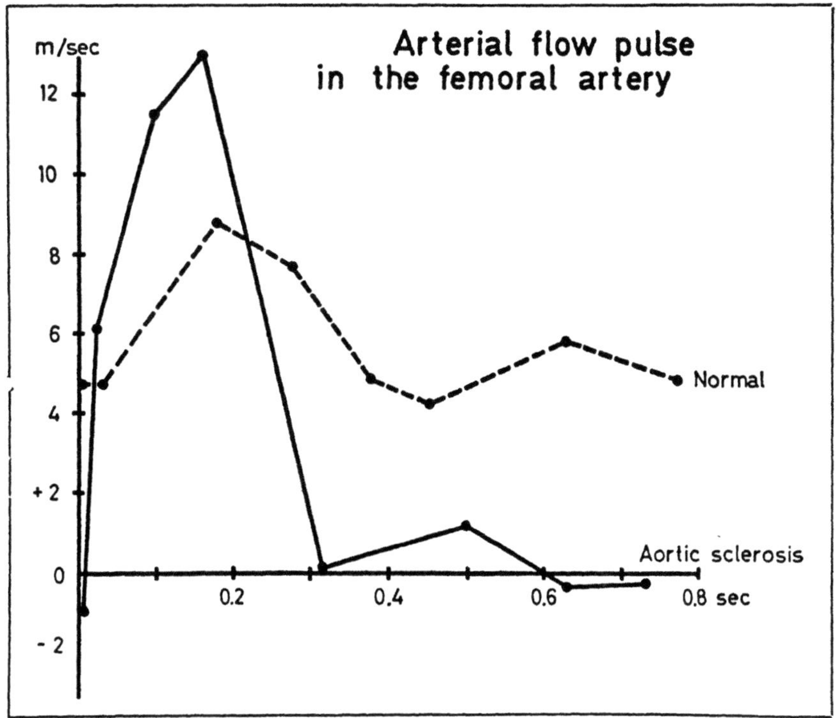

FIGURE 13. Flow pulsations in femoral arteries of a normal subject
and of a subject with aortic sclerosis.
(Anschutz, 1970)

     TABLE III compares the work load of hearts with normal and
sclerotic aortae. Blood pressure and ventricular stroke volume are
identical in both. Nonetheless, the total mass of blood moved during
systole is increased in the case of the sclerotic aorta from 70 ml
to 370 ml; and velocity of flow from 0.4m/sec to 0.8m/sec. Due to
the fact that blood pressure and cardiac stroke volume are the same
in both cases, factor 2 as defined by Evans and Matsuoka (Evans and
Matsuoka, 1915) is unchanged. Factor one however, is increased a
hundred-fold or more. The work load of the heart is thus considerably magnified.

     The increase of the work load of the heart in aortic sclerosis
becomes still more pronounced when strain is extraneously imposed on
the circulatory system. In FIG. 14 measurements of the work of the
heart of a patient with aortic sclerosis are compared with corresponding values obtained from a normal person.

TABLE III

HEART WORK WITH NORMAL ELASTIC RECOIL FUNCTION OF THE AORTA AND IN

AORTIC SCLEROSIS

Normal		Aortic sclerosis
120	Blood pressure (P)	120
70	Heart stroke volume (Vs)	70
70	Mass moved (m)	370
0.4 m/sec	Blood flow velocity (v)	0.8 m/sec
0.14 mhg	Heart work factor 1.(PxVs)	0.14 mhg
0.00057 mhg	Heart work factor 2.($\frac{1}{2}$ mxv^2)	0.018 mhg
0.14057	Heart work factor 1 + 2	0.158
670 mhg	Work performed per h	760 mhg

(Anschutz, 1970)

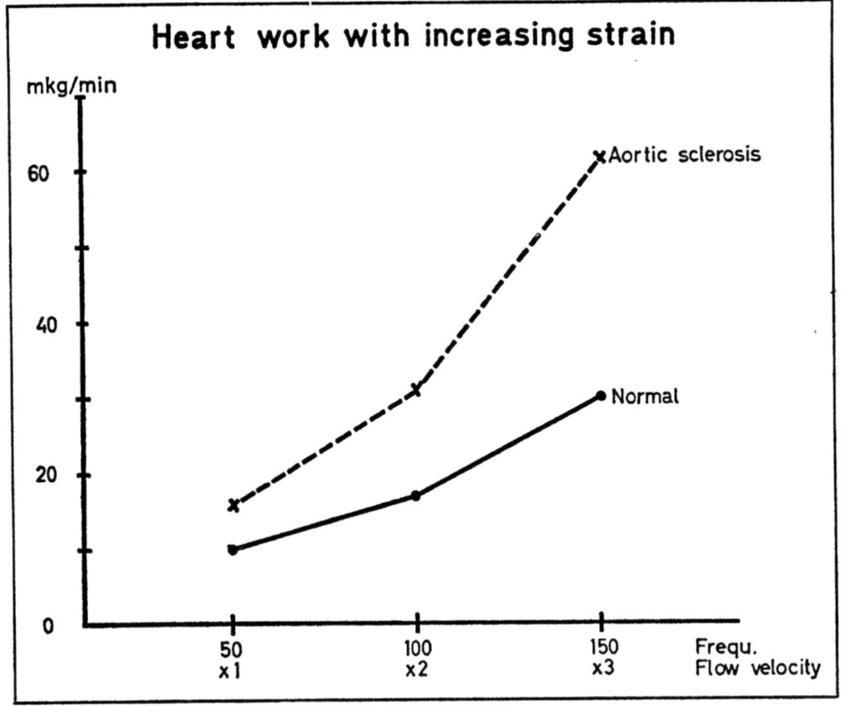

FIGURE 14. Effect of 'cardiac strain' upon work of heart with normal and sclerotic aorta, respectively.
(Anschutz, 1970)

COMMENT

Dr. Robert Schneider entered the discussion by reviewing studies on the axon dilation reflex (Lewis, 1930) as measured by plethysmography and thermometry of the thumb during 30 minutes immersion in ice water (0°C) and 10 minutes thereafter. Great variations were seen from person to person and from time to time in the same person (FIG. 15) but of special interest were the results on a student with labile hypertension whose skin temperature and digit volume went **HUMAN** down lower and stayed down longer than individuals of his same age who were normotensive (FIG. 16). Similar reactions were often seen in patients with chronic tension headaches who had a tendency to lose their normal vascular "hunting phenomenon." Such findings suggest that nervous controls above the axon reflex may also be at play in these conditions.

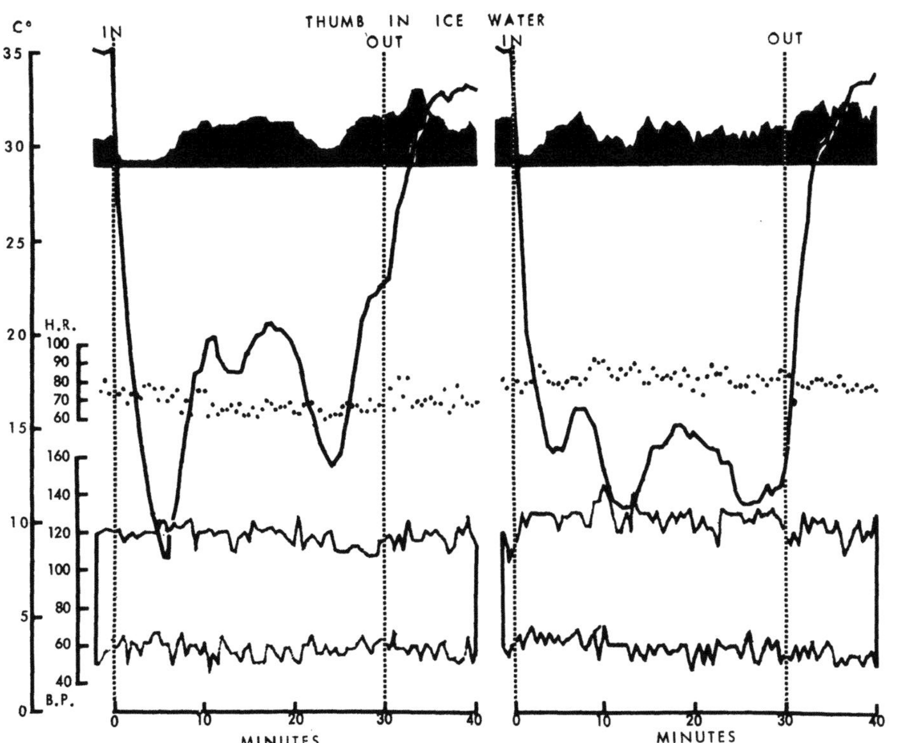

FIGURE 15. Two studies two weeks apart on the same 33-year-old man whose thumb temperatures were essentially the same on the two occasions prior to immersion. The thumb plethysmograph is shown in solid black, the thumb temperatures as a solid line. Blood pressures and heart rates (dots) are recorded every 30 seconds.

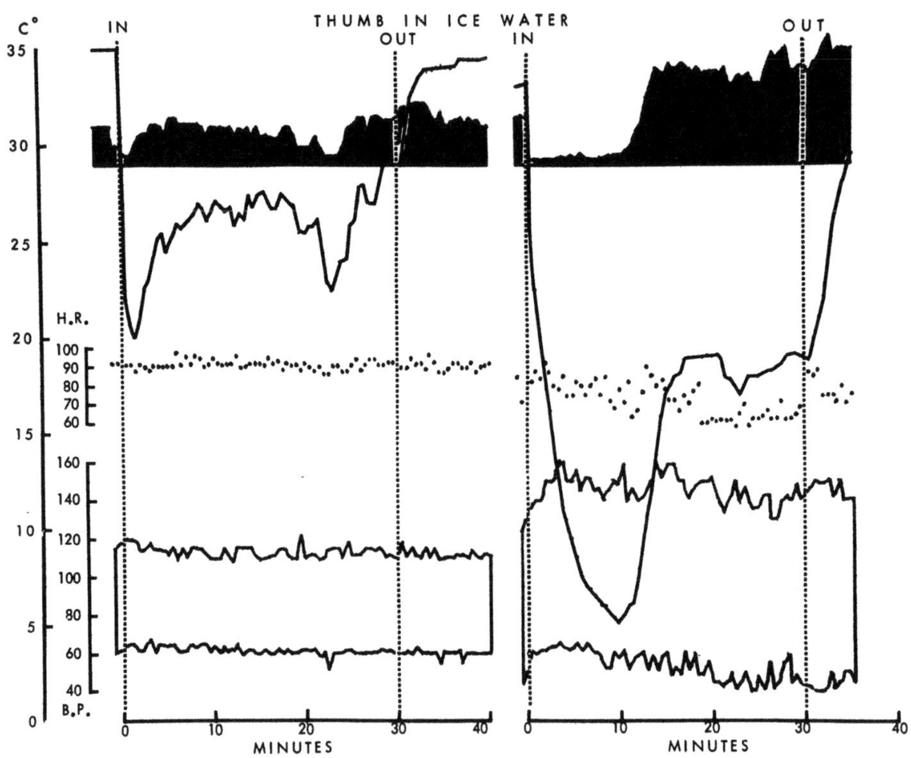

FIGURE 16. Studies (see FIG. 15) on a 21-year-old student on the
left who was normotensive and on a 22-year-old student on the right
who was being followed for labile systolic hypertension.

Based on experiments with injected ^{35}S-sulfate, Dr. Hauss reported enhancement of metabolism in the sulfated mucopolysaccharides
of the arterial wall following electrical stimulation of the hypothalamus in rats (FIG. 17 A and B). Tritiated thymidine was injected
for either three days or one hour before beginning the electrical
stimulation. In the former case labeled mononuclear cells were found
infiltrating the adventitia of aorta, coronary and intercostal vessels.
From the discussion that followed it appeared that the labeled cells
infiltrating the vessel wall came from the lymph nodes rather than
the marrow (Hauss, 1964).

Dr. Friedman presented data on "neurogenic hypercholesterolemia"
induced by making lesions in rats in the ventro-medial nucleus of
RAT the hypothalamus. The hypercholesterolemia that then followed cholesterol feeding greatly exceeded the results from cholesterol feeding
of non-operated rats (500-600 mg% vs 180 mg%). Examination of the
pituitary gland in such hypothalamically damaged animals revealed
loss of TSH and GH producing cells.

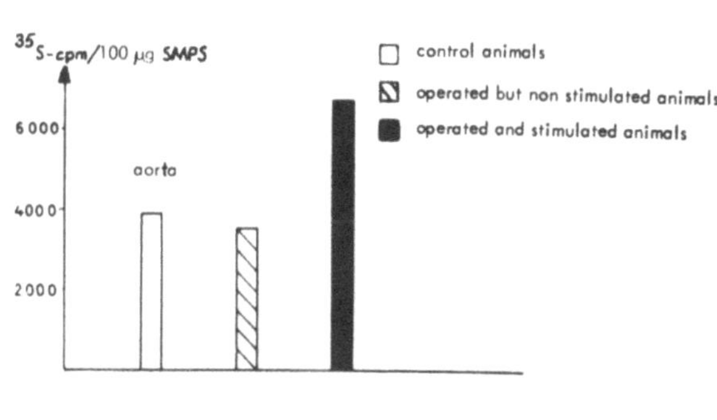
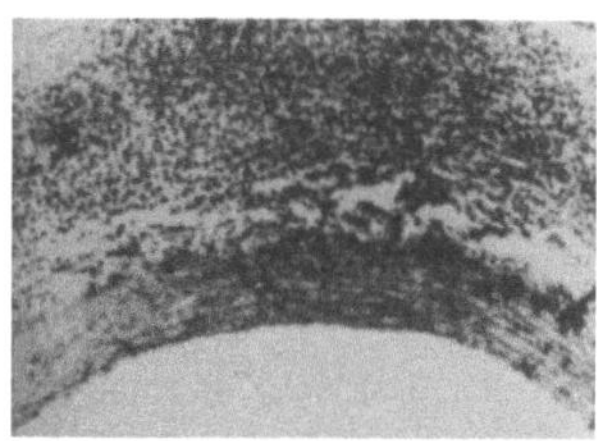
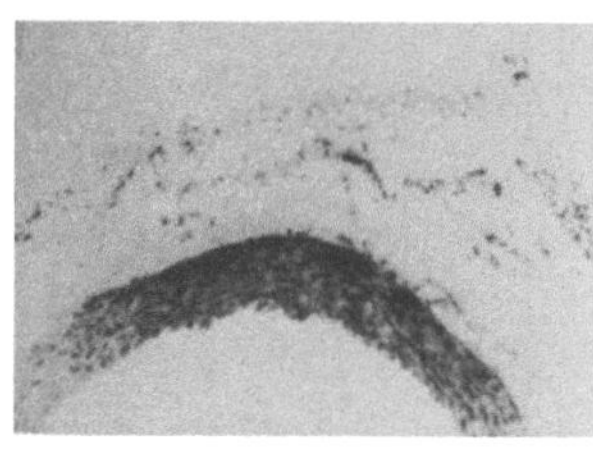

A   B

FIGURE 17. Effect of electrical stimulation of the hypothalamus
(7 days) on aortas of rats.
      A: Increase of ^{35}S-sulfate incorporation in the SMPS of
         aorta after electrical stimulation of the hypothalamus.
      B: above – Aorta of a stimulated rat: A great number of
              mononuclear cells is to be seen in the adventitia
              of the aorta.
       below – Aorta of a control rat.

DR. FRIEDMAN: We discovered that the hypophysectomized animal's
serum cholesterol is primarily elevated because it lacks growth hormone. In other words, we have found growth hormone to be absolutely
indispensable for the maintenance of a normal blood cholesterol. When
either thyroid hormone or growth hormone are given the serum cholesterol of hypophysectomized animals falls to normal (FIG. 18).

QUESTION: Dr. Friedman, could you get changes in other blood
lipids, too?

DR. FRIEDMAN: We have found no change in the serum phospholipid
or triglyceride of these animals. We have not measured the serum
growth hormone after the administration of growth hormone itself.
What wasn't reported was that growth hormone was essential to the
cholesterol control.

QUESTION: No, but I mean the other report that the administration of growth hormone increases serum free fatty acid.

DR. FRIEDMAN: Yes it does, very rapidly, within a minute or
two afterward. You're absolutely right. Dr. Li, having seen our

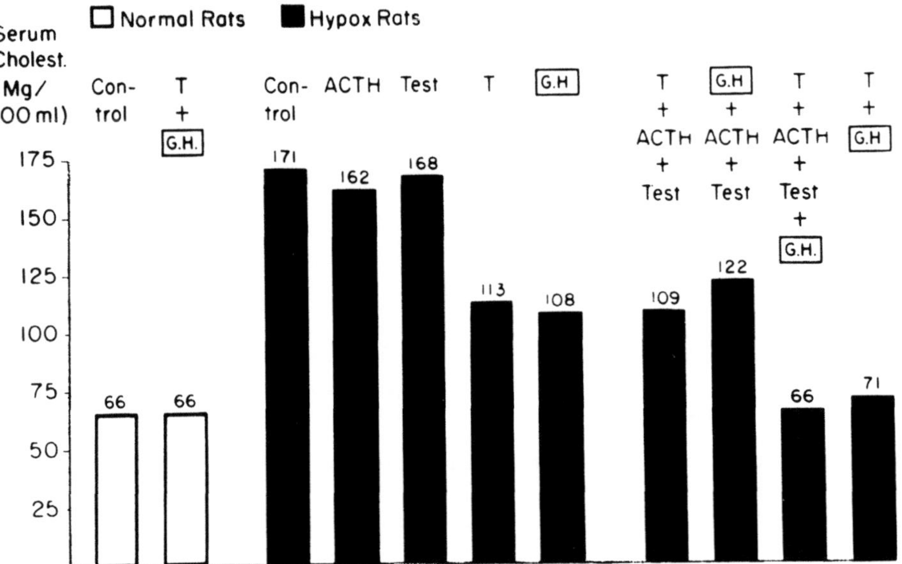

FIGURE 18. Rise of serum cholesterol in the hypophysectomized rat and its persistence despite the administration of ACTH and testosterone. Administration of thyroid extract (T) or growth hormone (G.H.) markedly inhibited this rise and prevented it entirely when both substances were administered together. The administration of both ACTH and testosterone together with either T or G.H., however, did not inhibit the serum rise in cholesterol more than the sole administration of either of the latter two hormones.

results, suggests that we increase our administration of growth hormone and give it more frequently, namely three times a day and we now give 300 micrograms of bovine growth hormone three times a day. FIG. 19 shows the data from a thyroidectomized rat and as you all know the serum cholesterol goes up, particularly on a high cholesterol diet in three weeks to about 350 mg/100 ml. When you take thyroidectomized rats and give them thyroid extract the cholesterol falls. When the thyroid extract is discontinued, the cholesterol again rises. When one takes thyroidectomized rats and gives them growth hormone only, one prevents the hypocholesterolemia of the thyroidectomized rat. If growth hormone is then discontinued, cholesterol rises. What I'm saying here is that the main reason that thyroid hormone is controlling blood cholesterol, is that it is maintaining the output of growth hormone. Growth hormone is probably far more important than thyroid hormone in the maintenance of a normal blood cholesterol. However, the administration of excess growth hormone to a normal cholesterolemic animal will not reduce its blood cholesterol. Just as the administration of a moderate amount of thyroid hormone given to a normal rat will not particularly reduce its already normal blood cholesterol. I'm bringing up the subject of growth hormone because later, when we talk about the matter of behavior pattern and its possible relationship to coronary disease, I would like to talk to you about growth hormones.

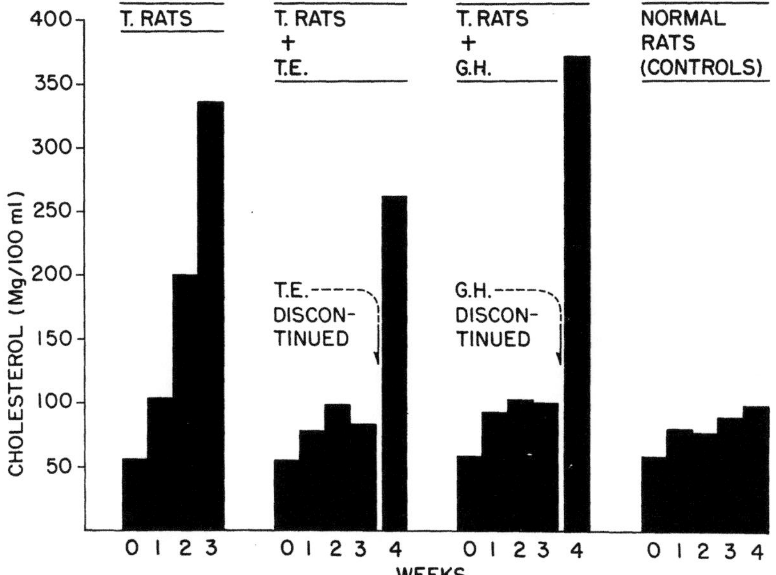

FIGURE 19. Plasma cholesterol rise of thyroidectomized (T) rats; of thyroidectomized rats given thyroid extract (T.E.); of thyroidectomized rats given growth hormone (G.H.) and normal rats. Note that administration of growth hormone is as efficacious as thyroid extract in preventing the otherwise expected cholesterol rise in thyroidectomized rats. Note also the sharp plasma cholesterol rise in the thyroidectomized rats after discontinuance of either thyroid extract or growth hormone.

DR. GUNN: It is clear from what has been said that autonomic mechanisms are capable of modulating arterial wall metabolism. I mentioned earlier the effects of denervation and hence presumably adrenergic hypoactivity on arterial wall lipid metabolism and atherogenesis. I also suggested that by different mechanisms adrenergic hyperactivity may also lead to arteriosclerosis in experimental animals. Several years ago Drs. Friedman, Byers and I carried out

stereotaxic stimulation of certain areas of the hypothalamus in cholesterol fed rabbits and found that we could not only greatly elevate
serum cholesterol but also accelerate the process of atheroma (Gunn
and Friedman et al., 1960), as shown in FIGURE 20. Dr. Friedman has
referred to more recent studies with his co-workers (Friedman and
Byers et al., 1969). Gutstein (Gutstein and Schneck et al., 1969)
has also seen the hypothalamic induced lipidemia; Somoza (Somoza,
1965) and Ueda (Ueda and Ebihara et al., 1965) have confirmed the
centrogenic atherosclerosis using slightly different techniques.

Chronic stimulation of peripheral adrenergic nerves to an artery
has also produced pathological sclerotic changes in intima and media
(Gutstein and LaTaillade et al., 1962) similar to those seen after
repeated intravascular epinephrine infusions (Shimamoto, 1960). Increased CNS and peripheral adrenergic stimulation to the arterial
walls thus appears to produce pathological arteriosclerotic responses
similar to a variety of irritative mechanisms and, especially in the
presence of increased blood cholesterol, atherosclerosis may result.

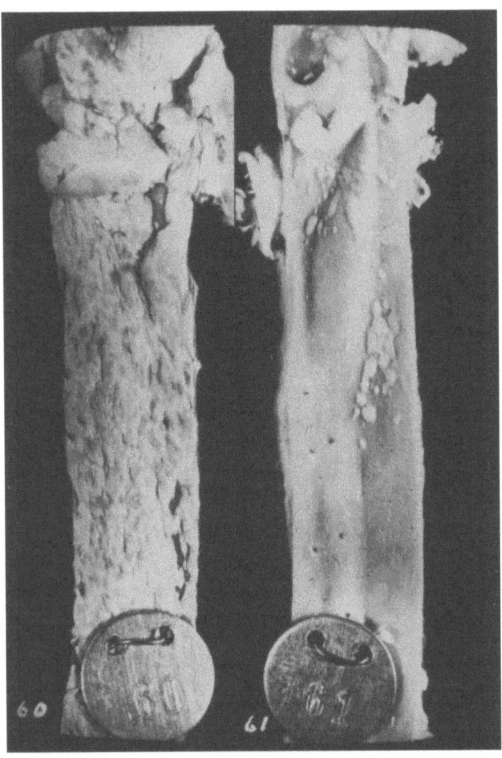

FIGURE 20.

Chapter 3

LIPID METABOLISM IN THE HUMAN ARTERIAL INTIMA WITH

AGING AND WITH ATHEROSCLEROSIS

Opening Address by Elspeth Smith, Ph.D.

Department of Chemical Pathology, University of Aberdeen, Scotland

In preparing these introductory remarks to the discussion on chemical changes in the human artery wall with aging and with atherosclerosis I have made no attempt to provide a comprehensive review. Furthermore, I will talk primarily about lipids and touch only lightly on the connective tissue components, as these can be discussed much better by the experts on the panel. What I hope to do is to highlight some of the areas which I personally feel are particularly in need of discussion.

Normal Intima In Different Age Groups
With increasing age the normal intima increases greatly in its thickness and in its lipid concentration, and to a much smaller and not significant extent in its collagen concentration. Total MPS concentration tends to fall a little, at least after age 20-30, and Klynstra and Bottcher (Klynstra and Bottcher et al., 1967) found slight changes in the proportions of hyaluronic acid and chondroitin sulphate C.

In lesion free aortic intima there is a steady increase in the lipid concentration with age (FIG. 1). Free cholesterol, phospholipid and triglyceride increase rather slowly, and more or less in parallel, but cholesterol ester increases much more rapidly, and from being the smallest component in children, becomes the largest component after about age 30 (Smith, 1965a). In children the lipid composition is very similar to the lipid composition in tissues such as skeletal or heart muscle - phospholipid is the major component, and most of the cholesterol is in the free form; these are probably the basic endogenous lipids of the cell, presumably mainly constituents of membranes. It is thought by Stein (Stein and Eisenberg et al., 1969) that, with age, changes may occur in these endogenous lipids themselves.

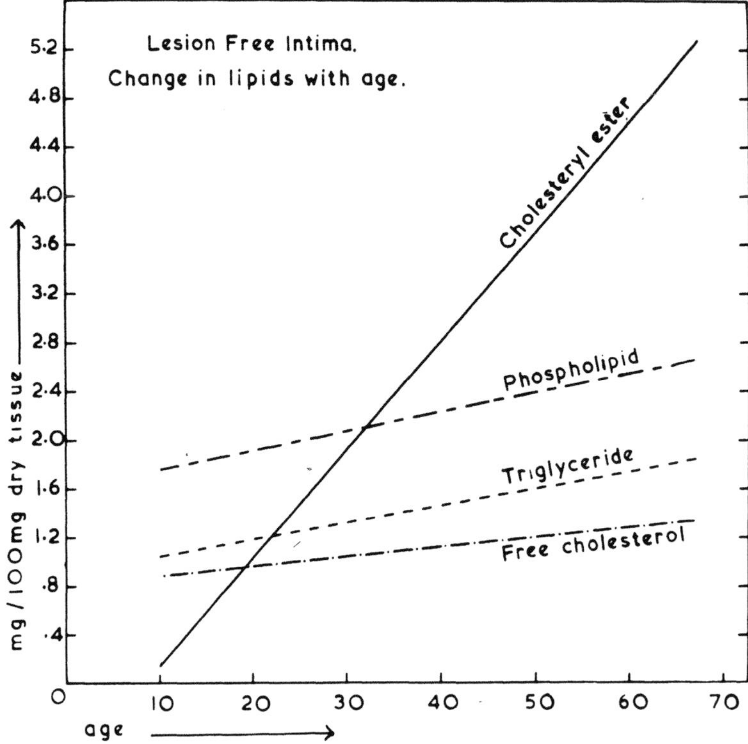

FIGURE 1. Regression lines for the change in concentration of each
major lipid fraction with age in macroscopically normal intima.
(Smith, 1965a)

The increasing proportion of cholesterol ester with age is accompanied by an increase in its linoleic acid content (TABLE I). In the
under 30 age group 26% of the lipid is cholesterol ester, of which
28% is the linoleate; in the 40-59 group total lipid has doubled,
but cholesterol ester has quadrupled to 42% of the lipid, and contains 38% linoleate. By age 70 the lipid is very similar to the
S_f0-12 lipoprotein of plasma, both in overall composition and in cholesterol ester fatty acid pattern. This accumulation seems to start
at a young age, but useful data are extremely scanty. If one assumes
that ester cholesterol is indicative of exogenous accumulation in
areas free of fatty streaks, it looks from our data as if measurable
accumulation starts somewhere between age 5 and 10, and this is in
agreement with Stein's findings (Eisenberg and Stein et al., 1969a).

Morphologically this accumulation of lipid correlates with the
accumulation of increasing numbers of fine, extracellular sudanophilic
droplets which lie between the cells, and seem to be oriented along

collagen and elastic fibers; we have called this perifibrous lipid
(Smith and Evans et al., 1967).

TABLE I

SERUM LIPOPROTEIN COMPARED WITH LIPID
IN LESION-FREE INTIMA

Age Group	Intima With Perifibrous Lipid			Serum S_f0-12 Lipoprotein
	Under 30	40-59	Over 70	
Total Lipid	5.6 mg%	10.8 mg%	16.0 mg%	————
% Composition				
Cholesterol ester	26.6%	42.3%	57.2%	58.2%
Free cholesterol	19.9%	13.0%	10.5%	11.6%
Phospholipid	42.6%	29.3%	17.2%	20.0%
Triglyceride	10.9%	15.4%	15.1%	10.2%
% of CEFA				
18:1	34.5%	28.0%	27.4%	24.1%
18:2	28.0%	38.6%	40.0%	46.8%
20:3	1.2%	1.0%	0.9%	trace
20:4	5.1%	5.3%	5.2%	5.2%

(Smith and Evans et al., 1967)

The simplest interpretation of these findings is that this accumulating perifibrous lipid is derived from plasma S_f0-12 lipoprotein, and the changing lipid pattern with age results from the
superposition of increasing amounts of plasma lipoprotein on the
endogenous tissue lipid. This idea receives support from the immunofluorescence studies of Walton and Williamson (Walton and Williamson,
1968) who find strands of specific immunofluorescence corresponding
with the perifibrous lipid.

Fatty Streaks

Chronologically, the earliest lesions to be detected macroscopically are fatty streaks. The relationship between juvenile fatty
streaks and mature plaques is controversial and confused, but one
thing is certain - unless a rigorous definition of fatty streak is
agreed on and adhered to by different workers the confusion will continue. In my laboratory we define a fatty streak as a lesion in
which most of the lipid stainable by Sudan dyes is in the form of
intracellular droplets which largely fill the cytoplasm of the cells.

In practice, in macroscopic fine flecks the fat-filled cells are
generally separated from each other, or scattered, whereas in the
typical slightly raised fatty streak they tend to be in confluent
masses.

The lipid composition is extremely characteristic (TABLE II)
with a high proportion of cholesterol ester containing 50% or more
oleic acid, very little linoleic acid and a great increase in
eicosatrienoic acid. This is strikingly different from the cholesterol
ester fatty acid (CEFA) pattern in plasma lipoprotein, or in intima
in the same age group which contains only perifibrous lipid (Smith
and Evans et al., 1967).

TABLE II

PLASMA LIPOPROTEIN AND AORTIC LIPID IN NORMAL INTIMA
AND FATTY STREAKS FROM SUBJECTS   AGED 40-59

	Perifibrous lipid (age 40-59)	Plasma S_f0-12 lipoprotein	Fat filled cells
Total Lipid mg/100 mg d.t.	10.8	--	38.7
% Composition			
Cholesterol ester	42.1	58.2	67.9
Free cholesterol	13.0	11.6	9.8
Phospholipid	29.3	20.0	15.8
Triglyceride	15.4	10.2	6.5
% of CEFA			
18:1	28.0	24.1	50.3
18:2	38.6	46.8	14.0
20:3	1.0	trace	4.0
20:4	5.3	5.2	3.4

Using a technique of microdissection from thick cryostat sections
we have isolated areas of the smaller, scattered fat-filled cells and
compared them with large, confluent cells (TABLE III). The cholesterol
in the scattered cell samples is lower, as one would expect, and the
percentage free is slightly higher; in both groups the proportion of
cholesterol oleate is extremely high and not statistically different,
thus their lipid characteristics are very similar, and do not appear
to change in relation to the age of the subject. This lipid pattern
is not unique to intimal fat-filled cells, but is found in even more

extreme form in skin xanthomata and in adrenal cortex, both of which
contain cells filled with lipid droplets which look very similar to
the droplets in intimal cells (TABLE III). Preferential esterification of cholesterol with oleic acid has also been demonstrated in
human intestine by Blomstrand and co-workers (Blomstrand and Gurtler
et al., 1964), which suggests that this is a commonly occurring
pattern; possibly it is the liver which is unique in producing cholesterol esters with a high proportion of linoleic acid.

TABLE III

COMPARISON OF THE LIPIDS IN SMALL, SCATTERED FAT FILLED CELLS AND
LARGE, CONFLUENT FAT FILLED CELLS FROM PLAQUES, AND IN SKIN XANTHOMATA
AND ADRENAL CORTEX

	Small, scattered fat filled cells	Large, confluent fat filled cells	Skin xanthomata	Adrenal Cortex
	8 samples	21 samples	5 samples	4 samples
Total Cholesterol mg/100 mg dry tissue	22.3	51.4	20.2	22.1
Ratio $\frac{cholesterol}{phospholipid}$	3.6	4.7	3.8	1.4
Percentage of Cholesterol Free	35.3	29.4	'22.6	19.8
CEFA % oleic acid (18:1) in combined 18:1 and 18:2 fraction	75.8	69.9	77.5	94.0

There seems to be little doubt that there is very active esterification of cholesterol within intimal fat-filled cells, but the
origin of the cholesterol itself is less certain. In most reports
on de novo synthesis the rate seems rather slow, but much of the work
has been done on cholesterol fed animals and it is possible that a
feedback inhibition is operating. Attempts to measure the uptake of
labeled cholesterol from plasma are confused by the rapid exchange of
free cholesterol between plasma lipoproteins, cell constituents such
as membranes, and other lipoproteins (Hagerman and Gould, 1951; Gould
and Wissler et al., 1963; Ashworth and Green, 1964; Graham and Green,
1967). This is a major confusing factor in trying to assess the contribution of plasma cholesterol to both intra- and extracellular cholesterol accumulation, as has been demonstrated by Hashimoto and Dayton
(Hashimoto and Dayton, 1966) and Newman and Zilversmit (Newman and
Zilversmit, 1966). Recent work by Dayton and Hashimoto (Dayton and
Hashimoto, 1968) is beginning to clarify the situation.

Thus it appears that in normal intima and early lesions, two
distinct types of lipid can accumulate - extracellular lipid which,
from its composition, appears to be derived from plasma low density
lipoprotein, and intracellular lipid which appears to be wholly or

partly synthesized in situ, and which has a highly characteristic
cholesterol ester fatty acid pattern.

Raised Lesions
    Sphingomyelin. Turning now to raised lesions, some of the ear-
liest detailed analyses of large plaques were made by Buck and Rossiter
in 1951 (Buck and Rossiter, 1951). They demonstrated the general similarity between the plaque lipids and serum lipids, and drew particular attention to the very high proportion of sphingomyelin in the phospholipids. This high proportion of sphingomyelin is such a striking
feature of plaque phospholipids that it has received a large amount
of attention, possibly disproportionate to its significance.

The increasing proportion of sphingomyelin with increasing
severity of atherosclerosis is shown clearly in TABLE IV, which
summarizes results from Bottcher and van Gent (Bottcher and Woodford
et al., 1960; Bottcher and van Gent, 1961). In the last column I
have calculated from their data the ratio of total cholesterol to
sphingomyelin. Although the percentage of sphingomyelin in the
phospholipid fraction doubles in severe atherosclerosis, cholesterol
increases at an even greater rate, so that sphingomyelin actually
constitutes a smaller proportion of the total lipid than in normal

TABLE IV

SPHINGOMYELINS IN INTIMA-PLUS-MEDIA PREPARATIONS OF WHOLE AORTAS

Stage of Disease	Number	Average age	Percentage of sphingomyelin in total phospholipid	Ratio* Total cholesterol / sphingomyelin
0	5	7	34.8	0.53
I	6	29	53.3	0.65
II	6	51	59.4	0.84
III	5	61	62.5	1.64

*Calculated from the authors' data

(Bottcher and van Gent, 1961; Bottcher and Woodford et al., 1960)

aortas. In TABLE V lesions are compared with normal intima from the
same aortas (Smith, 1965a). In fatty streaks and nodules the sphingomyelin content of the phospholipids does not differ significantly
from adjacent normal intima. There is, however, a very large increase
in cholesterol so that sphingomyelin provides a much smaller proportion
of the total lipid than in the controls. In fibrous plaques the phospholipid contains a much higher proportion of sphingomyelin than the

controls, and it increases with increasing plaque maturity, but the
ratio of cholesterol to sphingomyelin remains above the controls.

TABLE V

THE "SPHINGOMYELIN PLUS LYSOLECITHIN" FRACTION IN LESION-FREE INTIMA
COMPARED WITH LESIONS OF DIFFERENT TYPES FROM THE SAME AORTAS

		No.	Av. Age	Percentage of sphingo + lyso in total phospholipid	Ratio Total cholesterol / Sphingo + lyso
Fatty Streaks	Control	12	44	42.4	3.1
	Lesion			45.8	6.1
Raised Fatty Nodules	Control	4	49	44.1	3.5
	Lesion			52.1	8.3
"Early" Fibrous Plaques	Control	9	51	44.5	3.1
	Lesion			61.0	4.0
"Advanced" Fibrous Plaques	Control	9	51	40.0	3.8
	Lesion			70.0	5.9

(Smith, 1965a)

Sphingomyelin has a lower rate of synthesis and longer turnover
time than lecithin in all tissues examined. This has been shown repeatedly - for example, in the intact aortas of eviscerated rabbits
by Zilversmit and co-workers (Newman and McCandless et al., 1961);
in perfused rabbit aortas by Bowyer (Bowyer and Howard et al., 1968)
and by Vost (Vost, 1969); in human lesions by Chobanian and Hollander
(Chobanian and Hollander, 1964), and in isolated foam cells by Day,
Newman and Zilversmit (Day and Newman et al., 1966). There seems
to be no evidence to support the idea that sphingomyelin is playing
an active role in atherogenesis. Presumably it accumulates more than
lecithin because it is chemically and metabolically inert, and is
left behind. This is supported by the Steins' work on phospholipases
in aortic wall (Eisenberg and Stein et al., 1969) - they find that
lecithinase activity increases with increasing age, but sphingo-
myelinase does not.

Cholesterol and Cholesterol Esters
Very large quantities of cholesterol and cholesterol esters accumulate in large fibrous plaques, and it is difficult to visualize
a mechanism by which such large quantities of highly localized lipid
can accumulate from plasma without the intervention of cells. If,
however, the lipid mass were formed by disintegration of fat-filled
cells, then some very radical transformation would have to occur in
the cholesterol ester pattern. We have tried to obtain information
about this by studying a series of raised lesions of different types
and stages which were defined by careful histological control (Smith

and Slater et al., 1968). Histologically, the lesions seem to fall
into three rather distinct types:

(1) <u>Raised fatty lesions</u>. The earliest stages resemble enlarged
fatty streaks; they contain little extracellular lipid and large
numbers of cells filled with lipid droplets. In lesions presumed to
be in a more advanced stage small areas of "amorphous" lipid appear
in the center and deep layers ("amorphous lipid" is the term used for
the finely granular extracellular lipid mass without structure or
orientation, familiar in the center of large plaques; in larger lesions
it may contain crystals and larger lipid droplets). In advanced fatty
plaques a thin cap containing numerous fat-filled cells covers a large
central area of "amorphous lipid".

(2) <u>Fibrous plaques</u>. The earliest stage is presumed to be a
sharply raised mass, apparently consisting of collagen and smooth
muscle cells, which may show practically no lipid staining, or to
be suffused with a faint, uniform sudanophilia, or contain fine perifibrous lipid droplets. In the presumed next stage the fibers in
the deep central area seem to break up into a network coated with
larger lipid droplets, and in the advanced lesions there is a thick
collagen cap sharply demarcated from a large central area of amorphous
lipid.

(3) <u>Mixed lesions</u>. Many of the largest plaques were found to
be of this type, with a thick collagen cap containing numerous fat-
filled cells overlying a large central area of amorphous lipid.

We have equated increasing areas of amorphous lipid with increasing lesion development, but this may, of course, be wrong. During the
progression from presumed early to presumed late stage lesions (as defined here) the way in which the lipids change differs in fatty and
fibrous lesions.

The changes in the fat-filled cell group are conveniently illustrated in the series of small lesions from a single aorta shown in
TABLE VI. There is little change in the total concentration of cholesterol, but there are highly significant changes in the proportion
of free cholesterol, which doubles over the series, and in the CEFA
pattern. Where all the lipid is within fat-filled cells only 23% of
the cholesterol is free, and oleic acid accounts for 55% of the CEFA,
but in the lesion with a substantial area of amorphous lipid 44% of
the cholesterol is free, and oleic acid has fallen to 37%; there is
a steady progression between them.

This change in free cholesterol and CEFA pattern is so striking
that in FIG. 2 the percentage of the cholesterol free is plotted
against percentage oleic and linoleic acids, for both types of lesion;
the correlations are highly significant. In the fatty series oleic

acid falls and linoleic acid rises with increasing free cholesterol,
and in the fibrous series the reverse occurs.

TABLE VI

SMALL FATTY PLAQUES FROM A MALE AGED 48

Description of Lesion	Cholesterol		% of total CEFA	
	Total mg/100 mg	% free	Oleic	Linoleic
Superficial F.F.Cs. Extracellular lipid low	18.1 mg	22.7	55.0	15.9

F.F.Cs. at all levels
  Extracellular lipid +
  Amorphous lipid +
  Amorphous lipid ++
  Amorphous lipid +++
    (more collagen in cap)
	20.8 mg
	24.7 mg
	30.7 mg
	26.9 mg
		29.8
		28.6
		36.5
		44.1
			47.4
			44.3
			39.6
			37.2
				20.1
				21.1
				24.2
				27.4

(Smith and Slater et al., 1968)

There are some puzzling features about these correlations. The
most obvious suggestion is enzymic hydrolysis of cholesterol ester,
but the normal enzyme rules of rate proportional to substrate concentration are not being followed. One would have to postulate preferential hydrolysis of cholesterol oleate in fatty lesions, and of
cholesterol linoleate in fibrous lesions, which seems complicated,
and unlikely.

Different Components of Raised Lesions Separated by Microdissection
        This complicated situation might be clarified if the positions
in the lesions of maximum free cholesterol accumulation, and of maximum fatty acid change, could be localized. Mature plaques have
been separated into morphologically defined adjacent layers by microdissection of thick cryostat sections stained with Nile blue sulphate,
and the lipids in the fractions analyzed (Smith and Slater, in preparation). TABLE VII shows some of the lipid findings in the central
segments of pure fibrous plaques. Moving from the inner cap down
through the lesion, there is obviously a huge increase in cholesterol,
and it is accumulating much faster than phospholipid. There is a
significant increase in the percentage of free cholesterol but not
in CEFA.

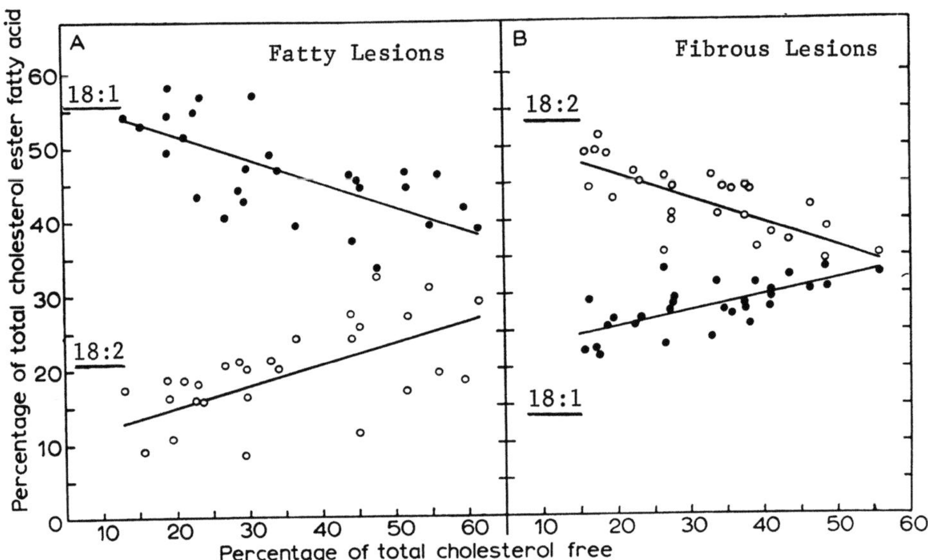

FIGURE 2. The percentage of linoleic acid (18:2) and oleic acid
(18:1) in the total cholesterol ester fatty acids plotted against
the percentage of cholesterol which is in the free (unesterified)
form.   Linoleic acid - O
                               Oleic acid   - ●
(Smith and Slater et al., 1968)

TABLE VII

LIPIDS IN SUCCESSIVE LAYERS OF FIBROUS PLAQUES WHICH CONTAIN NO,
OR VERY FEW, FAT FILLED CELLS

Layer	Surface of cap	Inner cap	Upper amorphous	Lower amorphous
	12 samples	7 samples	13 samples	12 samples
Total Cholesterol mg/100 mg dry tissue	2.7	7.9	65.8	94.8
Ratio $\frac{cholesterol}{phospholipid}$	1.2	1.7	3.4	4.2
Percentage of cholesterol free	47.9	35.8	42.1	49.8
CEFA % 18:1 in combined 18:1 and 18:2 fraction	41.2	37.0	39.7	40.6

Repeating the plot of percentage oleic acid against percentage
of free cholesterol for each separate layer gives the regressions
shown in FIG. 3. The cap and the lower amorphous have the same
slope, despite a 10-fold difference in cholesterol content, and
this is comparable to the slope found in whole lesions (FIG. 2);
there is, however, a constant difference in the free cholesterol
which is consistently about 10% higher in the lower amorphous.
In the upper amorphous the slope is different - compared with the
other two layers free cholesterol is changing more than oleic acid.
This seems to suggest that it is in this region just under the
intact fibrous cap, that free cholesterol is accumulating. I do
not, however, understand the linked variation of free cholesterol
and fatty acid pattern in the other two fractions. These regressions
do not represent changes in stage of lesion. Each regression is
the variation within a single, rather homogeneous fraction, and
the fractions were taken from lesions at a fairly similar stage
of development. I feel this must be telling us something about
the accumulation mechanism, but I cannot think what it is.

THE RELATIONSHIP BETWEEN THE PERCENTAGE OF OLEIC ACID (18:1) IN THE
COMBINED 18:1 + 18:2 FRACTION OF THE C.E.F.A. AND THE PERCENTAGE OF
FREE CHOLESTEROL, IN ADJACENT LAYERS OF FIBROUS PLAQUES

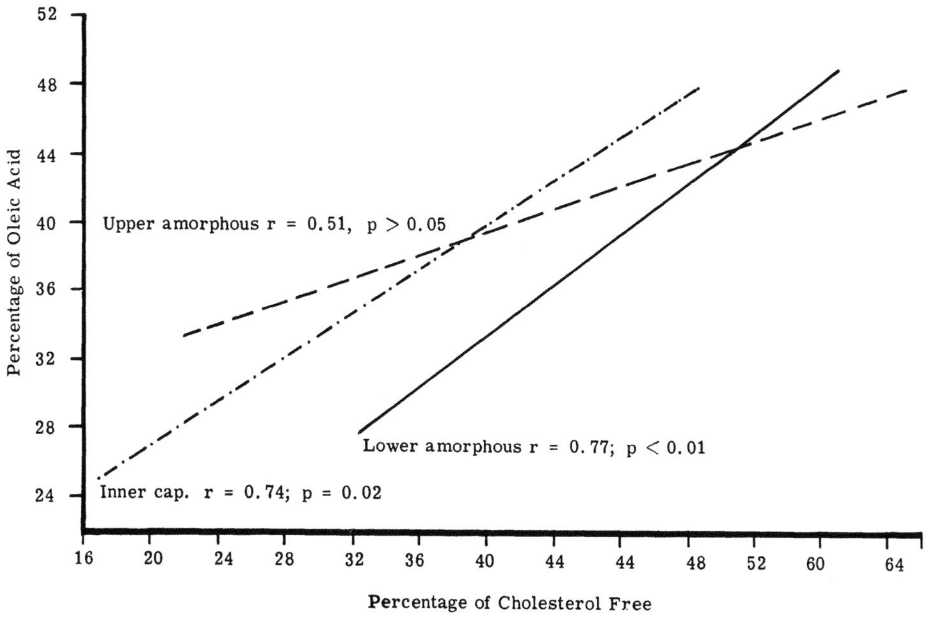

FIGURE 3.

Returning to the surface layers of the cap (TABLE VII) the free
cholesterol is very high. This might indicate preferential uptake,
but it is more probably related to the low total cholesterol level.

This becomes apparent from the plot of percentage free cholesterol
against total cholesterol (FIG. 4); the surface layers of the caps
lie on the same line as normal intima in the under 20 age group.
In the relationship between endogenous tissue lipid and accumulated
plasma lipid the surface of the cap seems to be behaving in the same
way as young normal intima. This is extremely interesting, but it
makes it even harder to understand the massive lipid accumulation
underneath.

THE RELATIONSHIP BETWEEN THE TOTAL CHOLESTEROL
CONCENTRATION AND THE PERCENTAGE OF CHOLESTEROL FREE

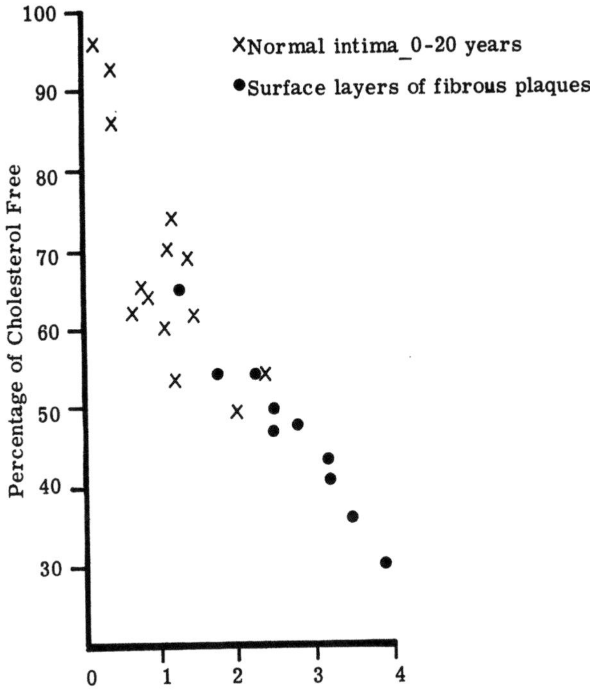

FIGURE 4.

Microdissection of Fat-Filled Cell Lesions

Microdissection of fat-filled cell type lesions was more difficult. Very small lesions did not give enough material for analysis,
but when larger plaques were serial sectioned they invariably turned
out to be of mixed type. We now think it is rare for larger lesions
to be derived purely from fat-filled cells, and the group of lesions
analyzed can only be described as "raised plaques with very numerous
fat-filled cells".

The analysis of adjacent layers is shown in TABLE VIII. Free
cholesterol reaches its maximum in the upper layers of the amorphous
lipid, and more recent work (Smith and Slater, in preparation)
suggests that the high level in the cap/amorphous lipid junction,
is associated with the amorphous lipid and not with the disintegrating
cells. Unlike the fibrous lesions, within each layer there is no
correlation between free cholesterol and cholesterol ester oleic acid,
but if all the layers are taken together they give a negative correlation comparable to that found in whole lesions. This suggests that
the observed fall in cholesterol oleate may be the result of dilution
with plasma cholesterol ester.

TABLE VIII

LIPIDS IN ADJACENT LAYERS OF SIX PLAQUES CONTAINING NUMEROUS
LARGE FAT FILLED CELLS

Layer	Intact FFCs.*	Disintegrating FFCs. + Amorphous	Upper amorphous	Lower amorphous
Total Cholesterol mg/100 mg dry tissue	56.5	142.2	172.3	83.5
Ratio $\frac{\text{cholesterol}}{\text{phospholipid}}$	4.5	3.6	4.4	3.5
Percentage of cholesterol free	32.3	46.5	52.7	44.6
CEFA % 18:1 in combined 18:1 and 18:2 fraction	64.6	47.8	42.1	37.3

*FFCs = fat filled cells

Summary of the Results of Lipid Accumulation

(1) In aging normal intima there are increasing numbers of
fine perifibrous lipid droplets with a high proportion of cholesterol
linoleate which suggests that they may be derived from the $S_f 0\text{--}12$
lipoprotein of plasma.

(2) In the fatty streaks from children of about age 7 upwards,
and from adults, lipid accumulates in droplets within cells, and is
particularly characterized by a high proportion of cholesterol oleate.

(3) In raised fibrous plaques there is a massive accumulation
of lipid with a chemical composition which is basically of the plasma
lipoprotein type, but differs from it in increased proportions of
free cholesterol and of cholesterol oleate, which seem to be correlated
with each other in each layer of the lesion.

(4) In small raised fatty lesions extracellular lipid may be
derived mainly from disintegrating fat filled cells, but in larger
plaques the decrease in proportion of cholesterol oleate, which is
not correlated with change in free cholesterol within each layer,
suggests that part of the extracellular cholesterol ester is coming
from the plasma.

(5) In both types of plaque there is a marked increase in the
proportion of free cholesterol, which seems to accumulate fastest
just under the cap; it is not clear if this is the result of hydrolysis or of preferential uptake.

Mechanisms of Lipid Accumulation
     In the last few minutes I want to raise the question of what
we know about the mechanisms involved in this lipid accumulation.
There seem to be three primary questions - firstly, what makes
intimal smooth muscle cells fill themselves with fat? Secondly,
why does perifibrous lipid accumulate in normal intima? And thirdly,
is there any information about the mechanism of accumulation of masses
of lipid under fibrous plaques in which fat filled cells cannot be
seen?

(1) What makes intimal smooth muscle cells fill themselves with
fat? Animal experiments suggest the very simple answer - high
plasma cholesterol - but in terms of human experience this does not
seem so clear. Streaks of fat-filled cells are found in the aortas
of very young children; according to Holman (Holman, 1961) all aortas
beyond the age of three have some degree of fatty streaking and this
increases rapidly from 3-12 years, and even more rapidly from 12-17.
But over this age range, serum cholesterol levels are at their lowest.
From the longitudinal studies of Lee (Lee, 1967) cholesterol appears
to fall from about age 4 until a year or two after the adolescent
growth spurt. The normal adult rise in serum cholesterol starts
about 18-20 (Lopez and Krehl et al., 1967), but there is little
further increase in the area of aortic fatty streaking after about
age 25 (Mitchell and Schwartz et al., 1964; Sternby, 1968; Vihert
and Zhdanov et al., 1969).

It might be postulated that the slight increase in mucopolysaccharide observed in fatty streaks (Klynstra and Bottcher et al.,
1967; Smith, 1965b) (TABLE IX) occurs before the development of fat-
filled cells, and causes local sequestration of plasma lipoprotein,
but in a recent study (Smith and Slater, 1970a) we have measured the
amount of immunologically intact plasma $S_f0\text{-}20$ lipoprotein which
could be extracted from aortic intima and were surprised to find
consistently low levels in tissue samples containing numerous fat-
filled cells (TABLE X). The lesions were significantly lower than
adjacent normal intima but even more surprisingly, the control intimas
were themselves significantly lower than all other normals in the

same age range. Thus fat-filled cells seem to be associated with low levels of plasma lipoprotein in the intima, both in their immediate vicinity and in the surrounding normal tissue.

TABLE IX

CONNECTIVE TISSUE COMPONENTS AND LIPIDS IN DIFFERENT TYPES OF LESION

Type of lesion	Number of cases	Concentration (mg/100 mg protein)				
		Hydroxy-proline	Calculated collagen	H + U[3]	Calculated MPS	Total lipid
Fatty streaks and nodules (average age 40)						
Normal	19	3.06	23.6	1.92	2.60	8.6
Lesion		3.41	26.3	2.25	3.02	30.6
Fibrous plaques[1] (average age 51)						
Normal	7	3.25	25.0	1.94	2.62	10.9
Lesion		5.32	41.0	1.83	2.47	47.3
Calcified plaques[2] (average age 53) with average of 64% calcium phosphate						
Normal		3.11	23.9	2.20	2.98	9.3
Lesion (based on protein)	5	7.90	60.7	0.91	1.21	109.0
Lesion (based on weight)		3.62	27.8	0.42	0.57	50.0

[1] No medial penetration or calcification

[2] With medial penetration in 4 cases

[3] H + U: hexosamine + uronic acid

(Smith, 1965b)

A study with interesting implications was that of Albrecht and Schuler in 1965 (Albrecht and Schuler, 1965). They fed rabbits on a high cholesterol diet for varying times and examined aortic cholesterol both during feeding and after the animals had been returned to a normal diet. Serum cholesterol and aortic cholesterol did not parallel each other. Serum cholesterol rose rapidly, reaching a maximum in about 20 days, whereas aortic cholesterol rose very slowly until about day 40, and then rose at a much faster rate, even when the animals had been returned to a normal diet, and serum cholesterol levels had fallen from their peak level. This suggests that the period of hypercholesterolemia initiated some process which continued even when the cholesterol level had fallen. Scott and co-workers (Scott and Jarmolych et al., 1970) have found increased cell death together with increased DNA synthesis in piglets after three days of cholesterol feeding. Possibly sporadic hyperlipemia could be a stimulus which triggers off fat-filled cell production in the young human.

TABLE X

COMPARISON OF TOTAL TISSUE CHOLESTEROL AND CHOLESTEROL IN
IMMUNOLOGICALLY INTACT AND TOTAL S$_f$0-20 LIPOPROTEIN IN LESIONS CONTAINING
NUMEROUS FAT FILLED CELLS AND ADJACENT NORMAL INTIMA, AND BETWEEN THESE
NORMAL CONTROLS AND NORMAL INTIMA FROM ALL OTHER AORTAE IN THE SAME AGE GROUP

Fat filled cell lesions	Number of samples	Cholesterol mg/100 mg dry tissue		Total in tissue
		S$_f$0-20 lipoprotein		
		Immunologic- ally intact	Total	
Lesion	15	0.148	0.517	15.25
Control		0.236	0.381	6.28
Difference		p = 0.01	p = 0.02	p = 0.001
Normal Intima				
Controls from above	15	0.236	0.381	6.28
Other normals	54	0.470	0.668	5.36
Difference		p = 0.001	p = 0.001	p = 0.005

(Smith and Slater, 1970)

(2) The accumulation of perifibrous lipid in normal intima.
Between the ages of 20-60 the intimal lipid concentration, particularly cholesterol ester, increases about 5-fold. There are small
changes in collagen, MPS and intimal plasma lipoprotein, and in the
cholesterol level of the plasma which bathes the intima, but the only
other obvious change of comparable magnitude is in intimal thickness,
which increases 2-3-fold. It seems reasonable to ask whether the
observed cholesterol ester accumulation is primarily associated with
age, or primarily associated with thickening.

The top part of TABLE XI shows the correlation coefficients
between intimal thickness and age, and cholesterol ester and age,
both of which are very high; and between cholesterol ester and
intimal thickness, where the correlation is considerably lower
(Smith and Evans et al., 1967). Presumably this indicates that
cholesterol ester is accumulating primarily as a result of aging
and not of intimal thickening, and conversely intimal thickening is
not primarily a response to cholesterol accumulation.

TABLE XI

CORRELATION COEFFICIENTS FOR THE RELATIONSHIP OF CHOLESTEROL FRACTIONS WITH AGE AND WITH INTIMAL THICKNESS IN NORMAL INTIMA WITH PERIFIBROUS LIPID

	Age		Thickness	
	r	p	r	p
Series 1, Total cholesterol ester in 62 samples				
Intimal thickness	0.698	0.001	–	–
Cholesterol ester concentration	0.746	0.001	0.370	0.01
Series 2, Total tissue cholesterol, and cholesterol in extracted lipoproteins in 79 samples				
Intimal thickness	0.837	0.001	–	–
Total tissue cholesterol	0.469	0.001	0.372	0.001
Immunologically intact lipoprotein	0.086	0.1	0.370	0.001
Total S_f0-20 lipoprotein	0.189	0.1	0.364	0.001

Surprisingly, the extractable plasma lipoprotein in the intima (Smith and Slater, 1970a), from which the accumulating cholesterol ester is presumably derived, is not significantly correlated with age, but is significantly correlated with thickness, although the correlation is not very high (lower part of TABLE XI). In this series there was again a highly significant correlation between cholesterol and age. Even more surprisingly, no correlation could be demonstrated between intact plasma lipoprotein in the intima and total intimal cholesterol, either in normal intima or in lesions. This leads to the question – what is the status of these perifibrous lipid droplets? If a droplet is deposited at age 30 does it remain intact for the next 30 or 40 years? This would seem incredible – compounds such as cholesterol linoleate and lecithin are not inert – but if the droplets are in a state of dynamic equilibrium with the intact plasma lipoprotein in intima, which is not increasing with age, why should there be accumulation?

(3) <u>Is there any information about the mechanism of the accumulation of the masses of lipid in large fibrous plaques which do
not contain fat-filled cells</u>? Although it is basically similar to
the lipid of plasma S_f0-20 lipoprotein, the accumulated lipid differs
from it in a number of ways and it is not clear if the changes are
a result of selective uptake or selective breakdown, or a mixture
of both. There has in the past been a strong feeling that binding
of lipoprotein by MPS might be an important factor in the development
of lesions. This was largely based on histological staining, but
quantitative measurement of MPS has really lent very little support
to this idea. TABLE IX summarizes our findings for total MPS in
lesions compared with normal intima from the same aortas (Smith,
1965b). There is a small but statistically significant increase in
fatty streaks. Here most of the lipid is within fat-filled cells,
the cholesterol ester is not of the plasma type, and intimal plasma
lipoprotein is particularly low. None of these observations supports
the idea of excessive sequestration of plasma lipoprotein.

In fibrous plaques, where increased binding of plasma lipoprotein might be expected, the total MPS is actually reduced; slightly
reduced in early plaques, and very greatly reduced in advanced plaques.
These results are in close agreement with those of Klynstra and
Bottcher (Klynstra and Bottcher et al., 1967), who further fraction-
ated the MPS and found some variation in pattern;·similar variations
were found by Kumar and co-workers (Kumar and Berenson et al., 1967)
using the whole aortic intima with different degrees of atherosclerotic involvement.

In spite of the negative MPS findings, it seems reasonable to
expect fibrous lesions to have a high affinity for plasma lipoprotein,
and in our recent studies on the amount of immunologically intact
S_f0-20 lipoprotein which can be extracted from intima (Smith and
Slater, 1970a) we examined early fibrous thickenings - these are
lesions which have not developed a definite amorphous center, and
which do not contain any fat-filled cells. The levels of plasma
lipoprotein cholesterol were higher in the lesions than in the
adjacent normal intima in all cases, but there was great variation
and no correlation with maximum thickness. In rather more than half
the lesions both immunologically intact and total S_f0-20 lipoprotein
were very high, whereas in the remainder there was minimal elevation;
the high and low groups are compared in TABLE XII.

In spite of a threefold difference in both immunologically intact
and total S_f0-20 lipoprotein there is no difference in the total cholesterol concentration of the tissue. There is no difference in the
proportion of the total S_f0-20 lipoprotein which is immunologically
intact and we could not recognize any consistent histological differences between lesions with high and low levels of plasma lipoprotein.
In the high group immunologically intact plasma lipoprotein accounts

for nearly 20 per cent of the total lesion cholesterol. This failure
to demonstrate any correlation between the concentrations of intact
plasma lipoprotein and of total intimal cholesterol is exactly comparable to the findings in normal, aging intima, and is very puzzling.

TABLE XII

COMPARISON OF TOTAL TISSUE CHOLESTEROL, CHOLESTEROL IN IMMUNOLOGICALLY INTACT AND TOTAL
S_f0-20 LIPOPROTEIN AND INTIMAL THICKNESS IN FIBROUS LESIONS WITH IMMUNO-β-CHOLESTEROL*
LEVELS ABOVE AND BELOW 0.65 mg/100 mg DRY TISSUE

Immuno-β Cholesterol	No.	Av. Age	Cholesterol mg/100 mg dry tissue			% immuno-β-cholesterol* in S_f0-20 fraction	Thickness of intima of µ
			Immuno-β*	S_f0-20	Total		
Above 0.65	9	49	1.214	2.457	7.23	49.5	820
Below 0.65	6	53	0.415	0.975	7.15	42.5	890
Difference			p = 0.001	p= 0.001	p>0.1	p>0.1	p>0.1

*Immunologically intact S_f0-20 lipoprotein

(Smith and Slater, 1970a)

The results of these detailed studies on intimal lipid in human
aorta strongly support the view that a substantial part of the lipid
is derived from plasma low density lipoprotein. However, simple
filtration cannot explain the observed facts, and the factors involved
in retention of lipid are still not understood.

Acknowledgement

Much of the work reported here was supported by the British Heart
Foundation, to whom the author is extremely grateful.

DISCUSSION

PARTICIPANTS: C.W.M. Adams, P.D. Lang, F. Parker, A.L. Robertson,
               D.D. Rutstein, P.J. Scott, E.B. Smith, N.T.
               Werthessen and S. Wolf

CHAIRMAN WOLF: we need to establish to what extent fat entering
the arterial wall is used for nutrition, and to what extent it is a
source of damage to the tissue. In considering the changes that are
associated with age, we're still having a bit of difficulty with
distinction between "normal" and "pathological." But we see from
the various earlier speakers as well as from Dr. Smith's presentation
that atherosclerosis involves intimal thickening, appearance of
muscle and elastic tissue above the basement membrane, increase in

lipid concentration in the intima, decrease in the dilatability of
the artery, and a loss of responsiveness to beta adrenergic agents.
To what extent are these changes related to physical forces brought
to bear on the artery, to what extent may they be related to a decrease in growth hormone, or perhaps to a loss of specific sympathetic
effect or other changes? I hope that in this and subsequent sessions
many of these and other questions brought out in Dr. Smith's lecture
will be dealt with.

COMMENT

Dr. Werthessen raised a technical point concerning the staining
of cholesterol ester with Sudan dyes. Dr. Adams answered the question
with data on twenty-three differently constituted lipids and forty
different staining methods that cholesterol esters, when unsaturated
and in liquid form do take the Sudan dyes while in the crystalline
state they do not.

DR. LANG: I would like to report briefly on some characteristics
of lipid droplets in arteriosclerotic fatty streaks of human aortas.
I have obtained these data in the laboratory of Dr. Wm. Insull, Jr.
from Case Western Reserve University in Cleveland, Ohio.

As you know, in fatty streaks thought by many to be the initial
lesion of human arteriosclerosis, lipid accumulates predominantly
in the form of intracellular droplets. The chemical composition
of these droplets has so far been only inadequately described, while
the composition of whole lesions has been extensively studied.

Around the turn of the century it had already been reported that
lipid droplets from superficial lesions of human intima polarize
light. But the fact that these droplets are predominantly anisotropic, has become the object of study only in recent years. As this
phenomenon seems to have important biological implications, for our
study we took the thoracic and upper abdominal part of the aortas
with extensive fatty streaking from 21 subjects, who had died suddenly and unexpectedly. None had metabolic disorders or debilitating
diseases. Most had died from acute trauma. The average time between
death and necropsy was 10 hours. Immediately after autopsy the
fresh aortas were processed. With the aid of a dissecting microscope
and ophthalmological surgical instru-
ments the fatty streaks were dissected
off the internal elastic lamina. All
Characteristics of
lipid droplets in   fatty streaks present in one aorta
fatty streaks   were pooled to obtain 200 to 500 mg
of tissue, that amount needed for analysis. Histological studies with
the light microscope were done on each aorta to show that the streaks
were confined to the intima and were free of fibrosis.

The dissected fatty streaks were thoroughly minced with fine
scissors and the mince gently homogenized with water at 22°C. The
pale yellow layer of droplets floating on the top of the homogenate
upon centrifugation was drawn off with a glass syringe, resuspended
in water and centrifuged again. This washing procedure was repeated
twice to obtain the droplet fraction. The sedimented residue,
containing nuclei, cytoplasm, membranes, etc., and the supernatant
fraction were not separately analyzed and this fraction is hereafter
referred to as residue preparation. The final preparations were
checked for purity by phase contrast microscopy, the droplet fraction
for particulate contaminants, the residue fraction for lipid droplets.

The droplet preparation consisted of a mixture of isotropic and
anistropic droplets. Both forms had average diameters of about 1.8µ,
with a range of 0.5-5.0µ. The optical distinction between these two
forms was done by using polarizing filters and a first order red
quartz plate. We have not been able to separate the two forms to
determine their quantities and chemical composition. We have therefore developed a method to determine the relative volumes of the two
forms in a given mixture by classifying them according to the presence
of anisotropy or isotropy and size. This was done with the polarizing
microscope, a bacteria counting chamber, an eyepiece micrometer, and
a warming stage for controlling the temperature. The latter is necessary because of the temperature dependency of the proportion of
anisotropic droplets. The proportion of anisotropic droplets is at
maximum and constant over a temperature range of 4 to 25°C. They
decrease from there on with increase of the temperature, as individual
droplets change their form. Anisotropic forms averaged 83.7% at
22°C and 37.8% at 37°C, with isotropic forms being 16.3 and 62.2%
respectively. The anisotropic form is the initial form, for it is
predominant in younger individuals and in the early lesions.

For chemical analysis the neutral lipids and phospholipids were
analyzed by quantitative thin-layer chromatography (Amenta, 1964).
The data presented are given as the proportions of total lipids or
total phospholipids. Small but unavoidable losses occurring particularly during the preparation of the droplet fraction prevented
accurate determination of lipid concentration in the tissue.

TABLE XIII shows the proportions of various lipids in total
lipids of the droplet and residue fraction. The composition is
strikingly different among preparations, but markedly uniform within each preparation. The droplet lipid is largely cholesterol esters,
with minor proportions of triglycerides, free cholesterol and phospholipids. In the residue the lipids are constituted largely of
equal proportions of cholesterol esters, of pholpholipids, a moderate
proportion of free cholesterol, and a small proportion of triglycerides. Droplets and residue each supply on the average about 50%
of total lipids, so 2/3 of the cholesterol esters and 1/3 of the

triglycerides are found in the droplets, and almost all phospholipids
and free cholesterol in the residue. The considerably varying droplet content of fatty streaks probably explains the rather large
variation in the lipid composition of whole lesions. It should be
pointed out here, and this is true also for the data presented later,
that the composition of the residue fraction is very similar to that
reported for normal intima (Smith, 1965a).

TABLE XIII

PROPORTIONS OF VARIOUS LIPIDS IN TOTAL LIPID OF DROPLETS AND
RESIDUE OF FATTY STREAKS FROM 21 AORTAS

Lipids	Precent of Total Lipid by Tissue Preparation		Significance of Difference between Droplets and Residue
	Droplets	Residue	
Cholesterol Esters	94.9 ± 2.2*	38.7 ± 4.7	P < 0.01
Free Cholesterol	1.7 ± 0.6	18.6 ± 2.0	P < 0.01
Phospholipids	1.0 ± 0.7	38.7 ± 3.8	P < 0.01
Triglycerides	2.4 ± 1.3	4.0 ± 1.3	P < 0.01

* Mean ± Standard Deviation

TABLE XIV shows also the proportions of the individual phospholipids - with the exception of lysolethicin, the smallest component -
to be different in the two preparations. Most of the phospholipid
in the droplets were lecithin and cephalins, and in the residue
lecithin and sphingomyelin.

The fatty acid composition of the cholesterol esters as determined by gas-liquid chromatography is seen in TABLE XV. These 8
acids contained 97% of the acid mixture. The droplets contained
more 16:1, 18:1, and 20:3, the residue had more 16:0, 18:2 and 20:4.
The sum of the proportions of oleic and linoleic acids was the same
in both preparations, while the droplets had more oleic and less
linoleic acids than did the residue. This difference between
residue and droplets in their ratios of these two acids is the same
difference as has been observed between normal and arteriosclerotic
pigeon aortas (St. Clair and Lofland et al., 1968), and between
normal intima and fatty streaks of human aortas (Smith, 1965a; Geer
and Malcolm, 1965). This suggests that the difference between normal
and diseased tissue is due to the presence of these droplets. The
fatty acid mixture of the droplets does not resemble the fatty acid

mixture found in cholesterol esters of any of the lipoprotein classes
of human plasma (Goodman and Shiratori, 1964), so simple infiltration
and deposition of unaltered plasma lipids in the form of droplets is
an unlikely process. If not synthesis at least the selection of the
cholesterol ester fatty acids must be very specific because of the
remarkable uniformity of the composition of the various droplet
preparations.

TABLE XIV

PROPORTIONS OF INDIVIDUAL PHOSPHOLIPIDS IN TOTAL PHOSPHOLIPID OF
DROPLETS AND RESIDUE OF FATTY STREAKS FROM AORTAS

| Phospholipid | Percent of Total Phospholipid by Tissue Preparations | | Significance |
	Droplets (17 Aortas)	Residue (20 Aortas)	between Droplets and Residue
Lecithin	39.5 ± 9.4*	46.9 ± 4.9	P < 0.01
Lysolecithin	8.3 ± 9.9	6.0 ± 2.2	N.S.
Sphingomyelin	17.1 ± 11.9	27.7 ± 5.3	P < 0.01
Cephalins	35.1 ± 9.6	19.4 ± 5.0	P < 0.01

N.S. Not significant

*Mean ± Standard deviation

A great number of correlations between the parameters observed –
including age and standard body weight of the subjects – were computed,
but none can be easily interpreted. So I will not go into this here.

The observation that these droplets are prominent in the morphology of the fatty streak lesions, and the fact that their high content
of oleate-rich cholesterol esters is similar to that reported for
analysis of the whole lesion (Smith, 1965a; Geer and Malcolm, 1965),
suggests that the droplets may play a central role in the pathogenesis
of the fatty streak lesion of atherosclerosis in man.

We believe that one can postulate a mechanism in the lipid filled
cells which specifies fixed proportions of the various lipids for
deposition in the droplets. Stoichiometric relationships might
exist between the various lipids to cause the physical structure
necessary for the anisotropic state of
Relation of intra-   the droplets. Conceivably this structure
cellular lipids to   is crucial for active metabolism at the
aqueous cytoplasm   interphase between the droplet and the
                            cytoplasm and possibly within the droplet,
as a lammelated ultrastructure of alternating lipid and aqueous layers
has been reported (Weller, 1967).

TABLE XV

PROPORTIONS OF VARIOUS FATTY ACIDS IN CHOLESTERYL ESTERS OF DROPLETS

AND RESIDUE OF FATTY STREAKS FROM 21 AORTAS

| Fatty acid | | % of total fatty acids by tissue preparation | | Significance of difference between droplets and residue |
Common name	Short hand*	Droplets	Residue	
Myristic	14:0	1.06 ± 0.36†	0.96 ± 0.22	NS
Palmitic	16:0	8.93 ± 1.76	11.15 ± 1.91	P < 0.01
Palmitoleic	16:1	5.91 ± 0.67	5.26 ± 1.13	P < 0.05
Stearic	18:0	1.96 ± 0.84	1.60 ± 0.57	NS
Oleic	18:1	50.37 ± 3.51	38.04 ± 3.98	P < 0.01
Linoleic	18.2	15.18 ± 3.24	27.61 ± 4.54	P < 0.01
Eicosatrienoic	20:3	7.04 ± 2.01	4.69 ± 1.49	P < 0.01
Arachidonic	20:4	6.55 ± 1.88	8.15 ± 2.06	P < 0.01

NS = not significant.
* Number of carbon atoms: number of double bonds, per molecule
† Mean ± standard deviation

(Lang and Insull, 1970)

The further progression or regression of the lesion may therefore
depend on the physical structure of these intracellular droplets, as
the milieu of the droplets, i.e., the residue, does not appear to be
qualitatively different from that of undiseased intimal tissue.

DR. ROBERTSON: Dr. Smith raised several questions relating to
cytological characteristics of cell types preceding foam cell formation. Using human intimal cells (atherocytes) (Robertson, 1965a;
Robertson, 1965b) isolated from short
Formation of foam   term organ cultures of arterial seg-
cells from smooth   ments obtained during direct coronary
muscle cells   artery surgery, we have been greatly
                          impressed by the striking morphological
changes occurring during the in vitro incorporation of serum lipoprotein fractions. The majority of these cells fulfill all histochemical and ultrastructural criteria of smooth muscle cells and may
be cloned to obtain homogenous cell populations FIG. 5. However,
their cytological characteristics (A) are rapidly modified following
short term incubation with homologous low density serum lipoproteins
(LDL). Their transformation to typical macrophage type cells (B),
monocytoid elements (C) or intermediate stages (D) has also been followed by time lapse cinematography. The findings suggest that morphological criteria alone may be inadequate to identify the origin of the
heterogenous cell population usually found in proliferative lesions
encountered in spontaneous "early" atheroma. Furthermore, functional
characteristics and rate of incorporation of extracellular lipids may
be quite variable depending upon the stage of cytoplasmic "transformation" and intracellular lipid storage in an individual arterial cell.

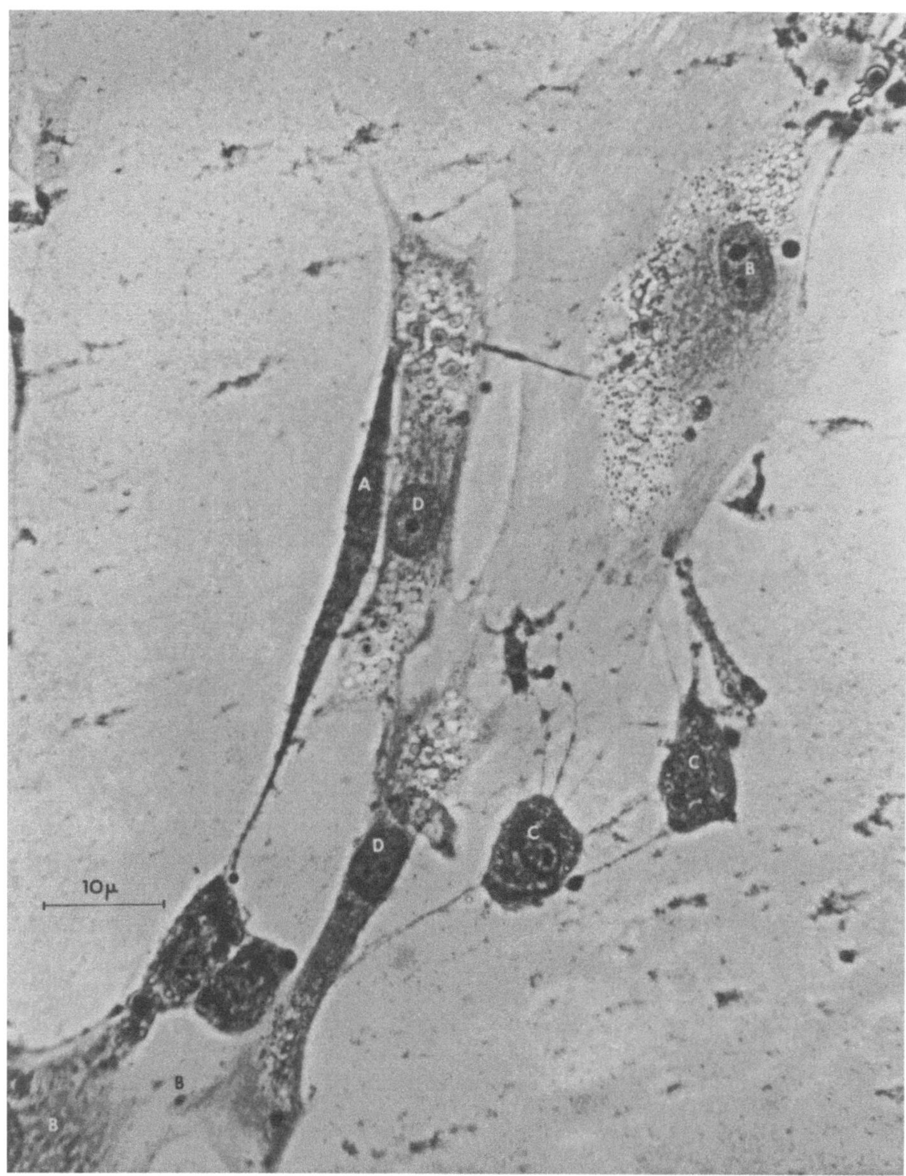

FIGURE 5. Acute morphological changes occurring with cultures of
human intimacytes following short-term incubation with homologous
low density lipoprotein (see text).
    A. Normal atherophils
    B. Monocytoid-macrophage transformation
    C. Monocytoid cells
    D. Intermediate cells

We have also attempted to identify at what rate incorporation of specific lipid fractions occurred. TABLE XVI. Matching suspensions of intimal cell cultures were incubated with medium 199 (Morgan) supplemented with 10% normocholesterolemic (TC 220 mg%, CE 184 mg%) or 10% hypercholesterolemic (TC 384 mg%, CE 286 mg%) pooled human serum. Average incorporation rates for 18 cultures each, showed that although both triglycerides (TG) and free cholesterol (FC) concentrations increased (2-3 times) following incubation in hypercholesterolemic serum for 60 minutes. The highest increase occurred in the cholesterol ester (CE) fractions (20 times). Parenthetically, labeled mevalonic acid

TABLE XVI

HUMAN ARTERIAL INTIMAL CELLS

INTRACELLULAR LIPID CONCENTRATIONS

	Cells in 199 + 10% NS (*)	Cells in 199 + 10% HS (**)
TRIGLYCERIDES	46	112 µg L/mg CP
FREE CHOLESTEROL	75	180
CHOLESTEROL ESTERS	24	420
C/CE RATIO	3.30	0.43

^{3}H MEVALONIC	% Total Lipids	Average dpm/µg L	% Total Lipids	Average dpm/µg L
FREE CHOLESTEROL	84	549	5	21
CHOLESTEROL ESTERS	8	86	74	132

18 cultures each incubated at 37° C

(*) Pooled Normolipemic Human Serum: TC 220 mg %
                                       CE 184 mg %

(**) Pooled Hypercholesterolemic Human Serum: TC 384 mg %
                                               CE 286 mg %

Cholesterol trans-
port, storage and
synthesis
utilization also increased particularly
in the CE fractions both as percentual
total lipids and specific activities.
These results would indicate a para-
doxical response of arterial intimal
cells to extracellular lipid incorporation, with both increased storage of CE and simultaneous acceleration of de novo intracellular
sterol synthesis.

We have yet to measure release rates of free cholesterol during
storage of cholesterol esters. Preliminary data would suggest that
free cholesterol, in contrast to cholesterol esters, is easily
carried across the cell membrane in both directions, to and from
the intracellular compartments. The fate of extracellular cholesterol in vitro seems to depend upon the amount of intracellular
lipid in surrounding intimal cells, once released by lysis of a "foam
cell" or atherocyte (Robertson, 1965a) it may be rapidly incorporated
or "reutilized" (Robertson, 1965b) by surrounding cells. These cytological findings could explain apparent discrepancies between serum
cholesterol levels and severity of atherosclerosis in some patients.
Temporary elevations (such as post-prandial increases) in serum
lipids could thus suffice to initiate as a trigger mechanism, self
sustaining arterial cell damage due to inability of the arterial
wall to readily release back cholesterol into the circulation.

DR. RUTSTEIN: I should like to summarize some of our work on
comparative gas liquid chromatography of fatty acids in the extracts
of the tissue culture cells and of the specimens of serum added to
the culture medium in which the cells were incubated (Rutstein and
Castelli et al., 1969; Rutstein and Castelli et al., 1964).

Tissue Culture Method
The cultures consisted of strains of diploid cells (L-809-15)
and (MAF) from human embryonic skin and muscle tissue in which lipid
deposition parallels that of human aortic cells in tissue culture.

The culture medium was the same as that used in our earlier
work--human blood serum (40%), chick embryonic extract (2%), and
Hanks' balanced salt solution (58%). The human blood serum provided nutrition to the tissue culture cells and acted as the carrier
for the serum lipid present when the specimen was collected. Each
specimen was tested at least in sextuplicate. Every experiment was
begun on tissue culture cells which had been transferred from pre-
scription bottles to roller tubes 7 days previously.

In each experiment, the culture tubes were coded and randomly
ordered before the human serum specimen was added. At the end of the
experiment they were read blindly before the results were decoded.
The cells were incubated for 5 days with the culture medium being re-

moved and replaced half-way through the experiment on the third day.
Deposition was read and graded as before from 1 (minimum) to 9 (maximum), except that the finding of cells so filled with lipids that
the cell membrane was ruptured in the experiments with hypercholesterolemic serum, led us to extend our lipid deposition scale to grade
10. Readings were made on the unstained cells and after staining
with Sudan black B. Previous work had demonstrated that stained and
unstained readings of the same cells showed similar trends and this
report, except in the deposition reversibility experiments, is limited to the readings of stained cells. Serum specimens were collected
at strategic times to determine changes from the baseline due to test
meals, the prolonged fasting state, and the intravenous injection of
10,000 units of heparin.

Effects of serum   Consistent findings were obtained.
composition on   The proportion of palmitic and stearic
incorporation of   acids (saturated) was always higher in
lipids into cells   the cells than in the serum, while that
in tissue culture   of linoleic acid (polyunsaturated) was
                                    always higher in the serum than in the
cells (TABLE XVII). These differences persisted and remained consistent under the varying conditions of the experiment, including the
time of specimen collection, the test meal, and the prolonged fasting
state. However, in the postheparin specimens, the differences in
relative saturation of fatty acids between cells and serum was clearly less than in the preprandial (control) or preheparin specimens.
The individual results, with minor exceptions in the concentration
of palmitic acid (16:0) for each of the three subjects revealed the
same differences as the mean values (TABLE XVII).

When the data were analyzed separately for cells or serum, there
were consistent changes in the fatty-acid patterns of each after the
injection of heparin. In every instance in the cells, there was a
drop in mean value after the injection of heparin in the proportion
of myristic, palmitic, and stearic acids (saturated) and a concurrent
steep rise in the concentration of linoleic and homogammalinolenic
acids (polyunsaturated) but not in that of arachidonic acid (TABLE
XVII). The changes in the proportion of myristic (p<0.05) and homogammalinolenic (p<0.01) acids are significant but their peaks on the
gas liquid chromatograph are very small and subject to greater error
of measurement. In contrast, after the injection of heparin, the
serum in the medium in which the cells were incubated showed only
slight changes in varying directions (viz., small increases or decreases in the proportion of myristic, palmitic, stearic, linoleic,
homogammalinolenic or arachidonic acids). Nevertheless, despite the
definitive changes in the cells, the sharp rise in the concentration
of the key unsaturated acid, linoleic acid, in the cells after heparin administration never attained its level in the serum.

TABLE XVII

EFFECT OF INTRAVENOUS HEPARIN ON FATTY ACIDS IN EXTRACTS OF TISSUE-CULTURE CELLS AND HUMAN SERUM IN
THE CULTURE MEDIUM AFTER TEST-MEALS AND IN PROLONGED FASTING STATE

Experiment	Specimen	Fatty acids (%)								Serum-N.E.F.A. (µeq./l.)	Deposition in cells (grade)
		14:0	16:0	16:1	18:0	18:1	18:2	20:3	20:4		
Safflower oil	Cells:										
	(a)	1.4	33.8	4.0	13.8	22.6	14.0	1.4	9.0		2.8
	(b)	1.7	32.6	3.0	14.0	20.5	17.9	0.2	10.1		2.8
	(c)	0.8	31.4	3.6	11.3	19.8	21.3	3.3	8.4		7.8
	Serum:										
	(a)	2.1	25.4	4.6	8.6	22.1	25.3	3.6	8.2	871	
	(b)	1.4	25.6	3.9	8.4	22.6	29.2	2.0	6.9	972	
	(c)	1.3	29.4	3.8	8.1	21.4	27.7	2.0	6.4	3338	
Carbohydrate	Cells:										
	(a)	1.6	32.5	4.3	15.1	18.6	12.5	1.5	13.8		2.9
	(b)	1.3	35.1	3.9	16.9	21.1	10.6	0.6	10.7		2.8
	(c)	0.7	32.3	4.0	13.6	23.6	14.0	2.6	9.1		6.1
	Serum:										
	(a)	1.1	26.5	4.0	7.6	24.9	27.6	2.4	5.9	950	
	(b)	1.1	24.6	4.3	8.0	23.9	27.2	2.7	8.3	606	
	(c)	1.3	27.3	4.0	7.7	23.0	26.6	1.9	8.3	2363	
Prolonged fasting state	Cells:										
	(a)	1.8	31.0	4.0	14.9	20.5	13.0	0.8	14.0		3.2
	(b)	3.4	37.3	3.3	16.0	24.4	7.8	0.6	7.2		3.4
	(c)	0.8	33.8	4.0	10.6	25.3	14.0	3.0	8.7		7.8
	Serum:										
	(a)	4.7	26.0	4.6	8.3	22.8	24.1	2.3	7.4	798	
	(b)	0.8	27.9	4.5	7.2	24.9	24.8	1.9	7.8	1478	
	(c)	3.8	25.4	4.2	8.3	23.1	24.5	3.3	7.5	3408	

Intracellular saturation of fatty acids

The results of the gas liquid chromatography studies indicate that the state of equilibrium of lipids within the cells is consistently at a higher level of fatty-acid saturation than that of the culture medium surrounding the cells. This equilibrium is shifted by the intravenous injection of heparin toward a greater proportion of unsaturated acids within the cells. This shift in the fatty-acid pattern must be interpreted in the light of the sharp increase in intracellular lipid deposition (from 2.8, 2.8, and 3.4 to 7.8, 6.1, and 7.8) observed in such preparations (TABLE XVII).

These results may be explained by any one of several mechanisms. There may be a mechanism by which the fatty acids become saturated as they are incorporated within the cell, or the effect may result from a selective transfer of saturated acids across cell membranes, or the immediate catabolism of the transferred acids within the cells may contribute to intracellular synthesis of saturated acids. Any one or all of such mechanisms could operate consistently throughout our experiments except that they would be relatively inefficient under conditions of extreme intracellular lipid deposition, as occurred in specimens of serum following the intravenous injection of heparin.

DR. SCOTT: Dr. Smith made some analyses on xanthomas in humans.
In untreated insulin dependent diabetics and in some patients with
prolonged heavy alcohol intake, there is often an elevation of plasma
prebeta and beta lipoprotein levels, corresponding to the type IV
pattern of Fredrickson (Fredrickson and Levy et al., 1967). In
some of these patients, xanthomas may develop quite rapidly. Following satisfactory treatment and dietetic adjustment, these xanthomas
rapidly disappear, with no subsequent fibrosis. At biopsy several
weeks later, light microscopy may reveal no abnormality in previously
xanthoma-bearing skin. Perhaps in our considerations of tissue
lipids we are concentrating too much on various extractable lipid
components and products of lipid catabolism, rather than looking
at the clues provided by the total plasma and extravascular lipoprotein situation. Thus, in the areas of xanthomatosis referred to
above, there must be some mechanism by which lipid can be rapidly
accumulated, and also a mechanism for its rapid removal.

Removal of lipid in xanthomas of different types and with different serum lipid patterns An entirely different situation occurs in human Type II hyperlipopro-
teinemia where the lesions in skin and tendons develop gradually and re-
solve extremely slowly following suc-
cessfully maintained lowering of blood
lipid levels. The mechanism for lipid deposition, exchange and removal must be different in these two types of human xanthomatosis
(Scott and Winterbourn, 1967). Moreover, the tissue response in
terms of fibrosis and residual scarring differs, as do the predominant anatomical sites for the lesions. It is possible, and perhaps
probable, that the types of lipoproteins circulating in the patient
and their levels influence the nature, extent and natural history
of lipid deposition in tissues other than skin, including artery
walls. It therefore seems important that in studies such as these
quoted by Dr. Smith, the site and type of the lesion, and the nature
of the lipoprotein pattern associated with the xanthomatosis should
be stated. Can Dr. Smith give us more information concerning the
xanthoma from which she isolated the lipids mentioned in her paper?

DR. SMITH: These were xanthomas taken from the elbows of four
patients with Type II hypercholesterolemia. Histologically, they
appeared to consist of intact fat-filled cells. I have not had the
opportunity to examine any of the hyperlipemias. I should like to
very much indeed.

DR. SCOTT: One further question. Were there cholesterol clefts
in the lesions which you examined?

DR. SMITH: No, I do not think there were. They seemed to be
quite intact fat-filled cells, but I must say, our histology was
not very good.

DR. PARKER: We have been very interested in examining xanthomas
in humans on the assumption that perhaps alterations in the vasculature of human skin might possibly reflect similar events in the
atherosclerotic process in the large vessel wall. In eight diabetic
patients with eruptive xanthomas large increases in serum triglyceride were seen, and when we subfractionated this triglyceride,
on the average, 70% of the triglyceride was found in chylomicron
particles as determined by a PVP flocculation method. It is
interesting to note that although total cholesterol was also increased in the plasma, very little was carried in these chylomicron
particles, and the total cholesterol of the plasma was relatively
less in each individual case than the triglyceride elevation. So
that these patients have primarily a chylomicronemia carrying 70%
of the total plasma triglyceride. When the eruptive xanthomas
were biopsied and sampled within two to eight weeks after they
first appeared, the major lipid in these xanthomas was found to be

	triglyceride rather than cholesterol,
Xanthomas in	the major lipid found in Type II
diabetics	xanthomas.

When the triglyceride fatty acids in the xanthomas were compared
with the total plasma triglycerides and the chylomicron triglycerides,
all the fatty acid patterns were found to be similar, suggesting
that the chylomicrons were contributing to the triglyceride accumulating in the xanthomas.

With oil-red O stains, lipid droplets were seen within and precisely outlining the capillary walls of the dermal vessels within
the xanthomas. By electron microscopy one could see numerous droplets, with a grey central core and a particulate outer surface,
within the basal lamina of the capillary wall between the endothelial and perithelial cells. The droplets measured approximately
2,000 Å ± 1,000 Å in diameter and looked identical in both size and
configuration to isolated circulating chylomicron particles taken
from these patients.

When the patients were first placed on a low-fat diet and subsequently on insulin the xanthomas disappeared. Both low-fat diet
and insulin also decreased the circulating chylomicrons. The major
initial decrease in xanthoma lipids was in triglyceride. Thus,
whereas the erupting xanthomas were triglyceride rich, the resolving
lesions were converted into cholesterol rich xanthomas, suggesting
that it is more difficult to remove free and esterified cholesterol
from these lesions than it is to solubilize the triglyceride in the
dermal lesions. There was no change in the fatty acid patterns of
the triglyceride and the cholesterol esters during the course of the
disappearance of xanthomas. In other words, there was nothing to
suggest that certain triglyceride or cholesterol ester fatty acids
were getting out at any greater rate than any others.

QUESTION: What do you think the droplets in the vessel walls
represent?

DR. PARKER: I think that the major thing that we see, but I
am not sure, is triglyceride in these droplets. It is the major
lipid and it does seem to take some sort of a stain. I think most
of the cholesterol, whether free or esterified, is totally washed
out in preparation when prepared for electron microscopy.

QUESTION: How do the chylomicrons get through the vessel wall?

DR. PARKER: The only time these chylomicrons are seen is out
in the basal lamina and cellular space up against histocytes. I
never have seen chylomicrons between endothelial cells or within
endothelial cells. I do not know how they get across the endothelial cell walls.

DR. SCOTT: It is clear that there are very real limitations
imposed by techniques which inherently limit observations to either
localized areas of anatomy, or to restricted periods of time. It
is no criticism of these methods that they should be thus restricted,
but it is important that we try to develop methods which will give
us some insight into continuing processes which may be relevant to
atherogenesis.

Some of the points raised by Dr. Elspeth Smith might receive
partial answers by dynamic studies of the metabolism of intact lipoproteins which is the form in which lipids other than free fatty
acids circulate in plasma. At the outset, I would point out that
our group does not retain any simple concept of a lipoprotein filtration process through arterial walls, such as envisaged by Page
and Lewis (Page, 1954), some years ago. We do not believe that the
evidence exists at present to suggest that lipoproteins are either
the initiating or even the major sustaining factor in atherogenesis.
We do believe however, that until adequate dynamic studies of lipoprotein metabolism and its relevance to vascular physiology have
been devised and undertaken, we will never have an adequate answer
to many of the questions which have been raised in the earlier
phases of this conference.

Ten years ago we commenced work on lipoprotein metabolism in
humans because we believed that there was no adequate animal model
in which to do this. It is possible that a suitable primate may
be found for this type of work, but care will be needed in selecting
such a model. Our studies have shown us that some of the problems
we set out to investigate cannot be adequately solved by studies
in humans alone. However, we still believe that careful attention
to balancing human experiments against animal studies should provide
fruitful approaches to further investigations of atherogenesis.

There are very good reasons why so few groups have attemped
dynamic studies of lipoprotein, rather than concentrating upon
lipid portions of the molecule. Lipoproteins are extremely difficult
to isolate, they are sticky, fickle, stubborn molecules which are
very difficult to handle, in pure form. We believe that the only
non-exchangeable portion of the molecule is the peptide component,
and we also believe that some cholesterol ester and phospholipid
may remain attached to the peptide until the final catabolism of
individual lipoprotein molecules. This, however, remains an assumption in the human. Labeling procedures, using radioiodine sub-
stitution of hydrogen in the tyrosine aromatic ring is more difficult
than in the case of proteins such as albumin. This is not the place
to discuss the technicalities of protein labeling; we have described
our methods in three recent papers (Scott and White et al., 1970;
Hurley and Scott, 1970; Scott and Hurley, 1970).

The general techniques for plasma lipoprotein turnover study are
outlined in the papers describing our methods. Standard plasma protein turnover techniques are used and a number of methods of multi-
compartmental analyses are available for analysis of the plasma decay
curves obtained following the injection intravenously of radioiodinated lipoprotein. Our group has used the multi-compartmental
method of Matthews (Matthews, 1957).

The classical plasma decay curves following an injection of a
protein such as radioiodinated human serum albumin follows a biphasic
pattern in time. Using a semi-logarithmic plot, an initial curving
decline in radioactivity of plasma is followed by a rectilinear
phase of decay. In the case of lipoprotein studies, there are relatively few published reports showing plasma decay curves. If these
are studied carefully, a true rectilinear phase of decline in plasma
radioactivity does not occur in short term studies (FIG. 6). In
our own work we have found that this phase is not entered until the
third week following injection of labeled low-density lipoprotein.
There are difficulties in preparing satisfactory labeled low-density
lipoproteins of sufficient quality to permit studies beyond the three
week stage, and this factor has limited observations of the type we
are describing. However, it is of fundamental importance to our
understanding of low-density lipoprotein metabolism to know how long
it takes for intravenously injected, labeled low-density lipoprotein
to equilibrate with the various exchangeable pools within the body.
Moreover, Nestel's group in Australia (Nestel and Hirsch et al.,
1965), have shown in studies of cholesterol-ester metabolism that
it takes over three weeks to achieve equilibration for this component of low-density lipoprotein. It is of some considerable
interest that the form of our long-term low-density lipoprotein
study decay curves is almost identical to that of cholesterol ester
studies. This raises the possibility that the peptide component of
low-density lipoprotein and at least some cholesterol ester may

establish equilibration with some extravascular exchangeable pools
over similar time courses.

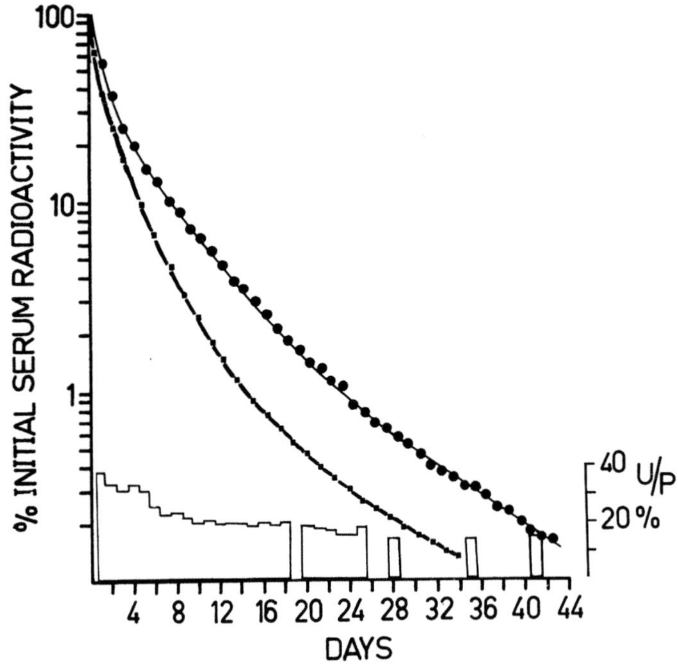

FIGURE 6. Decay curves following intravenous injection of radioiodinated low-density lipoprotein (S_f 3-9) into a 36-year-old normal
man (upper curve) and into a 64-year-old woman in coma (lower curve)
24 hour urine/mean plasma radioactivity ratio are plotted as per-
centages and recorded as block histograms corresponding to successive
24 hour collection periods plotted on the abscissa. Serum radioactivity showed a more rapid decline in the woman in coma, but the
general form of the decay curve is similar and an exponential phase
of decline in serum radioactivity was not entered until three weeks
had elapsed from the time of the intravenous injection of the radioiodinated lipoprotein.

By applying multi-compartmental analysis to our decay curves we
have concluded that the extravascular exchangeable lipoprotein pools
may be grouped into two categories, one group showing fairly rapid
equilibration, and the other a much slower time course for establishing
exchange equilibrium with the plasma compartment (Hurley and Scott,
1970). Our results suggest that about half of the total exchangeable pool of S_f 3-9 low-density lipoprotein lies outside the plasma
and that approximately equal amounts are distributed in the slowly
and rapidly exchanging groups of compartments respectively. The
possibility thus arises that plasma lipoprotein exchanges at different

rates with different tissues; the results also imply that S_f 3-9 low-density lipoprotein leaves the plasma compartment and may return to it without undergoing irreversible catabolism. Thus, the question remains open as to whether or not some lipid components reach extravascular tissues in the form of intact lipoprotein molecules.

We have investigated these possibilities further by recovering tissues from patients following injection of radioactively labeled low-density lipoprotein. For obvious reasons, one cannot undertake a series of biopsies from one particular person, and our results, therefore, represent a combination of information obtained by comparing tissue radioactivities from different patients at progressively increasing intervals between injection, and recovery of tissue specimens. Although we plan to carry out work of this type using surgical specimens, our data so far have been obtained from autopsy material. Details of this work have been published (Hurley and Scott, 1970; Scott and Hurley, 1970). FIGURE 7 shows results for liver and skin. The ordinate records tissue radioactivity per gram, expressed as a percentage of plasma radioactivity per ml at the time of death of the patient. The abscissa records the interval between injection of radioiodinated S_f 3-9 low-density lipoprotein and death of the patient. A wide scatter of results would be expected from work of this type, and the results can only be regarded as qualitative. Although showing a wide scatter, the results for liver suggest that equilibration is fairly rapidly achieved between the plasma compartment and lipid tissue. On the other hand, skin samples showed a rising ratio of tissue to radioactivity indicating that equilibrium had not been established for at least two weeks.

Similar results were obtained from the inner part of the artery wall. For these purposes, because tissue radioactivity levels were low, we were forced to study intima and the inner third of media together, and compare radioactivity from these combined tissues with that of the outer two thirds of the media (FIG. 8). As with skin, inner aortic wall (and inner coronary artery wall) may not equilibrate with plasma over the first 16 days following injection of labeled lipoprotein. FIGURES 7 and 8 comprise a combination of published and unpublished data. In two patients we have succeeded in obtaining satisfactory tissue counts at periods beyond 18 days from the injection of lipoprotein. The results of these two studies suggest that aorta and skin may eventually establish equilibrium with plasma in terms of the ratio of radioactivity derived from injected lipoprotein peptide. Our evidence that these observations on radioactivity have some meaning in relation to intact lipoprotein molecules, has already been published (Hurley and Scott, 1970; Scott and Hurley, 1970).

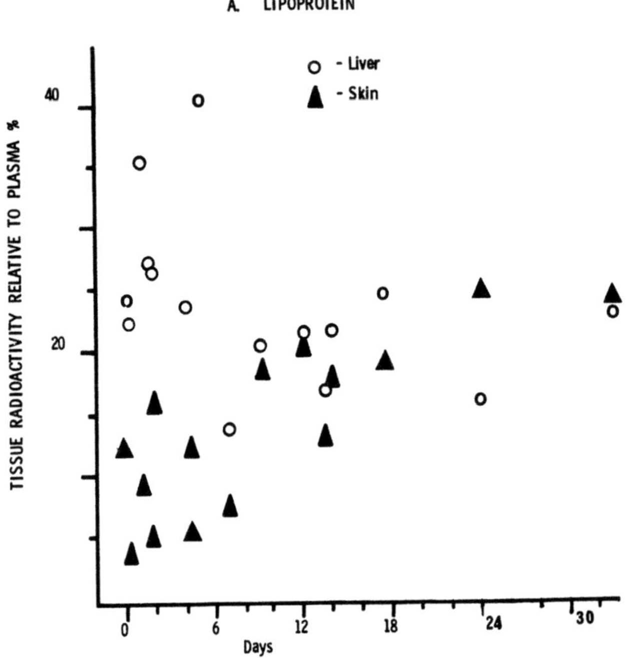

FIGURE 7. Radioactivity in samples of liver and skin relative to
plasma at increasing intervals of time after injection of radioiodinated S_f 3-9 low-density lipoprotein. The ordinate expresses
counts per gram of tissue as a percentage of the plasma count per
ml at the time of death. The interval between injection of radioiodinated low-density lipoprotein and death of a particular patient
is recorded in days along the abscissa. Each vertically placed pair
of results is thus derived from a different subject. The results
suggest a progressive rise in tissue radioactivity relative to
plasma for skin as the interval between injection and sampling of
tissues increases, whereas liver radioactivity relative to plasma
shows relatively constant ratios from about two-three days after
injection onwards.

As we have said, we regard our techniques as relatively crude
and our results as qualitative. However, we do consider that this
type of experiment can be extended considerably. For instance,
we have evidence that S_f0-20 (basically S_f 3-9) lipoprotein may
become incorporated within thrombi in the venous and arterial cir-
culations. Much higher concentrations of radioactivity will be
required to obtain histological evidence concerning the exact behavior of radioiodinated lipoprotein as it moves from the circulation
into blood vessel walls. In human studies it is not possible to
administer isotope in doses sufficient to obtain autoradiography.

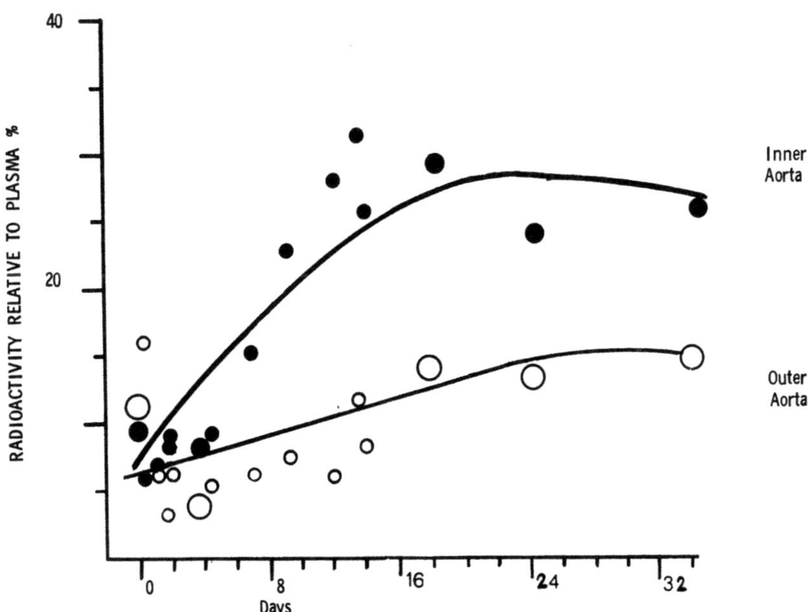

FIGURE 8. Tissue radioactivities relative to plasma for inner versus outer aorta plotted as for FIGURE 7. The solid circles show results for intima plus inner one-third of the media, and the open circles plot results for the outer two-thirds of the media. The lines are drawn free-hand to indicate suggested trends in alteration of tissue to plasma radioactivity ratios. These ratios were similar for the first few days following injection but thereafter the relative radioactivity in inner aortic tissue was higher than for the outer aorta. The results suggest that equilibrium does become established between aortic tissues and plasma during the third week following injection of radioiodinated S_f 3-9 low-density lipoprotein.

Professor Adams and his group have already undertaken work of this type but their studies have been of short duration. Had we limited our studies to only 4 days, we would not have observed the differences in behavior of skin and inner arterial wall on the one hand, and muscle and liver on the other. Like Professor Adams, we propose to study this phenomenon further in animals, and to compare the result of our animal experiments to human studies. In preliminary experiments on rabbit inner aorta, we found low tissue-to-plasma radioactivity ratios of between 1 and 2% six days after injection, as would be predicted from the results of Okisho (Okisho, 1961). We propose to use piglets in our future experiments.

It is of some interest that lipoprotein turnover studies have
also drawn attention to basic differences in metabolism of lipoprotein peptide compared with, e.g., albumin. With the exception
of thyroid disease (Walton and Scott et al., 1965), low-density
lipoprotein peptide metabolism follows a pattern similar to that
of IgM and fibrinogen in that the fractional catabolic rate for
the peptide appears to be relatively fixed. This leads to a situation where over-production is not compensated by a balanced increase
in catabolic rate. At present we do not know whether catabolic rate
determines the synthesis rate, or vice versa, but further studies
of this type may throw considerable light on the mechanisms underlying the various hyperlipoproteinemias (Langer and Strober et al.,
1969).

In summary, we wish to draw attention to a type of experimental
approach which may provide some answers to the source of lipids
in arterial intima. Studies of this type may provide evidence supporting both primary filtration and "encrustation" theories.

DR. ADAMS: With respect to Dr. Smith's question whether diffuse
extracellular intimal cholesterol ester accumulation is a matter of
age or thickening we have some data on human arteries taken at necropsy. Medial enzyme activity was studied in relation to lipid accumulation by means of the NADH-tetrazolium reductase - Van Gieson
histoenzymic method and ATPase - oil red O (Adams and Bayliss, 1969).
FIGURE 9 (A through D) illustrates that medial enzyme failure is
related to the degree of intimal thickening. The accumulation of
lipid, especially free and esterified cholesterol appeared subsequent
to the medial enzyme defects suggesting that intimal thickening may
partially block the diffusion of nourishment for the middle and inner
zones of the intima.

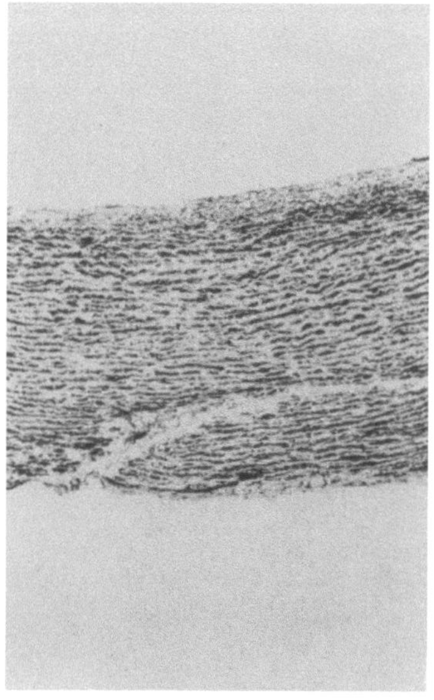

FIGURE 9 A. Aorta from a boy of 7 years to show intact medial muscle
fibers. NADH-tetrazolium reductase, x 49.
(Adams and Bayliss, 1969)

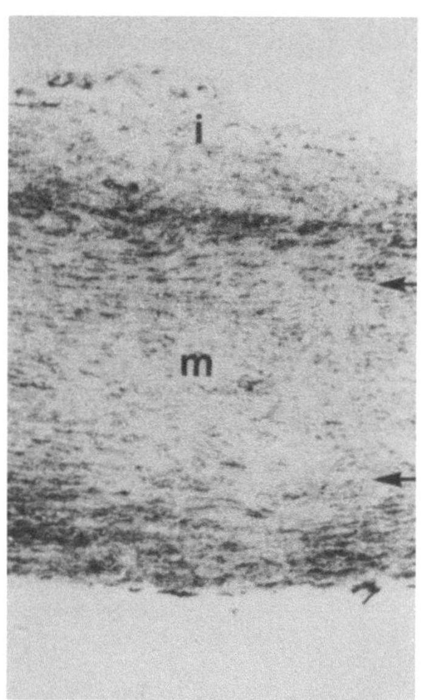

FIGURE 9 B. Aorta from a man of 27 years to show diffuse intimal
thickening (i) and mid-medial enzyme loss (m; arrows). Padykula-
Herman ATPase, x 49. (Adams and Bayliss, 1969)

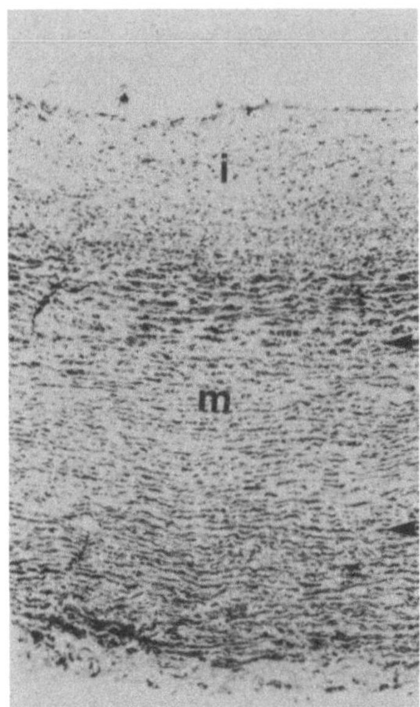

FIGURE 9 C.   Aorta from a woman of 41 years to show diffuse intimal
thickening (i) and mid-medial enzyme loss (m; arrows) NADH-tetrazolium reductase, x 49.   (Adams and Bayliss, 1969)

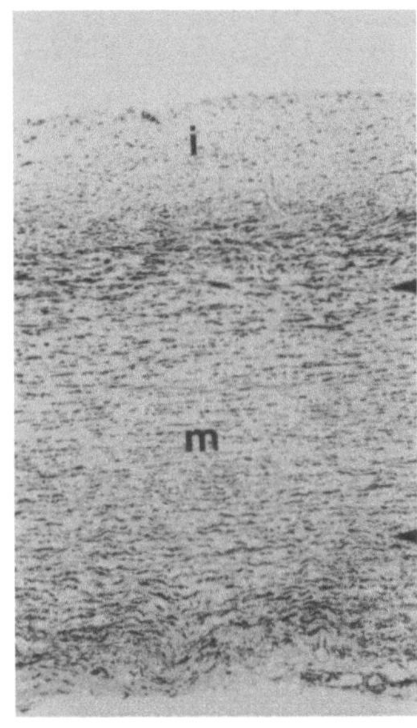

FIGURE 9 D.   As for FIG. 9 C but in a man of 50 years.
(Adams and Bayliss, 1969)

Chapter 4

LIPID TRANSPORT IN THE NORMAL AND ATHEROMATOUS

WALL OF EXPERIMENTAL ANIMALS

PARTICIPANTS: C.W.M. Adams, P. Alaupovic, G.V.R. Born, D.E. Bowyer,
P. Constantinides, A.J. Day, J. French, M. Friedman,
A.N. Howard, H.B. Lofland, K. Matthes, R.M. O'Neal,
A.L. Robertson, D.D. Rutstein, C.J. Schwartz, P.J.
Scott, E.B. Smith, Y. Stein, N.T. Werthessen and
R.W. Wissler

CHAIRMAN WERTHESSEN: May I ask Dr. Smith if there is a normal
accumulation of sterol esters in the arteries of animals that develop
spontaneous atherosclerosis that differs from those that do not, such
as the cow and the rabbit?

DR. SMITH: I do not know of any adequate published studies on
the chemical analysis of the lipids of normal intima from a range of
different animals. On a histological
Species differences   basis, fine extracellular lipid droplets, which may correspond to the
perifibrous lipid in aging normal human intima, have been described
in a number of species including baboons (McGill and Strong, et al.,
1960) ostriches, pigs, sheep and cows.

However, I doubt if it is valid to compare the intima of small
laboratory mammals, where the endothelium virtually sits direct on
the internal elastic lamina, with that of larger species in which
there is a sub-endothelial fibromuscular layer. It seems probable
that an age-related accumulation of plasma lipid could only occur in
the latter type of structure.

DR. ROBERTSON: I would like to comment on species differences
and the ability of their arterial cells to incorporate serum lipids.
Some time ago, we have compared in our laboratory, rates of incorporation of serum cholesterol fractions by vascular intimal cells
growing as monolayer cultures after their isolation from histologically normal arterial segments of several laboratory animals including rats, mice, rabbits, dogs, chickens, pigs and primates. As shown
on TABLE I, highest uptake levels expressed as dpm/mg wet weight were
found in microsomal/cell sap fractions of intimal cells obtained from
human, baboon and squirrel monkey arteries. All other species showed
considerably lower cholesterol uptake rates, the pig being a notable
exception to this rule. From these results we are tempted to speculate that these cytological differences may be a reflection of the
known increased susceptibility of some primates and swine to spontaneous or experimental arterial lesions. To find what factor or factors regulate sterol uptake at cell level in the less susceptible
species is of great potential therapeutical significance.

TABLE I

SPECIES DIFFERENCES ON INCORPORATION OF SERUM β-LIPOPROTEINS

BY NORMAL AORTIC INTIMACYTES IN ORGAN CULTURE

Average net DPM/μg wet weight cell sap fractions
24 Cultures Each

	1	3	5	7 HOURS
Chick	8–12	14–16	12–14	13–18
Rabbit	12–16	11–18	12–16	14–22
Dog	10–18	12–21	14–24	21–26
Swine	16–22	48–79	64–108	72–128
Baboon	14–26	104–128	146–179	158–184
Human	12–24	179–229	224–264	238–384

COMMENT

Continuing discussion emphasized the difficulty of transferring
data from one animal species to another and ultimately to man. There
was also the problem of the clinical signficance of some of the more
highly artificial experimental procedures, including the feeding of
unaccustomed diets to animals, and other more or less sudden and dras-
tic challenges to adaptive mechanisms. The main focus of concern was
the mechanism whereby lipid may accumulate in the arterial wall under
normal and pathological circumstances.

Most of the data indicated that the incorporation of lipid into the arterial wall is an active process and that whatever passive movement takes place is at least supplemented by a process of selective active transport. However, the transition from normal process in the arterial wall to atheroma remains obscure, and efforts to identify the form in which lipids are incorporated, and the degree to which they are altered within the wall have been inconclusive.

DR. DAY: I would like to raise the question of the role of active processes in the arterial wall with regard to the filtration of lipid. The filtration theory as originally envisaged implied that the arterial wall was simply a passive filter through which lipoprotein or other lipid particles could pass to a variable degree dependent on some physical entry or trapping mechanism. Newman and Zilversmit, (Newman and Zilversmit, 1962 and 1966) however, have demonstrated that the uptake of lipoprotein-free cholesterol by the atherosclerotic arterial wall is greater than that of lipoprotein-ester cholesterol and suggested that active trapping processes may be involved. These experiments, however, are open to the alternative interpretation that the greater uptake of labeled lipoprotein-free cholesterol may be explained in terms of physico-chemical exchange (Dayton and Hashimoto, 1966). I would like, therefore, to refer to some work that we have recently carried out in which we have investigated the passage of individual cholesterol esters from the serum of cholesterol-fed rabbits into the atherosclerotic arterial wall (Day and Wahlqvist, et al., 1970a). These experiments were carried **RABBIT** out in order to compare the relative entry rates of saturated, monounsaturated and polyunsaturated cholesterol esters into the atherosclerotic arterial intima and media. A single dose of ^{3}H-labeled cholesterol was given by mouth to cholesterol-fed rabbits. The free cholesterol was, of course, esterified in part in its passage through the intestinal wall and appears in the serum, therefore, as both ^{3}H-labeled free and ester cholesterol in the lipoprotein. Over the subsequent four days the free cholesterol and cholesterol ester specific activity rises to a maximum at 1-2 days and then falls (FIG. 1). As well as total cholesterol esters we also measured the specific activity of the individual groups of cholesterol esters - saturated, monounsaturated and polyunsaturated in the plasma over the four day period, so that we had some indication of the background to which the arterial wall was exposed over this time (FIG. 2). The animals were killed at the end of the four day period and the arterial wall was examined with respect to its labeled free cholesterol and ester cholesterol and also with respect to the labeled saturated, monounsaturated and polyunsaturated cholesterol esters that had entered during the four day experimental period.

Active lipid transport into arterial wall

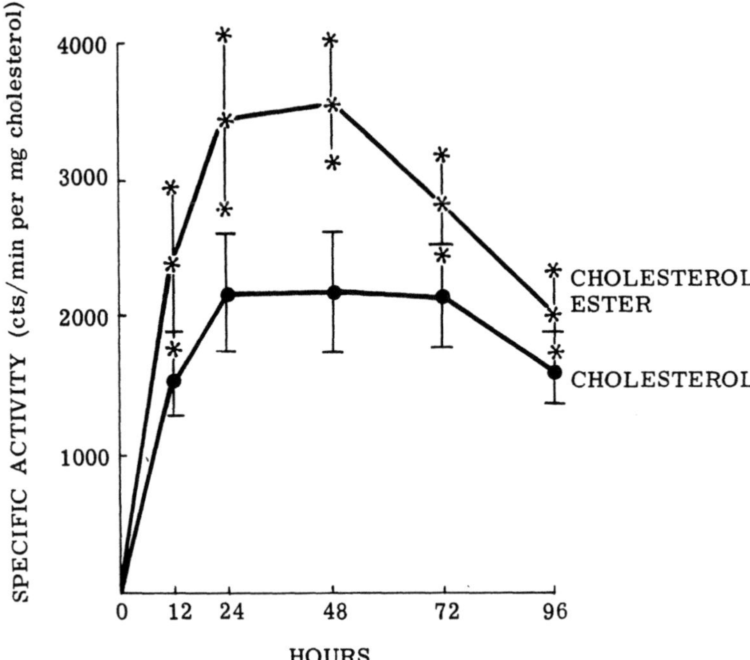

FIGURE 1. Specific activities of serum free and ester cholesterol following ingestion of ^{3}H-labeled cholesterol. Means of six experiments and standard errors of means are plotted.
(Day and Wahlqvist, et al., 1970a)

The cholesterol esters were separated into groups by argentation chromatography. In this way it was possible to separate both the serum cholesterol esters and the arterial wall cholesterol esters into three groups as indicated. They were not further identified. We used the specific activity measurements for the free cholesterol, cholesterol ester and for the three groups of cholesterol esters in the serum to derive a median specific activity in the serum over the four day period. By using this figure together with the amount of label in the arterial wall in the respective lipid groups, we were able to calculate the amount of these components (μmoles/hr) that had passed into the arterial wall. In agreement with the observations of other workers we found that the relative entry of free cholesterol exceeded that of ester cholesterol (TABLE II). However, this point is subject to difficulty in interpretation, as I have mentioned, because of the exchange of the serum lipoprotein-free cholesterol with the cholesterol in the arterial wall. Ester cholesterol, on the other hand, does not exchange and therefore differences in relative entry of the different groups of cholesterol esters can be considered in connection with the possibility of active entry. We found that the relative entry of monounsaturated cholesterol ester exceeded that of

saturated and polyunsaturated cholesterol ester. These data may be
taken to indicate differential entry presumably due to more active
filtration processes.

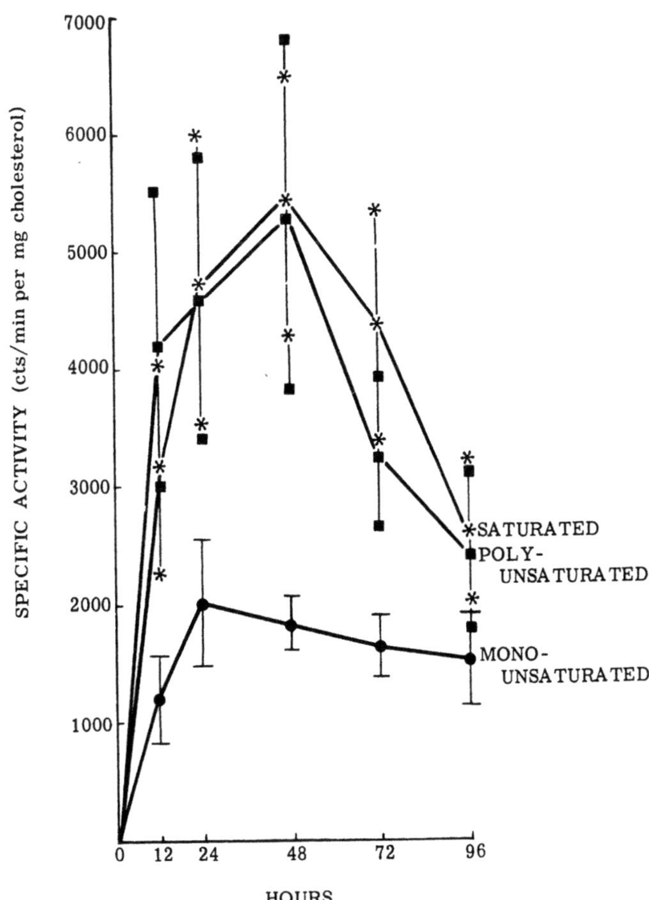

FIGURE 2. Specific activities of saturated, monounsaturated, and
polyunsaturated cholesterol esters in the serum following ingestion
of ^{3}H-labeled cholesterol. Means of four experiments and standard
errors of the means are plotted.
(Day and Wahlqvist et al., 1970a)

QUESTION: The cholesterol esters couldn't have been esterified
again?

DR. DAY: No, this possibility was specifically excluded in the
work I have described. I won't go into detail on this point, but
there was no significant esterification of the cholesterol demonstrable.

TABLE II

INFLUX OF LIPOPROTEIN [^{3}H] CHOLESTEROL AND CHOLESTEROL ESTERS
INTO CHOLESTEROL-FED RABBIT INTIMAL HALVES IN VIVO

	Influx		
	µg/day	µg/day per mg/ml	relative influx[c]
Free cholesterol[a]	179.1 ± 46.3	34.1 ± 6.8	1
Cholesterol ester[a]	224.8 ± 76.2	18.5 ± 4.2	0.54 ± 0.02[d]
Cholesterol ester[b]			
saturated	33.0 ± 5.1	15.4 ± 3.1	0.78 ± 0.11[e]
monounsaturated	108.0 ± 4.4	20.1 ± 3.8	1
polyunsaturated	30.6 ± 5.1	14.0 ± 4.5	0.68 ± 0.06[f]

[a] Means and standard errors of means of 6 experiments.

[b] Means and standard errors of means of 4 experiments.

[c] Relative influx is the ratio of the influx per mg/ml of serum cholesterol and cholesterol ester with respect to free cholesterol; or of the individual cholesterol esters with respect to monounsaturated cholesterol ester.

[d] Significant at < 0.1% level.

[e] No significant difference.

[f] Significant at < 2% level.

DR. STEIN: How extensive were the lesions you observed?

DR. DAY: The rabbits used were cholesterol fed from four to
five months so that the arterial intima investigated contained fairly
extensive lesions with the surface almost completely covered with
atheroma. We made no attempt to separate normal from atherosclerotic
intima.

QUESTION: What about the normal intima?

DR. DAY: We have no information regarding the relative entry
of individual groups of cholesterol esters in the normal intima.
There are, of course, other data available regarding the entry of
free and ester cholesterol, as a whole, which indicates that the
levels of entry of both free and ester cholesterol are much lower in
the normal intima than in the atherosclerotic intima. We have, however, in the present work sought to compare in the atherosclerotic
situation the entry of individual cholesterol esters. It would
certainly be of interest to make these observations in normal intima
and in intima with differing degrees of atherosclerotic involvement.

DR. LOFLAND: In experiments involving autoradiographic examination of plaques in rabbits after the ingestion of radioactively
labeled cholesterol we found that in all cases the cholesterol was

not deposited along the surface but, surprisingly enough, was deep
within the plaque and apparently associated with the area where there
was the most crystalline cholesterol. So, in our eyes at least, cholesterol does go into the arterial wall and into the relatively deep
layers.

QUESTION: How do we know whether cholesterol is going in or
just exchanging?

CHAIRMAN WERTHESSEN: The label was on the original cholesterol,
if I understand Dr. Day properly.

DR. DAY: That's right. We used ring-labeled cholesterol so that
the cholesterol remained labeled whether it was present as ester or
free cholesterol. However, as I have pointed out earlier, the data
with regard to the labeled cholesterol ester, I feel, is much more
valid than data with respect to free cholesterol, as it is less likely
that the labeled cholesterol ester will be exchanged by physico-chemical processes. For instance, if you incubate serum in which the
lipoprotein is labeled with free cholesterol, this free cholesterol
can be readily exchanged with added red cells. Ester cholesterol does
not exchange under these circumstances. I think the experiments,
therefore, using labeled cholesterol ester are much more valid than
are the experiments using free cholesterol.

DR. SMITH: I cannot agree that this is a valid argument because
there is no cholesterol ester in red cells.

DR. SCHWARTZ: As I see it one has the problem of specific activity in both the donor serum and in the recipient, the vessel wall.
The question of specific activity in the arterial wall and its importance presents some complex problems, and I would like to ask
Dr. Day to comment on this, particularly as we cannot make the assumption that the cholesterol in the donor or in the recipient is
necessarily all exchangeable or readily exchangeable. How can one
determine the size of the exchangeable pools in both donor and recipient, and is not the exchangeable cholesterol pool more relevant
than the total unesterified cholesterol pool in determining specific
activities?

DR. SMITH: I may have misunderstood. Were you actually putting
in cholesterol ester, or were you putting in whole labeled lipoprotein?

DR. DAY: If I could answer Dr. Schwartz' question first. I
agree that the question of specific activity in the arterial wall is
important. However, the data we present was concerned with the total
entry of cholesterol ester into the arterial wall and we used the
counts in the arterial wall in relation to the specific activity in
the serum to derive a figure for μmoles of cholesterol ester in the
three groups that were entering. With regard to pool size we do have

some information regarding the cholesterol pools in the arterial wall
and their relative turnover. We carried out experiments in which
atherosclerotic intima was labelled with cholesterol and cholesterol
ester in the way I have already indicated and then this intima was
removed and incubated in vitro and the efflux of cholesterol studied
in relation to time, both into an incubation medium containing Hank's
solution alone and one containing Hank's solution and serum (FIG. 3).

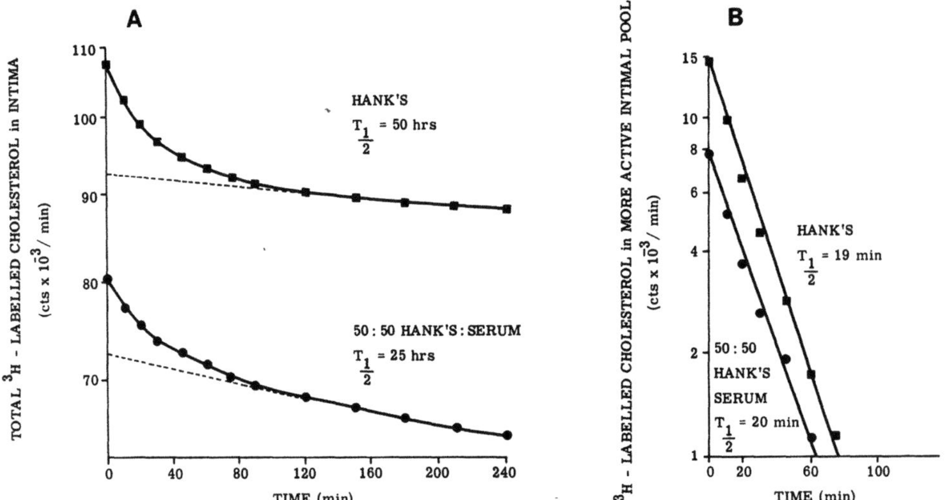

FIGURE 3. Efflux of ^{3}H-labeled cholesterol from atherosclerotic
intimal halves into either an incubation medium of Hank's solution
or 50:50 Hank's:hypercholesterolemic serum. Counts/min remaining in
the intima are plotted logarithmically in both A and B. Curves in A
have been resolved into two components. The more slowly removed
component (dotted line) has been subtracted from the composite curves
to yield a plot of the more rapidly removed component in B.
(Day and Wahlqvist et al., 1970a)

In this experiment it was possible to distinguish two pools of
intimal cholesterol, a rapidly exchanging pool which accounted for
the initial removal and having a half-life of 19-20 minutes when
either Hank's solution or serum were used. This may, in fact, be
a surface pool, as has been suggested by Dr. Stein earlier. There
is, however, a less readily exchangeable pool with a half-life of
approximately 25 hours when the incubation medium was Hank's solution
containing serum, but with a much longer half-life when Hank's solution alone was used.

With regard to Dr. Smith's question about the form in which the
labeled cholesterol ester was present in the original experiments,
we gave free cholesterol by ingestion and this was then esterified
in the intestinal wall and appeared in the plasma as labeled lipoprotein. We did check this by ultracentrifugation and it was pos-

sible to show that the bulk of the ^{3}H-labeled cholesterol was in the
very low density lipoprotein. Hypercholesterolemic rabbit serum contains most of the cholesterol and cholesterol ester in the very low
density lipoprotein. We can be confident, therefore, that both the
free and ester cholesterol was present in the lipoprotein.

DR. SMITH: I still don't understand how you know that it was
ester cholesterol going in and not free cholesterol that went in and
was esterified. Esterification has been shown to occur very rapidly.

DR. DAY: We specifically excluded this possibility by performing
a further series of experiments in vitro, in which we used cholesterol
labeled with ^{14}C in the free cholesterol and with ^{3}H in the cholesterol
ester. If you incubate lipoprotein with ^{14}C-labeled cholesterol in
vitro free cholesterol is readily incorporated into the lipoprotein.
If such lipoprotein labeled with only free cholesterol is then incubated with the artery wall, there is no conversion to cholesterol
ester. We were fairly confident, therefore, that we were not getting
esterification of the free cholesterol accounting for the apparent
entry of labeled cholesterol ester.

COMMENT FROM DR. SMITH: In retrospect, I still find these results
odd; Day himself has demonstrated extensive incorporation of labeled
fatty acid into cholesterol esters both in whole intima and in isolated
foam cells (Day, 1967; Day and Tume, 1970). Why, then, is there no
esterification in this system? If the conditions are not physiological, or there is no free fatty acid available this does not provide
a control for the in vivo part of the experiment. It is possible,
however, that this is telling us either that the incorporation observed previously was only turnover of prexisting ester, and did not
include de novo synthesis or that only cholesterol in certain sites
is available for esterification. Since the meeting this latter idea
has received strong support from the work of Lofland (St. Clair and
Lofland et al., 1970).

CHAIRMAN WERTHESSEN: I believe then from your work Dr. Day, that
you would like to conclude that if the filtration theory operates there
is a modicum of selectivity about it. And the comment is that the
panel would not disagree with that statement.

DR. FRENCH: Just for clarification in my own mind, I wonder if
I might ask Dr. Day if he is prepared to say where this selection is
taking place. Is this at the endothelial cell surface, or is it by
selection from components that enter the wall by the conventional
filtration theory? Is this something selected at the endothelial
surface? This is a metabolic process. Is it now introduced as a
modification of the filtration theory as far as cholesterol and its
esters are concerned? Is that what you're saying?

DR. DAY: I don't think I can speculate, as Dr. French wants me
to, in this regard. All I am suggesting is that there are changes
in the entry pattern. I don't think we have any data to suggest where
this occurs or by what mechanism. Presumably there is some active
trapping. However, the whole question of lipoprotein entry has not
been resolved and I am sure there will be further discussion later
in this regard.

DR. ALAUPOVIC: If cholesterol ester was soluble in this solution
it meant that it was part of a lipoprotein molecule.

CHAIRMAN WERTHESSEN: Which would mean therefore that the movement from the tissue into the pure Hank's solution would require that
the cholesterol be solubilized by a lipoprotein. Is that what you
were saying Dr. Alaupovic?

DR. ALAUPOVIC: Dr. Day does actually have the data showing that
the protein was present.

QUESTION: Did Dr. Day have any protein at all in the Hank's,
because it was just the protein itself, not the lipoprotein, that
could effectively serve as the receptacle for the cholesterol.

CHAIRMAN WERTHESSEN: Well, he did in the preparation where there
was serum added and it was obvious that the rates were faster.

DR. ADAMS: Could I raise a slightly different issue that perhaps
Dr. Day and Dr. Smith have commented on, namely, the exchangeability
of tritium labeled cholesterol with cholesterol already present in the
arterial wall. I do not think it is quite as simple as the biochemists
think. No doubt membrane cholesterol
and lipoprotein cholesterol exchange,
but I doubt if tritium cholesterol exchanges with large deposits of cho-
lesterol in the arterial wall. I have not got a slide here, but I
have an autoradiograph back in London which shows no labeling by tritium cholesterol over deposits of cholesterol crystals. In an atheromatous vessel I think there are three equilibria: cholesterol in the
plasma, cholesterol as lipoprotein in the arterial wall, and cholesterol that has been deposited in the arterial wall. I think the cholesterol that has been deposited in atheroma is not nearly so exchangeable as perhaps some people think. Even with this simple analysis,
there seems to be at least 3 clear-cut pools for cholesterol from
plasma to the arterial wall.

DR. Y. STEIN: I would like to comment on the point Dr. Adams
brought up, namely the exchangeability of cholesterol in the atheromatous aorta. We have attempted to study this problem by subcellular
fractionation in which rabbit aortic homogenates were separated by
ultracentrifugation into three fractions: a pellet, which consisted

RABBIT

Problems of
exchangeability

of cell membranes, nuclei, collagen and elastin, a supernatant and
a top fraction, which in the normal aorta consisted of a thin fatty
layer (Eisenberg and Rachmilewitz et al., 1970). The distribution
of cholesterol and phospholipids among the fractions is shown in
FIG. 4, and it can be seen that cholesterol feeding results in a

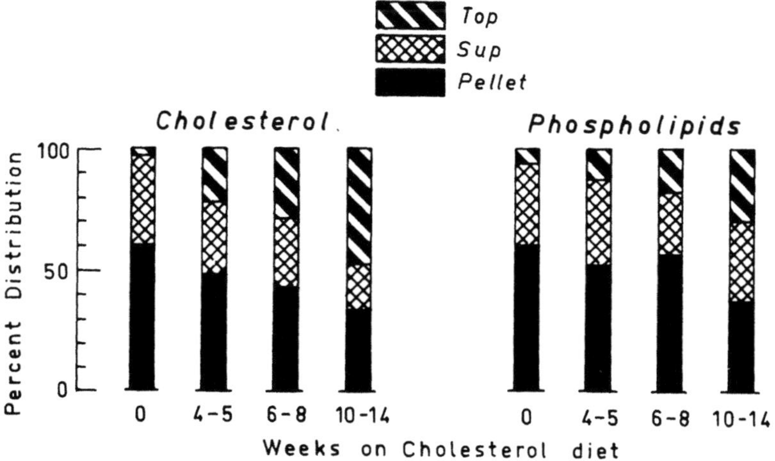

FIGURE 4. Distribution of cholesterol and phospholipids in fractions
of aortic homogenates of normal and cholesterol fed rabbits.

rapid enrichment of the top fraction in cholesterol and a somewhat
slower enrichment in phospholipids. In order to learn whether by
separation of the cholesterol and phospholipids into the three fractions one may detect the presence of different metabolic pools, aortic
lecithin was labeled by incubation with ^{3}H-choline and aortic cholesterol by incubation with rabbit serum containing ^{3}H-cholesterol.
FIG. 5 shows the ratio of specific activity of lecithin in the various
fractions, taking that of the pellet as 1.0. It can be seen that in
the normal aorta and even up to 4 weeks of cholesterol feeding the
lecithin of the pellet and supernatant have a similar specific activity. However, at later time intervals the specific activity of the
supernatant and especially of the top fraction is much lower than
that of the pellet. The same is true also when the specific activity
of free cholesterol in the pellet is compared to the top fraction
(FIG. 6). These findings indicate that in the atheromatous aorta of

rabbits the cholesterol is situated in more than one pool and that
the exchangeability of the cholesterol among these pools is not very
rapid.

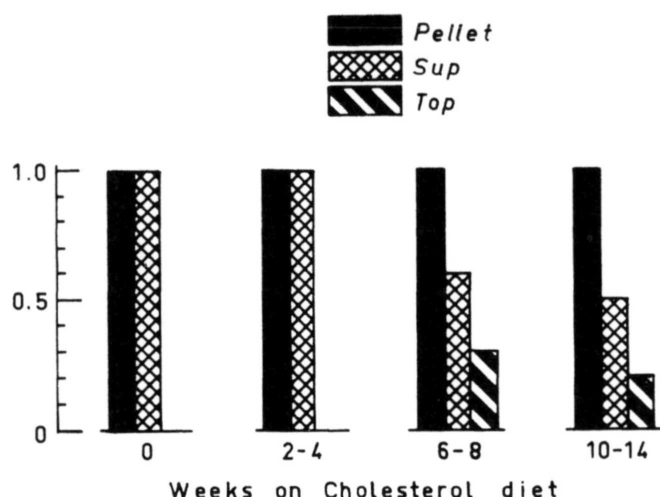

FIGURE 5. Specific activity of ^{3}H-lecithin in fractions of aortic
homogenates of normal and cholesterol fed rabbits.

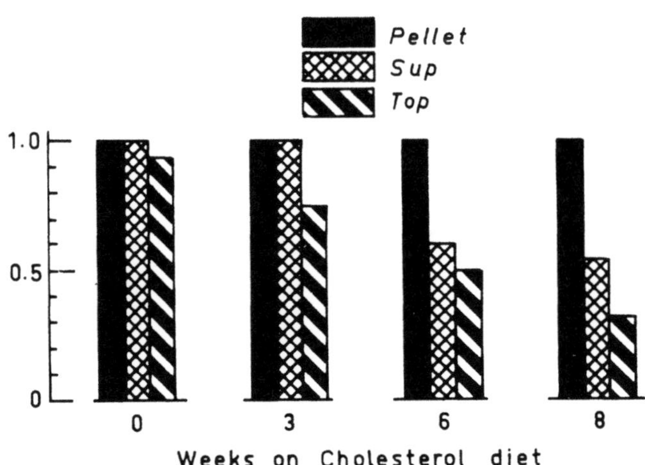

FIGURE 6. Specific activity of ^{3}H-cholesterol in fractions of aortic
homogenates of normal and cholesterol fed rabbits.

DR. HOWARD: Dr. Smith mentioned lipolytic enzymes in the arterial wall. Much of the work on this has been done by workers in Eastern Europe. In FIGURE 7, one can visualize that lipoproteins are entering the vessel wall and there they meet the lipolytic enzymes so that some of the lipids are metabolized, particularly by the phospholipases and lipases (Howard, 1968). Here, of course, the substrates are broken down to form water soluble or easily transportable metabolites. However in the case of cholesterol esters the picture is somewhat different. Either free cholesterol or its esters remain in the arterial wall, and these are very immobile. From our **RAT** work in rats and rabbits it has been found that in atherosclerosis **RABBIT** the enzyme which breaks down cholesterol esters is decreased and there is a preferential synthesis of cholesterol esters (TABLE III). Now one wonders whether or not the lipolytic enzymes are in the wall for some special purpose, and why there is such a high level present. Is it in fact to protect the arterial wall against lipid accumulation of cholesterol esters? We find in our studies that there is

Activities of lipolytic enzymes

an increase in cholesterol ester in the rabbit atherosclerotic lesion as there is in man (Patelski and Bowyer et al., 1968).

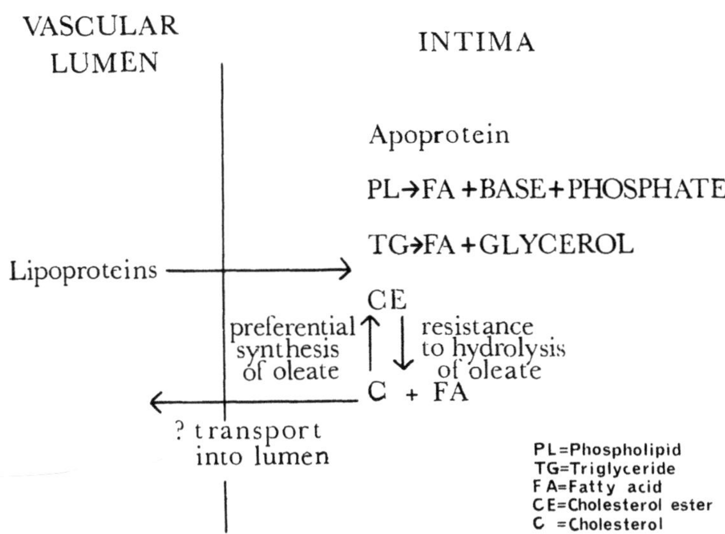

FIGURE 7. Metabolism of lipids in the arterial wall.

TABLE III

ESTERASE ACTIVITIES OF THE AORTIC WALL

Dietary Group		Number of animals	Time on Diet	Phosphatide acyl-hydrolase	Glycerol-ester hydrolase	Cholesterol-ester hydrolase
			Wks.	$mU^{1)}$, % change		
Rat	Control diet	5	20	1068 $\pm$ 415	627 $\pm$ 143	276 $\pm$ 31
	40% Peanut oil	5	14	198%	460% r = 0.89	25% (p $\leqslant$ 0.05)
	40% Butter	5	10	100%	199%	100%
Rabbit	Control diet	5	20-30	180 $\pm$ 44	148 $\pm$ 31	116 $\pm$ 32
	Atherogenic semi-synthetic diet containing 20% beef tallow	5	10	49%	142%	45%
		5	32	59%	100%	20%

1) mU - milliunits of specific activity, Mean $\pm$ Standard Deviation

2) Experimental diets contained 5% cholesterol and 2% cholic acid

One of the ways in which one can investigate the importance of
the enzymes is by changing their activity and there is a novel way
in which one can do this. Schrade and Bohle (Schrade and Bohle et
al., 1961) showed several years ago that the soya bean lecithin has
the peculiar property of stimulating lipase and clearing plasma containing chylomicrons. In our experiments (Patelski and Bowyer et
al., 1970) when soya bean lecithin is injected into the rabbit ear
vein the cholesterol esterase activity is normalized (TABLE IV).
The next question is what effect this has on the synthesis of esters.
^{14}C oleic acid was terfused in an atherosclerotic aorta in an animal injected with saline and there was an increase in colesterol
ester. When one gives the soya bean lecithin which normalizes the
lipolytic enzymes, one finds that this no longer occurs. So it may
be the case that the increased formation of cholesterol esters is
due to the decrease in lipolytic enzymes. Soya bean lecithin also
decreases the amount of aortic atherosclerosis and cholesterol deposition, but it is only a decrease and no complete protection
(TABLE VI).

It is interesting that the use of phospholipids in atherosclerosis research dates back to the work of Byers and Friedman (Byers
and Friedman, 1960), who found that the infusion of phospholipids
made the atherosclerotic lesions regress. It may be that the reason
for their remarkable results was the effect of phospholipids on lipolytic enzymes which we have seen demonstrated here.

TABLE IV

LIPOLYTIC ENZYMES IN AORTA OF RABBITS GIVEN AN
ATHEROGENIC SEMI-SYNTHETIC DIET

Diet	Time on diet (weeks)	Injection[a]	Number of Animals	Phospho-lipase A	Aortic lipase	Cholesterol esterase
Control	18	None	5	35 ± 4.1[b]	30 ± 2.4	24 ± 5.8
Atherogenic semi-	10	NaCl[1] 0.9%	5	41 ± 10.8	57 ± 12.8 (***)	6 ± 5.3 (****)
synthetic diet	10	Lipostabil[3]	5	42 ± 5.2	37 ± 11.4	18 ± 6.8
containing 20%	18	NaCl[2] 0.9%	5	48 ± 8.3 (*)	51 ± 16.4 (***)	8 ± 2.8 (****)
Beef tallow	18	Lipostabil[2]	5	34 ± 8.8	24 ± 6.9	19 ± 4.4

a (1)   Intraperitoneal injection of 1.0 ml six times a week.
  (2, 3)   Intravenous injections of (2) 0.5 ml and (3) 1 ml three times a week.

b Means ± standard deviations. The means were compared by Analysis of Variance. Where the values for means were different from control, the statistical significance is indicated by: (*) $P < 0.05$; (**) $P < 0.02$; (***) $P < 0.01$; (****) $P < 0.001$. The percentage changes of significantly altered means are tabulated. Glycerol-ester hydrolase and sterol-ester hydrolase were significantly negatively correlated, $r = -0.96$, $P < 0.01$.

TABLE V

THE INCORPORATION OF 1^{14}C OLEIC ACID INTO AORTIC LIPIDS

Diet	Time in diet weeks	Injection[a]	Number of Animals	Incorporation of 1^{14}C oleic acid μ μmoles/mg dry defatted tissue			
				PL	FFA	TG	CE[b]
Control	18	None	5	7.29 ± 4.46[c]	6.43 ± 3.15	4.70 ± 6.12	0.14 ± 0.06 100%
Atherogenic semi-synthetic diet containing 20% beef tallow	18	NaCl 0.9%	5	5.93 ± 0.79	6.14 ± 3.62	1.08 ± 0.53	0.46 ± 0.25 (+) 304%
	18	Lipostabil	5	11.22 ± 8.53	9.21 ± 6.35	2.24 ± 2.38	0.19 ± 0.27

a See TABLE IV

b PL = Phospholipids
 FFA = Free fatty acids
 TG = Triglycerides
 CE = Cholesterol esters

c Mean ± standard deviations. The means were compared by Student's t test. Where the means were different from control, the significance level is indicated by (+) $P < 0.05$; (++) $P < 0.02$; (+++) $P < 0.01$; (++++) $P < 0.001$.

TABLE **VI**

SEVERITY OF LESIONS AND LIPID COMPOSITION OF AORTAS

Diet	Time on diet weeks	Injec- tion[a]	Plasma Cholesterol mg%	Total No.of ani- mals	\multicolumn{4}{c}{Aortic Atherosclerosis No.of animals at each grade of lesion[b]}				\multicolumn{4}{c}{AORTA Phospholipids[c]}				Free Fatty acids	\multicolumn{2}{c}{Cholesterol}	
					0	1	2	3	PE	Lec	Sph	LL		Ester	Free
									\multicolumn{5}{c}{ng/mg protein}				
Control	18	None	114 ± 11.7	5	5	0	0	0	4.9 ± 1.56[d]	8.0 ± 3.20	5.9 ± 1.92	1.1 ± 1.26	4.6 ± 0.75	0.4 ± 0.26	2.4 ± 0.91
Atherogenic semi-synthetic diet containing 20% beef tallow	18	NaCl 0.9%	485 ± 217 (**)	5	0	2	1	2	5.6 ± 1.06	15.8 ± 6.90	7.2 ± 1.56	0.5 ± 0.38	4.1 ± 2.08	4.8 ± 1.33 (***)	6.6 ± 2.40 (***)
	18	Lipo- stabil	578 ± 139 (***)	5	0	3	2	0	5.9 ± 1.14	11.4 ± 3.60	8.1 ± 2.85	0.4 ± 0.11	3.7 ± 1.16	3.9 ± 2.41 (*)	5.6 ± 1.92 (*)

[a] For explanation, see TABLE V.

[b] Grade 0 = no lesions; grade 1 = 1%; grade 2 = 1-5%; grade 3 = 5% diseased aorta

[c] PE = Phosphatidyl ethanolamine
Lec = Lecithin
Sph = Sphingomyelin
LL = Lysolecithin

[d] Means ± standard deviations. The means were compared by Analysis of Variance. Where the values for means were different from control, the statistical significance is indicated by: (*) P < 0.05; (**) P < 0.02; (***) P < 0.01; (****) P < 0.001. The percentage changes of significantly altered means are tabulated. Glycerol-ester hydrolase and sterol-ester hydrolase were significantly negatively correlated, r = -0.96; P < 0.01.

DR. ADAMS: A point to consider is what effect cholesterol and
cholesterol esters have on tissues. Following subcutaneous implan-
tation of free cholesterol, there is a very substantial fibrotic reaction as can be seen in the Van Giesson stained sections. Not only
free sterol (cholesterol) but the more saturated cholesterol esters
do the same sort of thing. When one scores the amount of fibrosis
(sclerosis) around a subcutaneous lipid implant, the free sterol,
the more saturated and monounsaturated esters, have a high score.
However, the $\Delta 2$, $\Delta 3$ and $\Delta 4$ polyunsaturated cholesterol esters show
low scores and fibrosis is relatively slight. As regards tissue reaction, the polyunsaturated cholesterol esters are "good," whereas
the saturated esters and free sterol are "bad." Free cholesterol is
resorbed slowly (about 30% in 3 weeks). The saturated cholesterol
esters are also resorbed slowly, but
the really polyunsaturated (three
and four double bond) cholesterol
esters are absorbed much more rapidly.

Effect of exogenous
cholesterol on tissue

Now when Dr. Howard made the point at the Chicago congress that
free cholesterol may be the form in which sterols are removed from
atheromatous lipids, it occurred to me that it might be useful to
study what happens in a subcutaneous implant where one cholesterol
ester is radioactive and the other is cold. The implanted mixture
was three parts of cold cholesterol linoleate and one part of doubly labeled cholesterol linoleate (^{3}H-cholesterol-(1^{14}C)-linoleate.)
Without going into detail we have managed to extract extracellular
lipid with a very brief petroleum-ether wash. Intracellular lipids
are extracted with further washes of petroleum-ether and chloroform-
methanol. We have checked this histologically. The first wash re-
moves over 90% of total lipid; then there is about 5% or so of intracellular lipid that is extracted with the further extractions with
petroleum-ether and chloroform-methanol. If only free cholesterol
is taken up by foam cells, cholesterol esters would be hydrolyzed to
free cholesterol before being taken up by the cells. Reesterification
within the cell would result in randomization and the linoleate would
contain a hot sterol nucleus and vice versa. So you would expect 75%
randomization in the intracellular cholesterol esters. What we actually found is that the intracellular lipid was randomized only to the
extent of about 2%. This result implies that the cholesterol ester
had directly entered into these foam cells and had not been hydrolyzed
en route. This is evidence against Dr. Howard's view that cells can
only take up free cholesterol. I think possibly both free cholesterol
and polyunsaturated cholesterol esters can be taken up by cells.

DR. DAY: One of the objections to the work Professor Adams has
described is that the cholesterol and various cholesterol esters he
used were presented in an unphysiological form, so that uptake rates
may be related to differences in physical state rather than any more
fundamental difference. The question of relative removal of differ-

ent cholesterol esters from the arterial wall, however, is an important one and we have attempted to study this aspect by observing the
removal, from intimal lesions in cholesterol fed rabbits, of endogenous cholesterol esters labeled with different ^{14}C-labeled fatty
acids. Arteriosclerotic thoracic aortas from such animals were incubated in vitro with a mixture of ^{14}C-labeled palmitic, oleic and
linoleic acids (Day and Wahlqvist et al., 1970b). After an initial
2-hour incubation each of these fatty acids was incorporated into the
endogenous cholesterol esters as well as into the phospholipids and
triglycerides of the atherosclerotic intima. The aorta, so labeled,
was then incubated for a further 4-hours in non-labeled medium and
the specific activity of the labeled cholesterol esters, phospholipid
and triglyceride fractions followed for this period.

The reductions in specific activities of the triglyceride and
phospholipid groups were more rapid than those for the cholesterol
ester group. However, the specific activities of the ^{14}C-labeled
cholesterol palmitate, cholesterol oleate and cholesterol linoleate
were similar over the 4-hour incubation period. We would interpret
this data to indicate that, while cholesterol esters as a group are
removed more slowly from the atherosclerotic intima than either phospholipids or triglycerides, there is no difference in removal rate
of endogenously labeled cholesterol palmitate, oleate or linoleate
from the atherosclerotic intima.

CHAIRMAN WERTHESSEN: The question of movement of a sterol ester
across the cells of the intima is an important one. I believe we
were able to show in 1962 or 1963 that if you permitted a baboon to
synthesize cholesterol and fatty acids from acetate and then checked
the doubly labeled cholesterol esters in the plasma as compared to
those that were in the tissue, that you could only conclude that as
the ester went into the tissue it had to be split and then reorgan-
ized. I'd like to ask Dr. Lofland if he has any data which would
indicate that his normal intima can split the sterol esters, whereas
the lesion cannot. Do you have any information on that point? Because this would be an additional factor as regards the balance.

DR. LOFLAND: We have carried out a series of experiments using
atherosclerosis-susceptible White Carneau pigeons. We use these
particular pigeons because after cholesterol feeding, one finds, and
can excise from the same aorta, normal tissue, fatty streaks and
atherosclerotic plaques. So we have tried to measure the rates of
influx and efflux of ^{14}C-labeled cholesterol into these three different types of aorta preparations. We did this by feeding the birds
for relatively long periods of time, about 17 months, on a cholesterol-
containing diet. We then made diet radioactive with ^{14}C-labeled cholesterol for a period of 30 days in order to induce labeling of aortic
lipids, after which we removed the isotopic cholesterol from the diet
and observed the disappearance of the labeled cholesterol from aortas.

The concentration of cholesterol and especially cholesterol esters in atheromatous arterial tissue occurred during cholesterol feeding as Dr. Smith has pointed out, occurred in both fatty streaks and complicated plaques. There is an increase in free cholesterol, but more especially, an increase in cholesterol esters. This seems to be the hallmark of the disease in this and many other species. FIG. 8 shows the increase and decrease in cholesterol specific activity in the blood. The open circles represent our experimental data, the dotted lines with x's represent the theoretical curve which one should achieve by feeding a diet of this particular specific activity. As you see it increases, then declines in a linear fashion. We measured influx from the ascending portion

During the period of increasing radioactivity as well as the period of decreasing radioactivity we sacrificed subgroups of 8 birds each at weekly or biweekly intervals. In TABLE VII we show that the changes in analytical lipid composition which

TABLE VII

CONTENTS OF FREE CHOLESTEROL AND CHOLESTEROL ESTERS FROM

NORMAL ARTERY, FATTY STREAKS AND PLAQUES OF PIGEON AORTAS[a]

	Number of observations	Free cholesterol	Cholesteryl esters
Normal	66	2.2±0.08	0.84±0.05
Fatty streaks	67	5.1±0.34	2.30±0.23
Plaques	96	25.1±1.30	20.30±0.13

[a] Mean values in mg/g of wet tissue, followed by the standard errors of the means.
(Lofland and Clarkson, 1970)

of the curve at early intervals. Efflux was measured by calculating the slope of the descending portion of the curve after serum specific activity had reached low values, and multiplying this by the measured pool size. FIG. 9 shows the values obtained for normal tissue. The top line on the left hand side represents influx of free cholesterol followed by its rate of disappearance; the bottom line the appearance of labeled cholesterol esters in normal tissue. Note that this is a logarithmic curve so that in normal tissue there is an immensely greater influx rate of free cholesterol than of cholesterol esters.

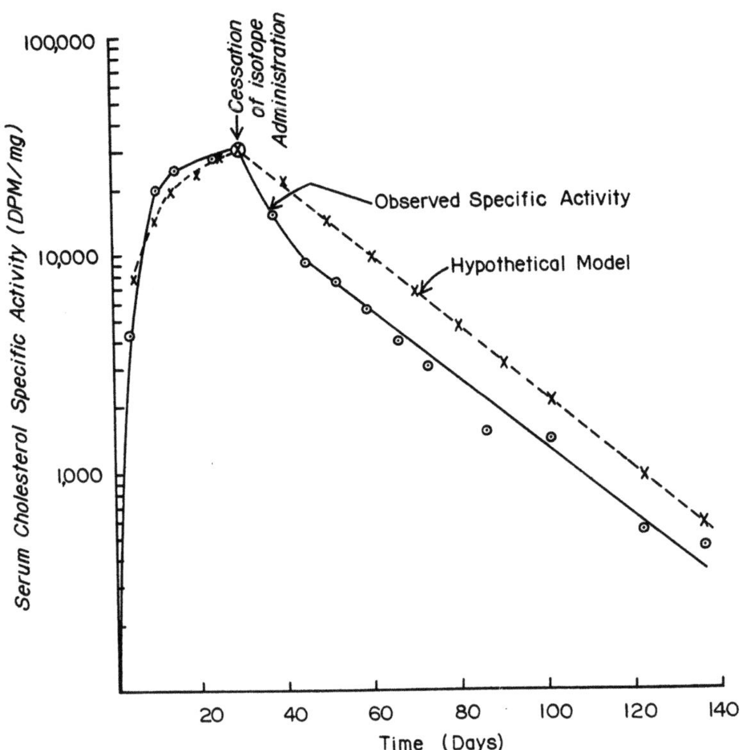

FIGURE 8.
(Lofland and Clarkson, 1970)

The situation in fatty streaks is somewhat different. FIG. 10 shows
that at practically every point observed over this more than 3½ month
period, the specific activities of free and esterified cholesterol
were almost identical which indicates that the rate of influx of cholesterol esters has increased to be equal to that of free cholesterol.
FIG. 11 shows what we observed in plaques. Here the situation is
completely different. At every point, with one exception, the degree
of labeling achieved by the cholesterol esters exceeds that of free
cholesterol. These data indicate that in normal tissue, fatty streaks
and plaques, there are both qualitative and quantitative differences
in the rates of influx and efflux of cholesterol and its esters. It
should be pointed out that the same hypercholesterolemic serum was
perfusing these areas of the aorta, since they all come from the same
pigeon. TABLE VIII shows that we are not dealing here with alterations
in specific activity due to different pool sizes. These values are
actual radioactivity (d.p.m.), and at any of the time intervals studied, there was more radioactivity in fatty streaks and plaques than
in normal tissue. TABLE IX shows that in normal aorta the rate of
influx is closely paralleled by the rate of efflux. The difference
was actually about 15 µg/day/gm of tissue in favor of efflux. The

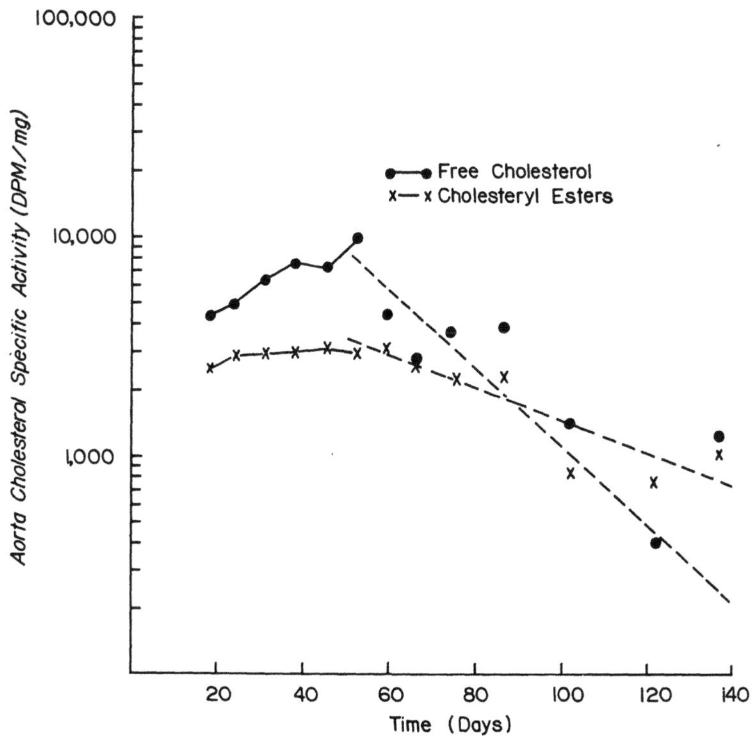

FIGURE 9.
(Lofland and Clarkson, 1970)

TABLE VIII

CHANGES IN FREE AND ESTER CHOLESTEROL RADIOACTIVITY IN NORMAL ARTERY, FATTY STREAKS AND PLAQUES AT VARIOUS TIME INTERVALS[a]

Day	Normal artery		Fatty streaks		Plaques	
	Free cholesterol	Cholesteryl esters	Free cholesterol	Cholesteryl esters	Free cholesterol	Cholesteryl esters
18	16727± 1081	2781± 492	24970± 2096	11478± 2787	54734±11680	59100±21003
24	17948± 1024	4859±1118	39310±11835	31702±15361	78917± 4567	125628±10391
31	20722± 3122	3832±1614	27526± 5178	8037± 2684	87075±27544	111325±52636
38	27456± 2010	5740±1228	36535± 5719	16414± 3161	93201±16883	134870±39021
52	43603±26566	3172±1548	37935± 6043	18442± 4424	123891±25581	178639±64723
66	14204± 569	8826±1750	27074± 4151	14808± 3479	86000±10132	118635±50337
86	8901± 1796	1597± 252	20274± 5949	8214± 4755	74858±17598	89098±25869
122	2072± 622	2067±1242	11572± 5025	4235± 2076	86660±19571	103732±24445

[a] Mean values (dpm/g of wet tissue) for 8 birds, at each time interval, followed by the standard errors of the means.

(Lofland and Clarkson, 1970)

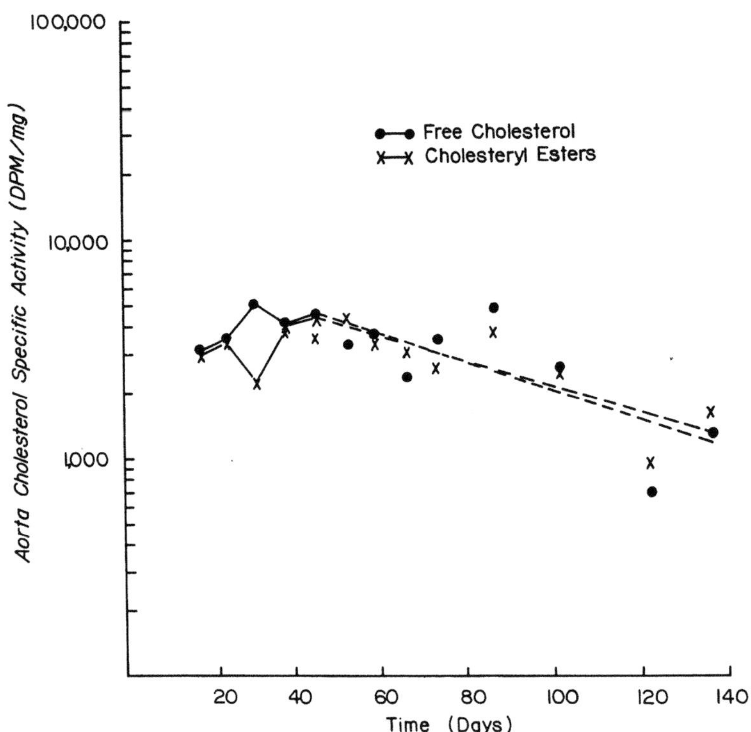

FIGURE 10.
(Lofland and Clarkson, 1970)

situation is different with fatty streaks, where you see that the influx appears to exceed slightly the efflux. This is even more marked
in plaques. So fatty streaks and plaques both appear to be in positive cholesterol balance, as surely they must be if cholesterol is
accumulating. I think this has some importance in that to me it represents confirmation of what Zilversmit postulated several years ago,
that is that very likely the normal aortic wall represents a metabolic
barrier and this may become destroyed as a result of injury such as
results from cholesterol feeding.

DR. BORN: This dynamic approach seems to be the right one.
Could I ask whether you have already tried to affect the influx –
efflux curve by drugs or by other means because your work seems at
last to open up the possibility of changing efflux and influx rates,
just as one can alter efflux and influx rates of ions, amino acids
or sugars by drugs. I would be very interested to know if there are
already results of this kind.

DR. LOFLAND: We have not tried this approach as yet. I think
that you are right. We are hopeful that this approach can provide
a means of evaluating the influence of diet or of therapeutic agents.

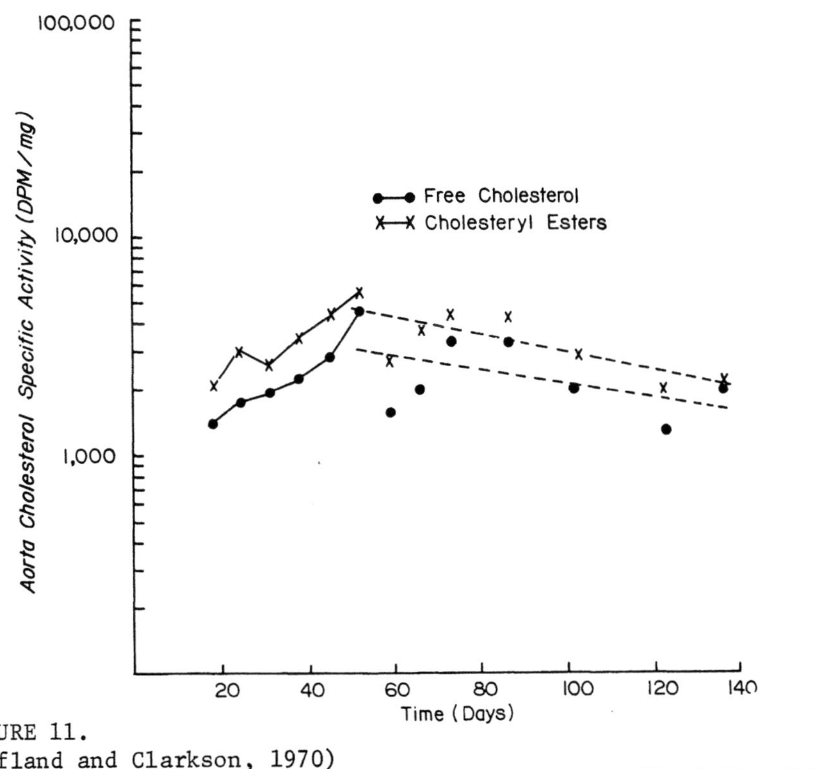

FIGURE 11.
(Lofland and Clarkson, 1970)

TABLE IX

INFLUX AND EFFLUX OF FREE CHOLESTEROL AND CHOLESTERYL

ESTERS IN NORMAL ARTERY, FATTY STREAKS AND PLAQUES[a]

	Free cholesterol			Cholesteryl esters		
	Influx	Efflux	Difference	Influx	Efflux	Difference
Normal aorta	71.3	86.4	-15.1	11.9	14.5	- 2.6
Fatty streaks	106.5	75.7	+25.8	49.0	29.6	+19.4
Plaques	198.0	167.0	+31.0	259.0	183.0	+76.0

[a] Values for influx and efflux represent µg cholesterol/g of aorta/day.
(Lofland and Clarkson, 1970)

QUESTION: Have you calculated the turnover rates of cholesterol? This would be enormously interesting in relation to the physiological situation.

DR. LOFLAND: I can't give you a figure for this except as it is reflected in our figures for influx and efflux. From data obtained in this way, however, one should be able to calculate turnover rates.

COMMENT

The question whether any or all of the lipid in atheromatous lesions was brought there by the macrophages was next approached, together with the question to what extent, if any, foam cells are macrophages. Dr. French asked the question - Drs. O'Neal, Friedman, Constantinides and Wissler commented.

DR. FRENCH: There is no doubt that in experimental animals and in man lipophages have been depicted half way in and half way out on the surface of the lesion. I don't **Role of** know whether they are entering the **macrophages** lesion, contributing to it, or whether some cholesterol is being excluded from the lesions. This is an important question. If anyone can answer it, it would be very useful indeed to know.

DR. O'NEAL: We have, as have many others, found it easy to ob- **HUMAN** tain light and electron microscopic pictures of lipophages in the **RAT** blood stream of experimental animals showing them half way into (or half way out of) the subendothelial space, and white blood cells more or less attached to the lining of the blood vessels. Circulating cells of man (Kim and Suzuki et al., 1967) and rats (Suzuki and O'Neal, 1967) do "transport" lipids of the types that are found in atheromatous lesions. But we don't have any evidence as to how important this is in the process of atheroma formation.

DR. FRIEDMAN: We were very much concerned about the traveling lipophage on the intimal surface and so we decided to produce a lesion in which there would be no circulating blood, namely a tied off carotid into which we instilled lipemic serum. After about 48 hours the only living cells in the preparation were endothelial cells. After 72 to 96 hours there occurred a typical foam cell accumulation. It was the endothelial cells that contained the lipid. Within a week there appeared a typical atheroma. There wasn't any question that endothelial cells had changed into foam cells so that a typical atheroma developed under these highly artificial conditions with no wandering lipophages present and with smooth muscle cells not contributing.

DR. CONSTANTINIDES: I used to think that lipophage migration
was a myth. But I was forced to see that it truly happens because
I found in injury experiments, that if you have a significant lipemia,
phagocytic cells in the blood will pick up lipid particles, approach
the arterial wall, get stuck to it, and crawl through the endothelium.
What Leary claimed many years ago Dr. O'Neal and Dr. Still and others
have proven to occur, and my own recent experience confirms theirs.
The problem now is whether this happens in man at all. I don't
think there is a reason why it should not happen in man under similar
conditions; I don't see why the human monocytes should not have the
properties of monocytes of most other mammalian cousins of man. The
only way to prove it would be to fix the aorta of very lipemic people
within a few minutes of death. Maybe then we will be able to catch
some lipophages in the process of entering a human artery.

DR. WISSLER: There may be two different kinds of pathogenesis
of atherosclerosis that we should be considering (Wissler and
Vesselinovitch, 1968). In the rabbit, the rat and the cockeral, many
of the cells in a plaque are derived from circulating foam cells accumulated in the intima of the artery. A typical plaque in these
species is mostly intimal and has very little necrosis and, generally
speaking, no thrombosis. This does not apply when the rabbit has
been fed intermittently in the manner Dr. Constantinides has used
so well.

The significance
of species
differences

In the monkey and the swine and
the rabbit who has been fed intermittently there are few if any blood-
derived foam cells involved in atheromatous plaques. In these animals the
low-density-lipoprotein largely accumulates in the arterial myointimal
or medial cells and this produces what we consider to be a plaque
like that seen in man with necrosis and thrombosis. In the primates
and swine as well as in man, low-density-lipoproteins are deposited
in smooth muscle cells. There has been confirmation of this recently from Becker and Murphy (Becker and Murphy, 1969). There are,
according to Imai et al. (Imai and Lee et al., 1966), two kinds of
cells in the rabbit lesion and with time there is much more conversion
to the smooth muscle lesion but in the early stages of the rabbit
lesion with very high cholesterol levels most of the cells are blood-
derived foam cells. The Cornell workers (Becker and Murphy, 1969)
have recently reported studies using, I believe, the best technique
that I have seen for fluorescence studies, the presence or absence
of actomyosin in the cells in human atherosclerosis. They have come
to the conclusion that virtually all the cells in the rather small
human lesion are smooth muscle containing cells. They do not describe
cells that fit the criteria of monocytes in the lesions that they
studied. Later on perhaps cells from the blood do come in. So, if
one wants to adopt a unitarian point of view then one could implicate

only one kind of cell in the development of the lesion. We know that
these cells proliferate, we know that they take up low-density-lipoprotein, we know that under some conditions such as peanut oil feeding they convert to increased collagen formation and we know that
they can undergo injury and death and thus contribute to the atheroma
with plaque ulceration thrombosis.

COMMENT

The association of endothelial injury with increased transport
of lipid into the aterial wall is discussed in Chapter 5 by Robertson
and by Astrup.

RAT DR. O'NEAL: In order to stain lipid-laden macrophages in the
blood smears of rats, it is necessary to fix the blood smear with
formaldehyde steam before it has had time to dry. With this technique lipid laden monocytes can be very easily demonstrated by the
oil red O stain. Up to ten percent of the white blood cells will
contain three or more fat vacuoles (Simon and Still et al., 1961).

MONKEY DR. FRIEDMAN: We tried to obtain the same kind of preparations
from hyperlipemic monkeys and we had rabbits as controls. We could
RABBIT find the lipid laden monocytes in rabbits consistently in large
numbers but so far we have not been able to find them in monkeys with
about the same degree of hyperlipidemia or hypercholesterolemia. I
am puzzled why there may be a species difference here. Showing monocytes that contain lipid granules is fine but I can show fat laden
hepatic cells in the cholesterol fed rabbit, but that doesn't mean
that because you have monocytes traveling in the blood that they are
part of the new atheroma. One has to find a reason why they are
sticking on and coming in. The picture that you referred to, Dr.
Constantinides, was, I think, in the Journal of Pathology and Bac-
teriology. They had to admit they didn't know whether that cell was
coming in or going out, at least the one I am talking about with
beautiful color. But if one can produce atheroma that replicates
what you find spontaneously in the cholesterol fed rabbit with the
complete absence of lipophages then I think the best you can say for
them is that they are adventitious travelers to the scene.

COMMENT

Dr. Matthes demonstrated enhanced accumulation of lipids in the
wall of the aorta in association with increased blood pressure. This
raised the whole question of filtration versus selective absorption
or active transport.

It was pointed out that if the distribution of lipids in the
arterial wall is found to be in the same proportion as those in the
blood, simple pressure filtration would not explain the findings, be-

cause, with simple pressure, small molecules would gain access to the wall more readily than the large ones. The discussion was continued by Dr. Bowyer, who alluded to the active process of breakdown and reconstitution of lipid molecules in the arterial wall itself as follows:

DR. BOWYER: When we are attempting to address the question of why lipids accumulate in the arterial wall, we must remember that we are referring to a large number of lipid classes. Thus, in fatty **RABBIT** streaks in man and in a number of experimental animals cholesterol oleate is one of the major lipids of the fat-filled cells, whilst in fibrous plaques much sphingomyelin accumulates.

In an attempt to make some synthesis of what we know about arterial lipid accumulation I should like to confine myself to considering the balance sheet for cholesterol esters. One must consider:

1. Transfer of cholesterol and cholesterol esters from the plasma lipoproteins.
2. Esterification of cholesterol in the arterial wall by fatty acid derived from the plasma and from in situ synthesis.
3. Transfer of fatty acid residue from lecithin or another complex lipid to cholesterol (analogous to the enzyme of plasma described by Glomset; see for example Abdulla et al. (Abdulla and Adams et al., 1969).
4. Catabolism of cholesterol esters by the hydrolases.

In an attempt to look at whether there is a selective synthesis of cholesterol oleate in fatty streaks, we perfused normal and atherosclerotic aortas of rabbits with ^{14}C-labelled palmitic, stearic, oleic and linoleic acids (see Chapter 5 for results).

As shown in TABLE X, there was a significantly greater incorporation of oleic acid than of the other three into the cholesterol ester fraction.

DR. DAY: The difference in incorporation of different fatty acids into cholesterol ester could also be explained by difference in uptake by the endothelial wall.

DR. BOWYER: TABLE X also shows the relative rates of uptake of the four fatty acids, in μμmoles/g wet tissue/hr in normal and atherosclerotic aortas.

In all cases the uptake was greater in the atherosclerotic than in the normal aortas. In the lesions the saturated fatty acids were taken up more than the unsaturated ones and thus a large preferential uptake of oleic acid does not explain the greater incorporation into the cholesterol ester fraction.

A more recent experiment, in which ^{3}H oleic acid and ^{14}C linoleic acids were perfused simultaneously showed conclusively that:

1. The rates of uptake of the two acids from plasma albumin into atherosclerotic rabbit aortas are very similar.

2. The rate of esterification of cholesterol with oleic acid is far greater than with linoleic acid.

TABLE X

INCORPORATION OF 1 ^{14}C LABELED FATTY ACIDS INTO THE FREE FATTY ACID POOL AND CHOLESTEROL ESTERS OF NORMAL AND ATHEROSCLEROTIC RABBIT AORTAS. FATTY ACIDS WERE PERFUSED SEPARATELY IN KREBS-BICARBONATE RINGER CONTAINING 4g/100 ml BOVINE SERUM ALBUMIN AT 0.1µE/ml FOR 1 HOUR

	\multicolumn{8}{c}{Incorporation, µµmoles/g wet tissue/hr}

	16:0		18:0		18:1		18:2	
	N	A	N	A	N	A	N	A
Free fatty acid	1200	3725	1441	6474**	647	2775*	575	1678*
Cholesterol Esters	25	404***	2	291***	18	1058***	17	345***

Mass percentage of arterial free fatty acid pool:

	16:0	18:0	18:1	18:2	Others
N	31.2	20.7	10.9	1.3	35.9
A	35.2	25.4	13.8	1.5	24.1

N – Normal, A – Atherosclerotic (fed a semi-synthetic hypercholesterol-emic diet for 24 weeks).
Significance levels * – P<0.05, ** – P<0.01, *** – P<0.001

COMMENT

The next point at issue was whether or not lipids enter the arterial wall as lipoprotein. Dr. Wissler reported observations on **MONKEY** intracellular droplets in the aortic wall of monkeys.

DR. WISSLER: I would like to discuss the question whether or not cholesterol enters as lipoprotein. We have used a modification of Bruce Taylor's classic diet for producing atherosclerosis in Rhesus monkeys. Added to a stock monkey ration is an abundant amount of cholesterol and saturated fats. We find that a mixture of coconut oil and butter fat is somewhat more atherogenic than butter fat alone. We find fatty streaks in coronary arteries as early as 30 days and one can see that most of the lipid is intracellular. There has already been some minor proliferation at this point in time and there is only a little lipid that is obviously associated with the elastic fibers.

Under electron microscopy we see the endothelium intact although it sometimes contains lipid droplets. Most of the lipid is in smooth muscle cells in the form of droplets. Later typical foam cells appear but these are modified myointimal cells.

Dr. Stamler suggested that we ought to review some of the evidence that lipoprotein can be found inside these cells that have lipid droplets. Actually the first evidence on this was produced by Herb Kayden using fluorescence microscopy and as far as I know he only reported it at an American Heart Association meeting (Kayden and Franklin et al., 1962). Then Dr. Harvey Watts produced similar evidence with fluorescence microscopy (Watts, 1963a) but took it one step further by labeling the antibodies to the lipoprotein with ferritin and showing with the electron microscope that the typical ferritin label could be found round the droplets in suitably prepared electron microscopic material in which the blocks were reacted with the lipoprotein antibody after slight disruption of the cell membranes by freezing (Watts, 1963b). We have done a considerable amount of work with fluorescence microscopy (Kao and Wissler, 1965; Knieriem and Kao et al., 1968; Knieriem and Kao et al., 1967) and I don't want to review this in detail except to say that we confirmed both Kayden and Watts and we found that the places where the lipoproteins accumulate on consecutive sections are the same places that one can find the lipid droplets when one uses the technique I described, so that the lipoproteins and the lipid droplets seem to be superimposable in consecutive sections. More recently, as I reported very briefly at the symposium in Chicago (Wissler, 1970a), we've been labeling the anti-lipoproteins with horseradish peroxidase. We're still in the early stages of these studies but we do find consistently that we can demonstrate the peroxidase reaction around the lipid droplets inside the smooth muscle cells. Even more recently, we have been doing experiments with tissue cultures of medial cells from arteries of Rhesus monkeys (Kao and Wissler et al., 1968; Dzoga and Jones et al., 1970). By removing the intima and adventitia we can obtain nearly pure cultures of medial cells. They grow quite well with about 80% of the cultures showing active growth. They can be used for various kinds of studies. Under the electron microscope they show the fibers that one expects to see in the smooth muscle cell. Upon introducing low-density-lipoproteins into the culture medium or by introducing serum from animals that have been fed with one or another of the atherogenic diets, a lipid accumulation appears in the cells. They also actively divide as seen by radioautographs. With horseradish peroxidase staining technique at the light microscopic level we can demonstrate in the medial cells the marker of the low-density-lipoprotein. I think this may be a useful technique with which to study the influx and efflux of lipoprotein molecules in the cells. I don't want to be misinterpreted. I do believe that lipids change markedly as they go into the cells. That there is deesterification and esterification of the cholesterol. Thus some lipid is synthesized in these cells, but I do believe that at least some of the lipid makes its way into the cell as lipoprotein molecules (Dzoga and Jones et al., 1970).

QUESTION: Dr. Wissler would it be fair to say that if these lipids go in in the form of lipoproteins, this would not exactly be filtration?

DR. WISSLER: I think filtration as it's usually used in this disease applies to the artery wall. And what this does do to support the filtration theory is that apparently intact lipoprotein molecules do make their way through the endothelium to gain contact with the medial cells, and these cells, somehow or other, some of them at least, take up intact lipoprotein molecules. Filtration is a bad word. I'm not trying to defend the filtration theory, but I think these kind of phenomena are what people have generally meant when they were talking about filtration.

DR. CONSTANTINIDES: By using tissue culture you can never demonstrate whether lipoproteins cross endothelium under normal conditions.

DR. WISSLER: I realize that, but, you see this follows work in three or more laboratories, where it was shown that the lipoprotein label appeared in sections of intact human arteries.

I would agree that protein might come in separately from the lipid or that the lipid and protein could be separated shortly after their entry. I think Abel Robertson has some excellent data suggesting that a great amount of protein at least is split off and may be at the cell surface or a short way beneath.

DR. ROBERTSON: Dr. Wissler's observations are indeed very interesting, particularly in describing the use of a new approach, that of utilizing electron markers of a small molecular size (m.w. 40-50,000) such as horseradish peroxidase, to demonstrate by immunotechniques the presence of intracellular lipoproteins. Since reference was made

HUMAN to our work on human arterial intimal cells in culture and their incorporation of homologous serum low-density (LDL) lipoproteins using dif-

Tissue culture of human arterial cells

ferent labels on their protein and lipid moieties, (Robertson, 1967), I would like to emphasize that such tissue culture studies showed differences in rates of incorporation of the two moieties of the lipoproteins. In other words, they demonstrated that the velocity of intracellular incorporation of the apoprotein and lipid portions of the lipoprotein were different, but that both occurred. In cells with very little or no lipid in their cytoplasm free cholesterol was incorporated faster than the corresponding apoprotein. Once the intimal cell or atherophil becomes

lipid-laden, however, the whole LDL lipoprotein molecule seems to be
rapidly incorporated into these cells. I would like to emphasize,
therefore, that it is possible to visualize that two different mechanisms of sterol transport across the cell membrane may be operational depending upon the severity of cell injury: One, selective for
faster incorporation of the lipid moiety of LDL fractions and another, occurring when the cell has lost its lipid regulatory capacity and becomes a foam cell, resulting in the indiscriminate uptake
of whole lipoproteins. We have evidence, for example, that inhibition of protein synthesis by puromycin or actinomycin D and even more
dramatically by cell hypoxia (Robertson, 1968) results in significant
increases in permeability of arterial wall cells to whole serum lipoproteins. In fact, we wonder if such increases in permeability of
the arterial wall may be operative in atherogenesis. A possible explanation of the very intriguing
studies presented by Dr. Lofland at
Relation of injury   this meeting, may be that differences
to rate of lipid   in rates of cholesterol efflux and
incorporation   influx that he showed us so clearly,
may result from variations in the
severity of lesions present at a given portion of the arterial wall.
In other words, intra- and extracellular lipids from lipid rich
lesions may exchange very rapidly with other lipid pools, whereas
cells from less or non-affected areas may handle lipid transport in
a more selective fashion. If this is the case, Dr. Lofland's findings may help to explain why the rate of atherogenesis both in man
and experimental animals seems to accelerate with age. Arteries
with fatty lesions would thus appear to be more susceptible to further lipid uptake. Hypoxia appears to be an important injurious
condition in the pathogenesis of atherosclerosis as emphasized by
Astrup.

COMMENT

Further findings from tissue culture were reported by Dr.
Rutstein.

DR. RUTSTEIN: Early experiments (Rutstein and Castelli et al.,
1964) demonstrated that intracellular lipid deposition in tissue culture following exposure to serum specimens collected after the administration of test meals was increased after the ingestion of fat and
in the prolonged fasting state, and was decreased after the ingestion
of carbohydrate.

Although there was a correlation between the increase in deposition after a fat meal and triglyceride concentration, serum lipid a-
nalysis revealed no consistent correlations between increases or decreases in deposition and the concentration of any of the lipid constituents measured, i.e., cholesterol, triglycerides and phospholipids.

Studies were then initiated in which another lipid constituent, the
non-esterified fatty acids, was included as an additional measurement
(Castelli and Nickerson et al., 1966; Rutstein and Castelli et al.,
1967). Now the situation became clear. There was a direct correlation between the concentration of non-esterified fatty acids and
the increases in intracellular lipid deposition following fat ingestion and in the prolonged fasting state and with the decreases in
intracellular lipid deposition after the ingestion of carbohydrate
and of protein.

Final confirmation on the correlation of intracellular lipid deposition in tissue culture and the concentration of non-esterified
fatty acids was obtained by studies of intracellular lipid deposition
produced from serum specimens collected before and after the administration of intravenous heparin which activates lipoprotein lipase
(Rutstein and Castelli et al., 1969). Serum collected after the administration of heparin demonstrated increased intracellular lipid deposition which correlated with the increase in the serum levels of non-
esterified fatty acids, but not with the decreased concentration of
triglycerides, cholesterol and phospholipids. This heparin induced
lipid deposition was more striking in hypercholesterolemic individuals.
Experiments in which the cells were first exposed to post-heparin and
later to pre-heparin serum demonstrated that intracellular lipid deposition in our model system is reversible.

Similar experiments are now underway using tagged cholesterol and
non-esterified fatty acids to measure the kinetics of lipid transport
in and out of tissue culture cells. Early results demonstrate a par-
allelism between visible lipid deposition and tagged lipid transport
and that increased transport of tagged fatty acids is associated with
increased tagged cholesterol transport into cells.

DR. ALAUPOVIC: Was this deposition in the form of lipoproteins
or lipids?

DR. RUTSTEIN: They're in the form of stainable lipid by Sudan
black B...

DR. ALAUPOVIC: Have you checked the protein moiety by any chance?
If this lipid deposit was in the form of lipoprotein, did you observe
an increase in the protein content of the cells?

DR. RUTSTEIN: No, it is a most important question. We have
been following the transfer of tagged free fatty acids across cell
membranes. We do know that the rate of transfer of fatty acids is
10 times that of albumin (Fredrickson and Gordon, 1958; Volwiler and
Goldsworthy et al., 1955). We are also studying the transfer of tagged cholesterol but have not yet been able to label the protein moiety, i.e., the lipoproteins to determine relative rates of transfer.

DR. SMITH: We have certainly been able to extract from normal intima intact lipoprotein in the S_f 0 to 20 group. It reacts with antibody to human low-density-lipoprotein, and electrophoretically it appears as beta lipoprotein. It can amount to nearly half the cholesterol in the total extract.

QUESTION: Could the cholesterol be combined with protein in the wall once it enters the arterial wall?

DR. SMITH: I suppose it could, but to me it seems more reasonable to suppose that it is filtered in the form of lipoprotein.

UNIDENTIFIED SPEAKER: We can confirm your findings from these extraction procedures. The fact that the lipid is still attached to the protein moiety in the arterial wall, and as such displays its original label, argues against the lipoprotein having been synthesized in situ.

QUESTION: Has anybody any evidence that lipoprotein is able to be synthesized in the arterial wall?

CHAIRMAN WERTHESSEN: None published that I know of. Have you looked for it in your cultures?

DR. WISSLER: Yes, the lipid droplets in the cultures will react immunologically with antibodies to Rhesus monkey low-density-lipoprotein.

In the artery without a lesion we cannot pick up detectable low-density-lipoprotein inside any cells. There's always a very slight amount of fluorescence. But not the kind of fluorescence that we call immunofluorescence.

CHAIRMAN WERTHESSEN: Would you say, Dr. Wissler, just to confirm it for the audience, that if you look at the early stage of feeding you cannot show the lipoprotein inside the wall, but you can show it with ease once you get to the point of atheromatosis.

DR. WISSLER: In our series of human studies we used all kinds of control material. New born, premature, normal areas from blood vessels, and so forth, and these were all reported in two papers (Kao and Wissler, 1965; Knieriem and Kao et al., 1967). What these control data say is that the fluorescent technique is a little bit more sensitive than the usual Oil Red O technique. We can see the fluorescence of lipoprotein in areas of the wall where we can just barely see sudanophilic droplets in the cells.

DR. ADAMS: We have investigated the site of protein entry into the arterial wall by studying the radioactivity concentration in multiple layers of rabbit aorta after injecting I^{125} albumin. We

found by well-counting and autoradiography that radioactivity in the
normal vessel is greater in the outer part than in the inner part
(outside-inward gradient). However, by the time a severe atherosclerotic lesion has formed, the gradient usually slopes the other
way (i.e., inside-outwards). We feel that this evidence shows that
albumin normally enters the aortic wall predominantly from the vasa
vasorum, but with severe atheroma it leaks directly from the intima
into the inner part of the arterial wall. This does not imply that
no plasma constituent filters into the normal arterial wall from the
lumen, but we think that most of it comes from outside. I would like
Dr. Wissler's comments on these results.

DR. WISSLER: I'd ask how do you explain your observations with
Duncan's data. After cutting the vessels he found that labelled
albumin and lipoprotein accumulated much more quickly in the intimal
areas than in the media and finally later in the adventitia.

DR. ADAMS: Some of Duncan's data (Duncan and Buck, 1962) do
actually match up with ours in the rabbit. He was using the dog   **DOG v**
which has an entirely different pattern of aortic vascularization.   **RABB**
When I visited Duncan he didn't disagree with these observations.
Furthermore, his samples were divided into intimo-medial and medio-
adventitial parts only, whereas ours comprise about 8 layers from
the intima to the media.

DR. WISSLER: He showed time studies, though, in which the highest concentration of his labeled protein appeared first in the intima.

DR. SCOTT: May I ask Dr. Adams, when were his animals killed?
I think I am right in saying that you have not done these studies
over an extended period of time. It cannot be assumed that initial
concentrations or apparent sites of entry of ^{125}I-albumin give a true
picture of normal or abnormal physiology. If a given protein requires a long interval to establish an equilibrium of exchange between a particular extravascular pool and the plasma, then the initial
concentration of the protein in the extravascular pool may be very low.
Hence, the gradient between inner and outer aortic wall over the first
few days may not be a meaningful indicator of events in this context.
Have you any results for the 10 to 21 day interval between injection
of your labelled protein and sampling of the tissues, and if so, what
were the ratios of radioactivity in inner to outer aortic wall after
these longer periods for equilibration between plasma and extravascular tissues?

DR. ADAMS: These results were at two or four days after pulses
of labeled albumin. All we are trying to ascertain is where the   **RABB**
protein enters, not where it accumulates. (Note in proof: - Studies
at 2 and 4 hours show an even steeper outward-inward gradient of ^{125}I-
albumin in rabbit aorta.)

DR. ALAUPOVIC: It is important to realize that human plasma lipoprotein density classes are heterogeneous, not only with respect to hydrated density and particle size, but also with respect to the protein moieties (Alaupovic, 1968). To formulate a chemical rather than an operational classification system I suggested that the specific protein moieties (apolipoproteins) be utilized as criteria for the classification and differentiation of lipoproteins. Accordingly, the plasma lipoprotein system consists of at least three polydisperse lipoprotein families, each of which is characterized by the presence of single, distinct apolipoproteins A, B and C, respectively. The human low-density-lipoproteins contain all three lipoprotein families (Lee and Alaupovic, 1970) in various proportions. Although the lipoprotein family characterized by apolipoprotein B is the major lipoprotein family of low density class the relative amount of apolipoprotein C-containing family may be as high as 20-25%. It is essential, therefore, that this protein heterogeneity of plasma lipoprotein system be recognized in all future studies of the lipoprotein composition of normal and diseased arterial walls.

Chapter 5

PARTICIPANTS: D.E. Bowyer, P. Constantinides, A.J. Day, G.A. Gresham,
               C.G. Gunn, W.H. Hauss, A.N. Howard, A. Keys, H.B.
               Lofland, G. Schlierf, C.J. Schwartz, J. Stamler,
               O. Stein, Y. Stein, N.T. Werthessen and R.W. Wissler

COMMENT

The question arose as to the nature of metabolic changes in
the arterial wall and the extent to which an increased concentration
of lipids during enhanced metabolic activity is attributable to
incorporation of lipid from the circulation, local synthesis within the wall, or both.

DR. DAY: I want to indicate the way in which foam cells might
contribute to the synthesis of lipid in the atherosclerotic arterial
wall. We have approached this problem in three ways. Firstly, by
isotope studies using homogeneous preparations of foam cells isolated
from atherosclerotic lesions; secondly, by incubating atherosclerotic
lesions with radioactively labeled lipid precursors and then isolating
the foam cells and other fractions for biochemical study, and thirdly,
by autoradiography in atherosclerotic lesions incubated with lipid
precursors. In TABLE I the incorporation of P^{32}-labeled phosphate
into phospholipid by isolated foam cell preparations is compared with
that of intact atherosclerotic intima incubated in vitro. The similarity in incorporation is readily apparent. In TABLE II the uptake
of ^{14}C-labeled acetate and its incorporation into various lipid components in foam cell preparations and in atherosclerotic intima incubated in vitro is shown. The relatively high proportion of acetate
converted to cholesterol ester in the foam cell preparation is apparent.

TABLE I

PERCENTAGE DISTRIBUTION OF P^{32}-LABELED PHOSPHOLIPIDS IN FOAM CELLS

AND IN WHOLE INTIMA FOLLOWING INCUBATION WITH P^{32}-PHOSPHATE

	Foam Cells	Intima
Origin	0.2	0.7
Lysolecithin	0.7	0.6
Sphingomyelin	2.3	1.2
Lecithin	65.4	64.1
Phosphatidyl inositol	20.7	27.0
Phosphatidyl ethanolamine	7.5	5.3
Front	2.4	1.2

(Data from Newman and Day et al., 1966; Day and Newman et al., 1966)

Where atherosclerotic arteries were incubated with either P^{32}-labeled
RABBIT phosphate, (Day and Newman et al., 1966) or ^{14}C-labeled oleate (Day
and Tume, 1970), the foam cells separated subsequent to the incubation,
were found to contain labeled phospholipid and cholesterol ester with
specific activities considerably in excess of that of other fractions.
These findings were interpreted as indicating that, of the synthesis
of lipid occurring in the artery, most was taking place in the foam
cells present. This conclusion was confirmed by autoradiography,
both in experimental lesions in cholesterol-fed rabbits and in human
lesions obtained from renal transplant donors. We used ^{14}C-labeled
oleic acid and studied the localization of its incorporation into
phospholipid and into cholesterol ester, the major components labeled
under such circumstances in both the human and experimental lesions.
We also used ^{14}C-labeled choline to study the synthesis of phospholipid in the experimental and human atherosclerotic lesion. Relatively little incorporation of oleic acid into lipid occurred in the media
HUMAN or in the intimo-medial junction, but considerable uptake and incorporation of oleic acid in the foam cells of the intima was found to
occur (Day and Wahlqvist, 1968). In human fatty streak and fibro-
fatty lesions we had a slightly more complicated and perhaps better
preparation inasmuch as there were several types of cells present
in the lesion, in addition to the large fat-filled foam cells. Relatively little oleic acid was taken up and incorporated into lipid
in the small round cells and spindle-shaped cells of the fatty streak
and of the fibro-fatty lesion in the human material studied, but relatively large amounts of oleic acid were taken up and incorporated
into cholesterol ester and phospholipid in the fat-filled foam cells
present, (Wahlqvist and Day et al., 1969).

TABLE II

PERCENTAGE DISTRIBUTION OF SYNTHESIZED ^{14}C-LABELED FATTY ACID BETWEEN
VARIOUS LIPID FRACTIONS AFTER INCUBATION OF EITHER WHOLE INTIMA
OR FOAM CELLS WITH ^{14}C-LABELED ACETATE

	Foam Cells*	Intima**
Phospholipid	41.0 ± 2.48	55.6 ± 1.29
Cholesterol	3.0 ± 0.32	2.6 ± 0.23
Fatty acid	4.5 ± 0.94	3.0 ± 0.52
Triglyceride	7.2 ± 1.38	10.1 ± 1.05
Cholesterol ester	44.3 ± 1.14	28.7 ± 0.92

*Mean of 5 experiments; duplicate batches of cells incubated separately in each.

**Mean of 6 experiments with SE of mean. Aorta halves were incubated separately in 4 of the 6 experiments and these have been treated as duplicates.

(Data from Day and Wilkinson, 1967)

TABLE III indicates the quantitation by grain counting of this situation in the human atherosclerotic lesion.

TABLE III

RADIOAUTOGRAPH GRAIN COUNTS (NO./100 μ^2)

		Intima				
Case No.	Lesion Type	Foam Cells	Nonsudanophilic Round Mononuclear Cells	Spindle-shaped Cells	Extra-cellular	Media
			Aorta			
1	Fatty streak	15.6	5.0		2.9	1.1
2	Fibro-fatty	15.3	4.9	4.1	2.5	1.1
3	Fibro-fatty	17.7	4.0	2.6	2.2	1.2
4	Fibro-fatty	18.7	5.8	4.7	4.1	4.4
			Renal Artery			
4	Fibro-fatty	15.2	3.6	4.5	2.4	3.6
			Iliac Artery			
4	Fibro-fatty	12.6	2.7	1.8	1.1	1.1

(Data from Wahlqvist and Day et al., 1969)

While considerable concentration of label appears over the foam cells much less label is concentrated in the non fat-filled mononuclears and in the spindle-shaped cells. Similar findings with respect to the role of foam cells were observed using ^{14}C-labeled choline as precursor, (Day and Wahlqvist, 1969; Wahlqvist and Day, 1969).

Dr. WERTHESSEN: Do you have any idea from your data as to the micrograms of fatty acid that were incorporated? Did you make that calculation?

DR. DAY: We have carried out a number of in vitro experiments in which the amount of oleic acid taken up by the artery and incorporated into lipid has been determined. When ^{14}C-labeled oleic acid was added to an incubation medium containing Hanks' solution and serum, a mean of 0.83% of the label present was taken up by the normal artery and of 4.48% by the atherosclerotic artery over a 4 hr incubation period (Day and Wahlqvist, 1968). In both the normal and atherosclerotic artery approximately 80% of the oleic acid was incorporated into combined lipid, mainly phospholipid and cholesterol ester during this period. More recently (Day and Wahlqvist et al., 1970b) we have attempted to determine the amounts in terms of µmoles of oleic, palmitic and linoleic acids taken up by the atherosclerotic artery incubated in vitro. These data were calculated from the measured specific activity of the respective fatty acids in the intimal pool, rather than of that in the incubation medium. In this way, we could obtain a more adequate indication of the incorporation of the respective fatty acid. An indication of the sort of data obtained is contained in the fact that a mean of 7.37 µmoles of oleic acid was incorporated into cholesterol ester per gram of dry defatted weight of the artery over the 4 hr incubation period. Data, however, were obtained for all three fatty acids and for their incorporation in vitro into cholesterol ester, triglyceride and phospholipid. They are given in the paper cited.

DR. O. STEIN: During the last two years we have been studying the localization and metabolism of aortic phospholipids (Stein and Eisenberg et al., 1969; Eisenberg and Stein et al., 1969a; Stein and Rachmilewitz et al., 1970). Recently we tried to apply high resolution radioautography to the study of phospholipids in normal and atheromatous rabbit aorta. To that end normal aortic segments were incubated with choline-H^3, which resulted in the formation of one labeled product, namely lecithin. At the light microscope level the radioautographic reaction was localized to the smooth muscle cells of the media (FIG. 1). The localization of the labeled lecithin was further confirmed by electron microscopic radioautography (FIG. 2). The silver grains were seen over the cytoplasm of the smooth muscle cells, but the extracellular material was not labeled. In the atheromatous aorta of cholesterol fed rabbits, concentration of the label was seen over smooth muscle cells of the media (FIG. 3). In the area of transition between the media and the atheroma, label was seen over smooth muscle cells containing numerous lipid droplets. Concentrations of the radioautographic reaction were seen also over foam cells in the atheroma and over extracellular material (FIG. 4). Electron

microscopy of a labeled foam cell revealed that the labeled lecithin
was localized mostly to the cytoplasmic septa separating the lipid
droplets (FIG. 5). These results have indicated that in the normal
aorta the bulk of lecithin is confined to the smooth muscle cells.
These cells participate also in the increased synthesis of phospholipids in the atheromatous aorta. This is a confirmation of an old
statement made by Dr. Parker and many others which I think shows very
well that the synthesis of phospholipids in the atherosclerotic arteries is not limited to foam cells; it certainly is carried out also
by smooth muscle cells and I would like to propose that most of the
foam cells are derived from the smooth muscle cells.

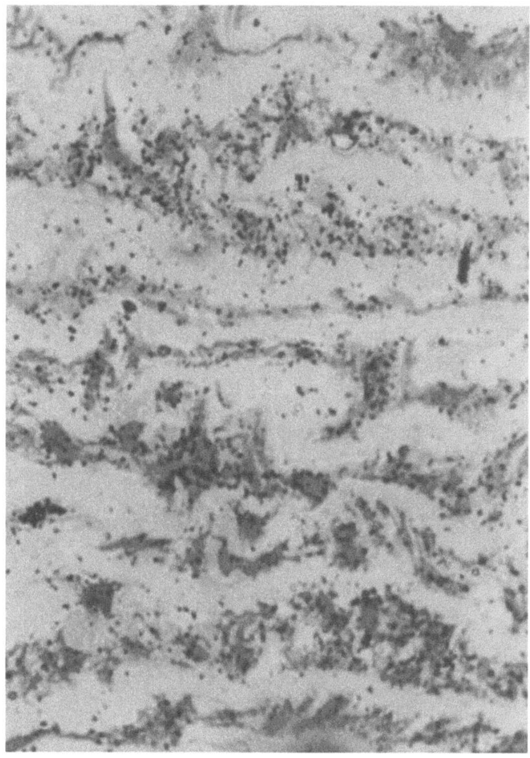

FIGURE 1. Section of normal rabbit aorta labeled by incubation with
choline-H^3. The radioautographic reaction which represents labeled
lecithin is concentrated over the smooth muscle cells of the media
(x 1,000).

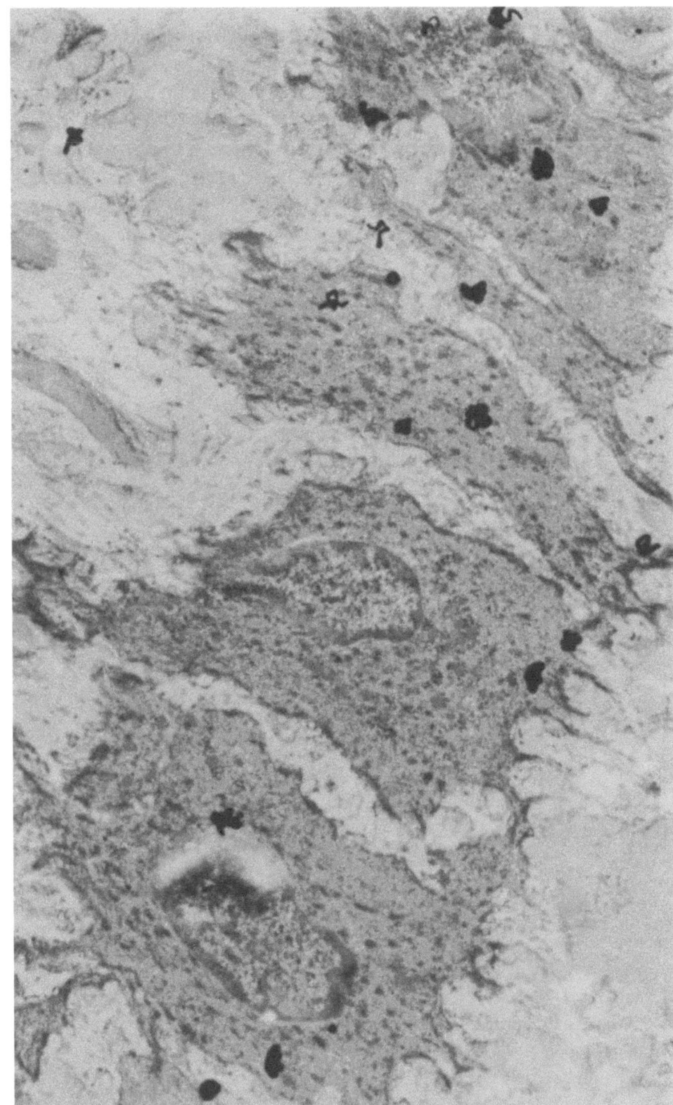

FIGURE 2. Electron micrograph of section of normal rabbit aorta
labeled by incubation with choline-H^3. The radioautographic reaction
is seen over the cytoplasm of the smooth muscle cells. There is no
label over the extracellular tissue (x 12,500).

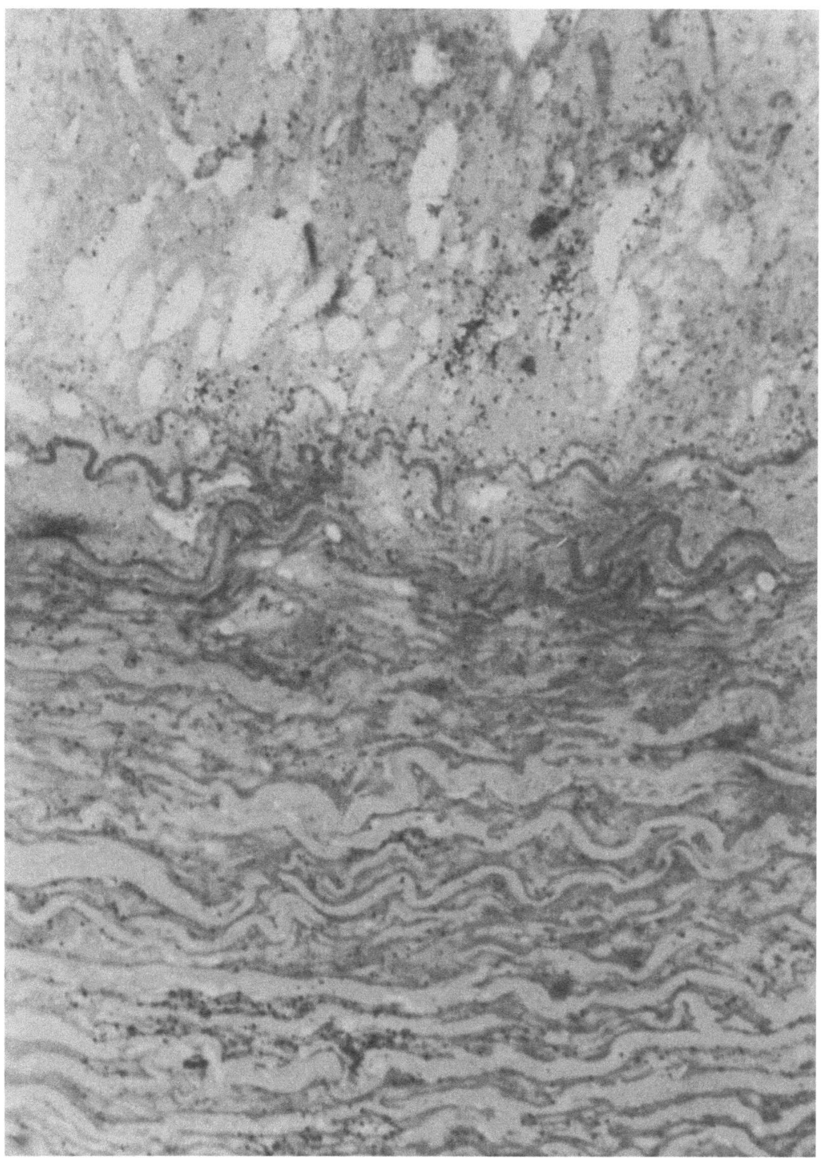

FIGURE 3. Section of aorta of cholesterol fed rabbit labeled by incubation with choline-H^3. Over the media, the radioautographic reaction is localized to smooth muscle cells and there are concentrations of label over some cells. In the atheroma there is both diffuse and focal labeling (x 1,100).

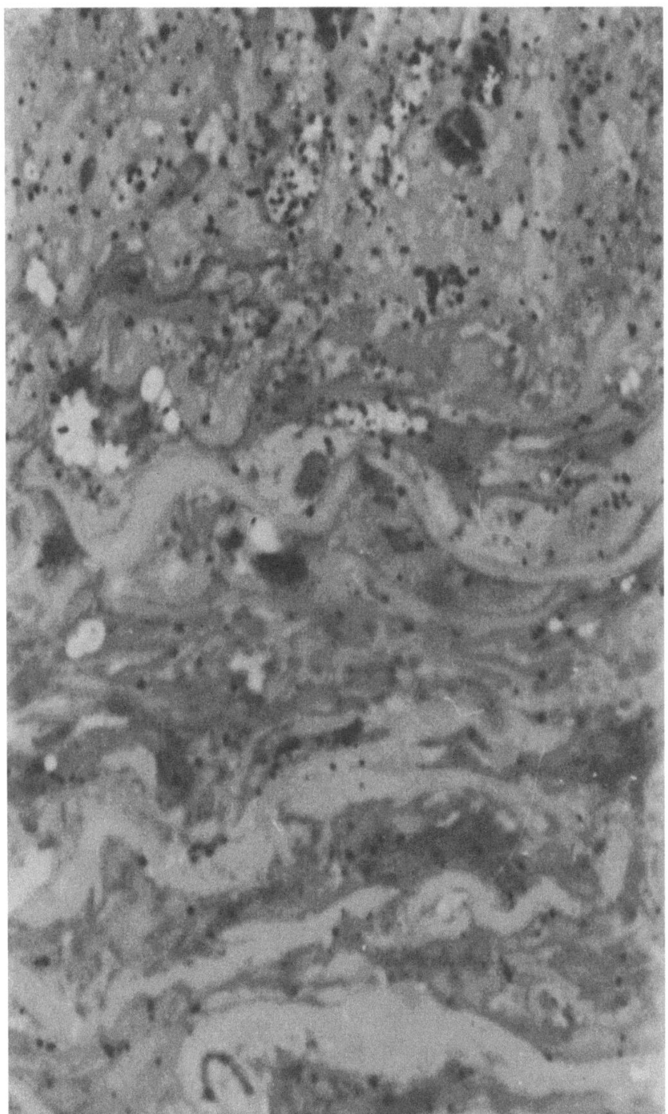

FIGURE 4. Another area from the preparation shown in FIG. 3. Smooth
muscle cells with lipid droplets and radioautographic reaction are
seen in the transition zone between the media and atheroma. In the
atheroma the focal concentrations of label are over foam cells (x2,000).
(Stein and Stein, 1970)

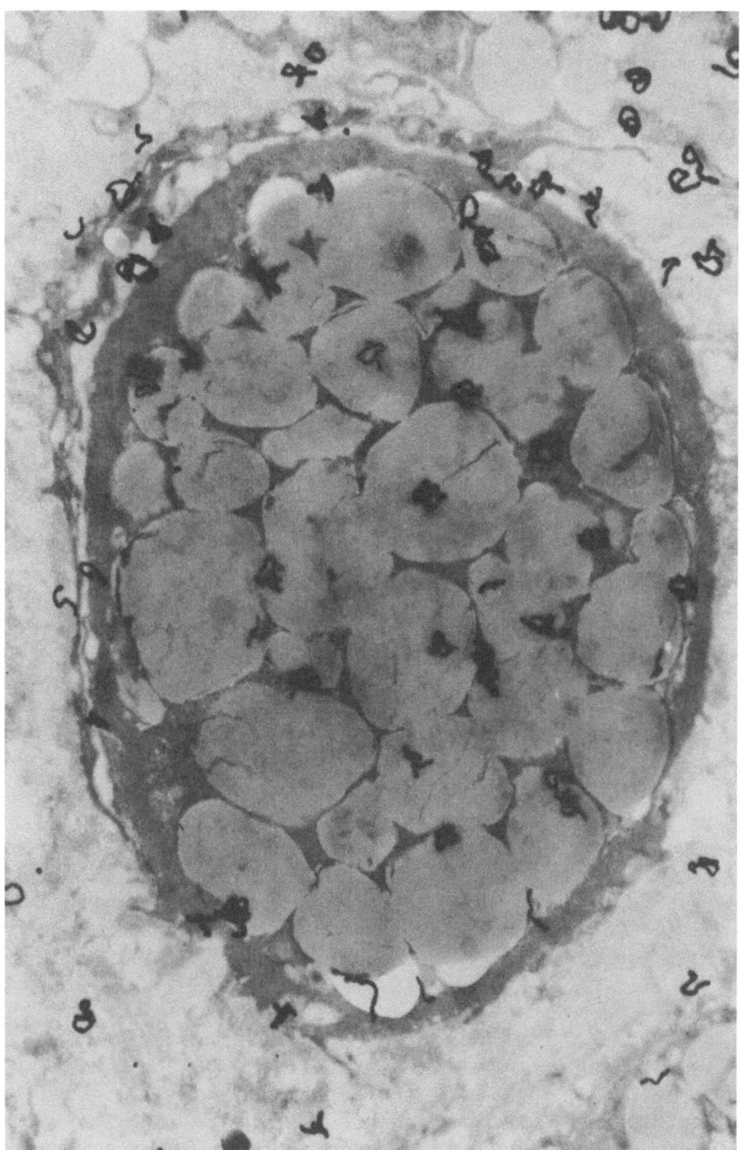

FIGURE 5. Electron micrograph of foam cell in the atheroma depicted
in FIG. 4. Note that the silver grains which represent labeled lecithin are localized to the cytoplasmic septa among the lipid droplets
(x 17,000).
(Stein and Stein, 1970)

DR. GRESHAM: Are there some shreds of elastin?

DR. O. STEIN: Well, this would be very exceptional.   On electron microscope radioautography one can show that the grains which might seem to be over elastin, actually are related to cytoplasmic projections of smooth muscle cells.

DR. WERTHESSEN: Am I correct, Dr. Stein, that this preparation is an incubation?

DR. O. STEIN: Yes.

DR. WERTHESSEN: Therefore the synthesis you see is due to uptake from the medium with no driving force other than that of the tissue, so to speak, "swallowing" the substrate.

DR. O. STEIN: Yes, but similar results were obtained in a combined heart-aorta perfusion system.

DR. LOFLAND: I wonder if I could ask Dr. Day and perhaps also Dr. Stein if they would relate their findings in some sort of temporal fashion to the development of atherosclerosis.   In other words, where are we in this process when you see these events taking place.   I ask this question because quite a number of years ago we observed synthesis of phospholipids and triglycerides and sterol ester fatty acids in isolated perfused aortas of pigeons and non-human primates. It was always our impression and still is that an enhanced synthesis of lipid is a consequence of a lesion already being present.   We have rarely been able to show increases in the early stages of the disease as compared with normal tissue or even slightly diseased tissue.   Perhaps you have a different experience, but I think it would be interesting to put this into some sort of time sequence.

DR. DAY: It would be of interest to carry out studies in which lipid synthesis in relation to different stages of the early lesion were observed.   Unfortunately, our own studies shed no light on this aspect.

DR. O. STEIN: I may try to answer your question.   We have studied the enrichment of rabbit aorta in phospholipids during the first weeks of cholesterol feeding.   We have found that at a time (2 - 4 weeks on 1% cholesterol in the diet) when aortic cholesterol increased from 2.3 to 3.7 mg/g wet weight, there was no increase in aortic phospholipids.   The increase in the latter became apparent only between 4 - 6 weeks of cholesterol feeding, when the cholesterol concentration was increased to 7.5 mg/g.   These findings would tend to support your suggestion that enhanced synthesis of phospholipids in the atheromatous artery is a consequence of the accumulation of cholesterol.

RABBIT

DR. WERTHESSEN: I would like to point out that as some of you
know I am an old hand in this local synthesis business, and as a
result I know that this is a very critical point - When does this
local synthesis occur? When there is a lesion present? In the beginning stages? Just when? Because this will determine the contribution of local synthesis to the development of the lesion.

DR. GUNN: I would also like to add further points to the question: Not only what stimulates or increases synthesis but what in-
hibits it. Does anyone have any information about that? I think it
is equally as important to understand inhibitory functions when talking about a long term process such as atherosclerosis as it is to
speak of excitatory functions.

DR. HAUSS: One of the major mechanisms of inhibition of lipid
synthesis is the presence of fatty acids in this tissue. This is
particularly true for the biosynthesis from acetate, for instance,
and it holds for fatty acids as well as for cholesterol, but mainly
for fatty acids. Cholesterol may be inhibited by the presence of
cholesterol itself. On the other hand, the biosynthesis of fatty
acids and cholesterol from basic material like acetate is very low
in the arterial wall, if you compare it with the amounts of fatty
acids and cholesterol present in the arterial wall in the normal
state and in the atherosclerotic state. I have done many experiments
on early conditions of atherosclerosis and on later conditions of
atherosclerosis and I have never seen fatty acid or cholesterol
synthesis from acetate that would exceed a few millimicromoles per
gram per day. That would mean any accumulation of fatty acids or
cholesterol in the aortic wall exceeding that of normal would take
months to years without any catabolism of these two compounds taking
place.

DR. O. STEIN: I would like to point out that acetate is a very
poor precursor for de novo synthesis of free fatty acids, triglycerides
and phospholipids within the arterial wall. Free fatty acids are
excellent precursors of triglycerides
and phospholipids in the aorta of all
Acetate a poor pre-   mammalian species examined so far (rat,
cursor of lipid   rabbit, guinea pig, dog, human, etc.).
synthesis   The incorporation of free fatty acids
into complex lipids was determined at physiological plasma concentrations of both albumin and free fatty acids as they occur in the different species (Stein and Stein, 1962; Stein and Stein et al., 1963; Stein
and Selinger et al., 1963).

We think that the reason we do not find rapid accumulation of
these lipids in normal aorta is the presence of intracellular enzymes
which hydrolyze these lipids (Eisenberg and Stein et al., 1969a;
Eisenberg and Stein et al., 1969b).

CHAIRMAN WERTHESSEN: With respect to inhibition of lipid synthesis, Dr. Siperstein, who has studied the cholesterol feedback control system, has informed me in a personal communication that while
this holds beautifully in the liver it does not work in the blood
vessel. There is another mechanism which he does not understand.
I'll leave this open but he is one of the authorities on the subject.

RABBIT
DR. BOWYER: In an attempt to illuminate the question of the
role of arterial lipid synthesis in atherogenesis, we have studied
the incorporation of ^{14}C acetate and ^{14}C fatty acid into the lipids
of normal and atherosclerotic rabbit aortas (Bowyer and Howard et al.,
1967; Bowyer and Howard et al., 1968). The aortas were perfused
with Krebs-Ringer bicarbonate buffer containing bovine serum albumin
and radioactive labeled fatty acid or acetate; a schematic diagram
of the apparatus is shown in FIG. 6. After 1 hr perfusion, the arterial lipids were extracted and separated on thin-layer chromatography
into individual neutral lipid and phospholipid classes. TABLE IV
shows the results in μμmoles of ^{14}C acetate incorporated per gram
wet tissue per hour, assuming no dilution of the acetate by unlabeled
endogenous acetate of the tissue pool, into normal rabbit aortas and
atherosclerotic rabbit aortas (animals fed a semisynthetic diet containing 20% beef fat for 24 weeks). The only statistically significant difference was the enhanced incorporation into cholesterol esters in the atherosclerotic aortas. This is in agreement with Clarkson
et al. using a similar system in pigeons and squirrel monkeys (St.
Clair and Lofland et al., 1968; St. Clair and Lofland et al., 1969).
In their experiments the newly synthesized fatty acid esterified to
cholesterol esters was oleic acid. In this experiment no enhanced
synthesis of oleic acid in the atherosclerotic aortas could be demonstrated. TABLE V shows the results of the incorporation of 1 ^{14}C
fatty acids into normal and atherosclerotic rabbit aortas, calculated
in μμmoles/g wet tissue/hr again assuming no dilutions of the fatty
acid by unlabeled endogenous tissue pool. 1 ^{14}C palmitic, stearic,
oleic and linoleic acids were perfused in separate experiments and
in each case the fatty acid concentration was 0.1μE/ml and the bovine
serum albumin concentration 4g/100 ml (0.6 μmoles/ml).

The most striking result is the highly significant increase in
incorporation of the fatty acid into cholesterol esters of the atherosclerotic aortas. Further, there is a greater rate of incorporation of oleic acid than of the other three. Other differences between
tissues are very small.

This result suggests that the turnover of oleic acid in the cholesterol esters of these lesions is greater than of other fatty acids.

A comparison of the rates of incorporation of exogenous fatty
acids into any of the complex lipids with the rates of in situ synthesis from acetate (assuming as a working hypothesis that the mass

of fatty acid synthesized is 1/10 of the acetate incorporation) shows
that de novo (from acetate) synthesis is much slower than 'assembly'
from fatty acid.

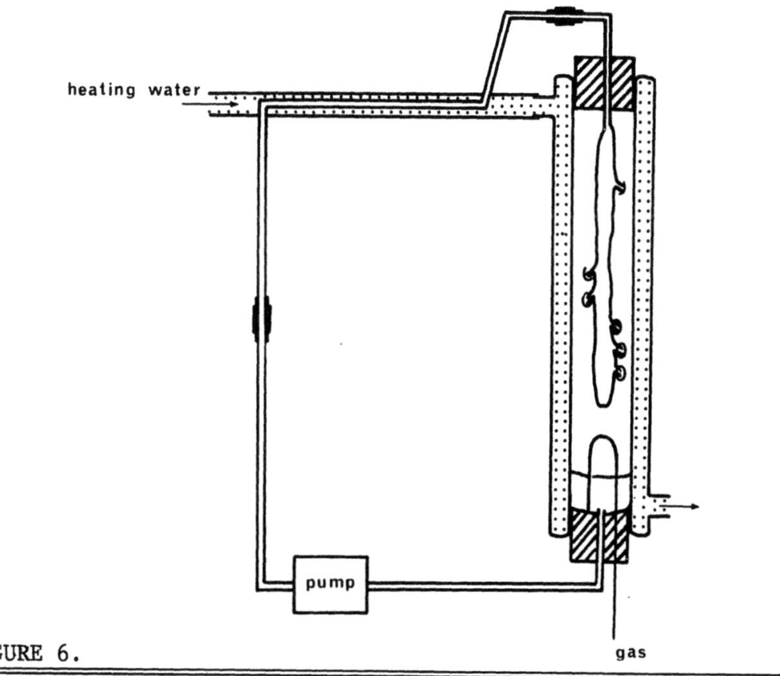

FIGURE 6.

DR. WERTHESSEN: Is it your impression that there could be significant contribution into the cholesterol ester pool by local synthesis.

DR. BOWYER: If we measure the rate of exogenous fatty acid
incorporation in a perfusion experiment and assume that the rate is
similar in vivo (a dangerous assumption) in 24 weeks we would expect
the synthesis of:

        1.3 mg per g wet tissue of cholesterol linoleate
        3.4 mg per g wet tissue of cholesterol oleate

In fact over this period of feeding an atherogenic diet the
amount of cholesterol esters which accumulated were (in mg/g wet
tissue):

cholesterol palmitate	2.0
cholesterol stearate	1.2
cholesterol oleate	9.6
cholesterol linoleate	0.6

It is possible, therefore, that 'assembly' of cholesterol esters
from cholesterol and free fatty acid (whether synthesized in situ or

derived from the plasma albumin) might contribute to the maintenance
of the cholesterol ester pool of a fatty streak. Net synthesis would
be favored in situations where the arterial precursor pool of fatty
acid is increased, such as in stress, after smoking, etc. The balance
sheet for cholesterol ester metabolism by the arterial wall deserves
our close attention.

DR. STAMLER: Does Dr. Bowyer feel that any of these data support
the notion that a fundamental source of lipid (and particularly cholesterol) in atherosclerosis is endogenous synthesis?

DR. BOWYER: The de novo synthesis of cholesterol itself in the
artery is clearly very small. The synthesis of cholesterol ester in
the artery from cholesterol plus fatty acid is larger.

TABLE IV

MEDIAN INCORPORATION OF 1 ^{14}C ACETATE IN μμMOLES/g WET

TISSUE/HR INTO PERFUSED NORMAL AND ATHEROSCLEROTIC RABBIT AORTAS

	Normal	Atherosclerotic	Significance of difference
Number of observations	6	6	
Sphingomyelin	44	76	[1]NS
Lecithin plus phosphatidyl inositol and phosphatidyl serine	3320	2116	NS
Phosphatidyl ethanolamine	213	161	NS
Diglycerides	454	409	NS
Free fatty acids	274	225	NS
Triglycerides	189	162	NS
Cholesterol esters	31	110	P < 0.05

[1]NS – Not Significant

% Radioactivity in newly synthesized fatty acid	14:0	5%
	16:0	66%
	18:0	29%
	18:1	Trace

TABLE V

MEDIAN INCORPORATION OF ^{14}C FATTY ACIDS IN μμMOLES/g WET

TISSUE/HR INTO PERFUSED NORMAL AND ATHEROSCLEROTIC RABBIT AORTAS

	16:0		18:0		18:1		18:2	
	N	A	N	A	N	A	N	A
Number Observations	6	5	6	4	6	5	6	5
Sphingomyelin	38	74*	18	52**	27	62	29	39
Lecithin plus phosphatidyl inositol and phosphatidyl serine	5871	3784	2891	2892	2056	2104	2568	1982
Phosphatidyl ethanolamine	245	203	178	397	269	331	240	283
Diglycerides	548	400	231	233	411	268	418	238
Free fatty acids	1200	3725	1441	6474**	647	2775	575	1678*
Triglyceride	181	615*	99	243	285	814**	289	297
Cholesterol esters	25	404***	2	291***	18	1058***	17	345***

N – Normal, A – Atherosclerotic (fed a semi-synthetic hypercholesterolemic
        diet for 24 weeks).

Significance levels * – P < 0.05, ** – P < 0.01, *** – P < 0.001

DR. Y. STEIN: I am afraid it is not possible to draw a conclusion as to the physiological relevance of these experiments, since
Dr. Bowyer has used a concentration of free fatty acid which is 4-5
times lower than that normally found in rabbit serum (0.1 μmole/ml
as compared to 0.4-0.5 μmole/ml). Since the rate of uptake of fatty
acid is dependent not only on its concentration but also on the fatty
acid and albumin ratio, one cannot extrapolate from the data obtained
what would have been the rate of uptake at physiological concentrations of the fatty acid (Stein and Stein, 1962).

DR. BOWYER: That would mean possibly that these rates would
come into a reasonable range to account for some synthesis, and may
I say that Hashimoto and Dayton (Dayton and Hashimoto, 1968) in an
experiment in which they used elaidic acid in vivo could clearly
demonstrate that about 30% of the cholesterol ester could be accounted for by incorporation of elaidic acid in the arterial wall.

DR. Y. STEIN: Which is an unnatural fatty acid.

DR. BOWYER: Yes, it is unnatural, I would agree with you, but
it lends just a little support to the idea that local synthesis of
cholesterol ester can account for about one-third of what we find.

DR. KEYS: Is there any reason to believe that the rate of degradation is of an order of magnitude different from the rate of synthesis? Presumably there is some degradation going on. Or is it
not conceivable that this quickly attains a state of equilibrium of
which synthesis and degradation are carrying on at about the same rate.

DR. WERTHESSEN: I don't think that our colleagues here can give
us a good number as to the contribution of local synthesis to total
amount of lipid in the lesion. Far less can they give us a good notion as to how much lipid the lesion is extruding. All we know is
that both are going on at once though I don't think we have any solid
data at the moment on the basis of quantity. Am I correct?

DR. HOWARD: I would like to ask Dr. Bowyer if he feels that
the apparent synthesis of cholesterol esters is purely a reflection
of a decrease in lipolytic enzyme activity. In our experiments with
polyunsaturated lecithin (lipostabil) we found that injections of
the drug not only normalized the cholesterol esterase but also the
incorporation of C^{14} oleic acid into the cholesterol esters.

DR. BOWYER: I am sure this question has plagued many people.
When you use radioactive isotopes what you do is to follow the turnover, as it is called, of that labeled compound by both synthetic
and catabolic enzyme systems. If you find an increase in incorporation of a compound you can't immediately say it is caused by
synthesis. It may in fact be caused by a decreased breakdown or by
an altered transport of that compound to the enzymes of the arterial
wall. On the presented evidence alone, it isn't clear which is the
case.

DR. SCHWARTZ: Mr. Chairman, I would like to ask you a question
concerning phospholipid synthesis. Is this a process which is ·specif-
ically involved in atherogenesis, or is it merely a generic response
of cells to injury in this situation? Are we referring basically to
the fact that in atherogenesis there is a population of injured cells,
and that as part of the repair process we have a membrane synthesis;
or is there something quite specific in terms of arterial phospholipid
synthesis?

DR. WERTHESSEN: There is evidence that 99.9% of phospholipids
within the blood vessel are locally synthesized.

DR. WISSLER: In line with Dr. Schwartz's comment the increased
rate of synthesis of connective tissue elements in the early lesions
is almost at the same site as the phospholipid synthesis.

DR. CONSTANTINIDES: As far as increased phospholipid synthesis
is concerned I think it makes very good sense. As Dr. Schwartz has
suggested, the injured and regenerating wall of the artery which is

manufacturing new cells needs a lot of phospholipid. It needs more
internal membranes to make new lysosomes, new enzyme charged membranes
which are presumably consumed. There may very well be a daily turnover rate of membranes. As membranes are consumed they must be re-
generated in a single cell. It would be exceedingly interesting to
carry out the experimental procedure referred to on a healing wound
or on a growing embryo which makes a lot of cells and also in phagocytic cells that you have stimulated by loading them with fat and
thus forced them to make a lot of lysosomes, to make sacks, to make
membranes. Furthermore, it seems to me that the arterial wall is not
so much an Alice in Wonderland tissue, but an intelligent and very
purposeful tissue. As Dr. Bowyer told us, if you load it with a lot
of cholesterol it is not stupid enough to start making even more cholesterol of its own, but it will make fatty acids to couple with the
free cholesterol, which may be toxic. On the other hand, when it is
charged with a lot of fatty acids it will start making glycerol to
neutralize the fatty acids.

DR. GUNN: May I remind the group of what I showed earlier,
namely, evidence that lipid accumulation, presumably lipid synthesis,
is enhanced by denervation. The rates of synthesis of lipid fractions
increased with denervation, including phospholipids which rose from
a control value of 128 counts/mg to 1513 in the denervated artery.
I would like some comment from people as to how the denervation, the
loss of neural control, has excited lipid synthesis. This excitatory
function may be important in the process of atherogenesis. Within
three weeks, one has certainly not produced atherosclerosis but there
is functional evidence of a change in biochemical activity in the artery wall.

DR. SCHLIERF: Is this increased synthesis or is it lack of
removal?

CHAIRMAN WERTHESSEN: There is accumulation manifest by increased count. One has to assume as a first approximation, not proven,
that there is increased synthesis. The work is too early.

If I may sum up, it would appear at this moment that local synthesis of lipid probably can contribute to the atheroma but as of
this time, I would quote a Scottish jury statement, "not proven."
We must leave it at that and perhaps we can delineate some of the
future experiments needed to set up the quantitation which is so
obviously necessary.

Chapter 6

THROMBOGENIC MECHANISMS IN ATHEROSCLEROSIS

PARTICIPANTS: G.V.R. Born, P. Constantinides, J. French, M. Friedman,
               G.A. Gresham, M.D. Haust, K. Laki, C.J. Schwartz,
               D. Sinapius, E.B. Smith, M. Vastesaeger, N.T.
               Werthessen and R.W. Wissler

     DR. SINAPIUS: May I present a few observations on the evolution
of fatty streaks in human coronary atherosclerosis.

     Microthrombi, consisting of platelets, erythrocytes and little
amounts of fibrin are a very frequent finding at the surface of
plaques and thickened intima. Most of these microthrombi contain
various and often considerable amounts of stainable (sudanophilic)
fat. Pure platelet thrombi may show a strong, diffuse sudanophilia,
indicating lipids in a very fine dispersion. Many microthrombi rich
in erythrocytes contain even more visible fat, forming droplets of
different size. There are thrombi with an extremely high fat content.
The components of such thrombi seem to be completely enveloped by
lipids.

     These lipids do not originate from the constituents of the throm- **HUMAN**
bi themselves; they are rather absorbed from the bloodstream. By
means of histochemical techniques cholesterol and phospholipids could
be demonstrated. These properties point to lipoproteins as the trans-
porting vehicles.

     In the early stage, extracellular lipids are phagocytized by
endothelial cells or (probably) by monocytes, thus being transformed
into lipophages. Occasionally clusters of such lipophages, surrounded by platelets and erythrocytes, adhere to the endothelial surface.

Microthrombi, lipophages and the remaining adsorbed extracellular lipids are covered by a new endothelium and thus incorporated. Absorption of lipoproteins with microthrombi, phagocytosis and incorporation seems to be an important if not the main process, which forms fatty streaks. Further investigations will be needed to clarify whether this mechanism of lipid entry into the vessel wall occurs in experimental atherosclerosis or lipidosis.

HUMAN

DR. SMITH: I do not think, from a chemical point of view, that it is possible for the platelet to provide the lipid which is found in fat-filled cells. TABLE I compares lipids in platelets with lipids in fatty streaks and isolated intimal fat-filled cells; the cholesterol content of the platelet is very low compared with the cholesterol content of fat-filled cells, but the phospholipid in the platelet is relatively much higher than the phospholipid in the fat-filled cells. If one postulates that the lipid in fatty streaks is coming from platelets it would mean that the fat-filled cells must ingest about 20-times their own weight of platelets in order to obtain enough cholesterol, and then somehow get rid of a vast amount of phospholipid and other platelet material.

TABLE I

COMPARISON OF LIPIDS IN WASHED PLATELETS AND IN WHOLE FATTY STREAKS AND

ISOLATED LARGE FAT-FILLED CELLS FROM HUMAN AORTIC INTIMA

	Concentration of lipid (mg/100 mg dry tissue)		
	Platelets	Fatty Streaks	Isolated Large Fat-filled Cells
No. of Samples	2	8	8
Cholesterol			
Total	3.07	24.4	61.5
Esterified	0.07	19.8	45.6
Free	3.0	4.4	15.9
Phospholipid	13.8	5.8	15.4
Triglyceride	1.3	3.2	7.8
Cholesterol ester[a]	0.1	33.2	76.5
Total lipid	18.2	46.8	115.6

[a]Calculated from the average mol. wt. of the CEFA and the amount of esterified cholesterol.

Furthermore, we have not really found that platelet thrombi seem to accumulate lipid from plasma. TABLE II illustrates the concentration of lipids in small thrombi in contact with ulcerated plaques (samples a and b) compared with portions of larger thrombi overlying intact intima (samples c and d). There is no evidence of lipid accumulation in samples c and d, which suggests that in a and b the lipid is coming from the underlying lesion.

TABLE II

LIPIDS IN THROMBI AND PLATELETS

	Washed platelets	Concentration of lipid (mg/100mg dry tissue) Platelet thrombi				Fibrin thrombi
		In contact with plaque lipid		In contact with intact intima		
		a	b	c	d	
Cholesterol						
Total	3.08	79.5	36.3	2.72	2.63	0.23
Esterified	0.07	30.7	13.3	0.08	0.25	0.09
Free	3.01	48.8	23.2	2.64	2.38	0.14
Phospholipid	13.80	18.4	12.2	10.30	6.00	0.55
Triglyceride	1.26	--	17.3	3.15	2.03	0.73
Cholesterol						
Ester*	0.12	51.4	21.9	0.13	0.42	0.15
Dry weight of tissue analyzed	152.8 mg	8.8 mg	19.4 mg	65.1 mg	19.7 mg	260 mg

*Calculated from the average mol. wt. of the cholesterol ester fatty acids and the amount of esterified cholesterol.

(Smith, 1967)

I think that Dr. Sinapius's observations are of extreme interest, because it makes one think that possibly the platelets on the surface are producing some substance which is stimulating lipid synthesis within the cells. Perhaps this answers my question of yesterday – what is it that makes fat-filled cells fill the cells with fat. Possibly it could be serotinin, or some other platelet material, which is arriving at the surface of the intima.

DR. VASTESAEGER: In connection with the presentation of Prof. Sinapius, such fatty-laden microthrombi may be specific to the pig, as at least I have never observed them in other species, and certainly not in man.

DR. BORN: An important question is whether blood platelets can adhere to absolutely normal endothelium or whether some kind of damage is always necessary. The experimental problem is to establish whether blood platelets adhere to vascular walls which are as nearly as possible undamaged. We apply very small quantities of chemical agents **HAMSTER** by the technique of iontophoresis to small blood vessels in the hamster cheek pouch (Duling and Berne et al., 1968). When ADP is applied to a small arteriole it constricts and, in both arteriole and venule, causes a small platelet thrombus to form. On recent electron micrographs we have found that there is no damage to the endothelial cells to which the platelets adhere other than a decrease in electron density of the cytoplasm. GDP has the same effect without causing the formation of white bodies (Begent and Born, 1970). This may answer Dr. French's question, namely that traces of an agent such as ADP can cause platelets to adhere to what looks like normal endothelium.

CHAIRMAN FRENCH: I would not be absolutely sure that platelets can adhere tenaciously to the surface endothelium, in spite of what Prof. Born has just said. Two problems are still present: first, are you altering the flow locally by inducing vascular spasm by your

injection? And secondly, are those endothelial cells after this treatment really strictly normal? Some of your endothelial cells don't look
quite right but rather pale. We all know that ADP will make a platelet
stick to another platelet. Do you think that ADP can make a platelet
stick to an endothelial cell on the surface of a perfectly normal
vessel?

   DR. BORN: Dr. French is right about the electron micrographs
which were made by his technician, Mr. Shepherd, and Mrs. Begent, who
works with me. I oversimplified: the endothelial cell is not normal
because the cytoplasm is not electron-dense as that of surrounding
cells, but that is the only abnormality one can detect at present.
There is no obvious lesion other than this "pallor" and the application of GDP under otherwise identical circumstances causes this also
without causing thrombi. As for spasm, the vessels are very big compared to the little adhesive white bodies that form in them. Moreover, there is undoubtedly a stationary layer of plasma nearest the
wall of the vessels and many questions now arise about the width of
this layer in relation to chemical agents coming from the wall and to
the size of the platelet. To these open questions we are trying to
find experimental answers. Could Dr. French indicate what pallor of
a cell might imply?

   CHAIRMAN FRENCH: Presumably endothelium can be defective in more
ways than one. It may be absent, thereby exposing basement membrane
and collagen. Then platelets will stick. There is the other possibility that the surface of an endothelial cell which is still in its
normal position may change. The question is, is there something special about the surface of a normal endothelial cell that has to be
maintained, otherwise platelets stick to it and thrombi form. I do
not think that we know this yet. Very tentatively I have suggested
that the layer stainable with ruthenium red may have something to do
with this but it would be nice to know whether that layer is still
present when a platelet appears to stick.

   DR. WERTHESSEN: Unpublished work of a colleague (Dr. Hahn), in
which both Dr. Friedman and I collaborated, showed that the electro-
static charge on glass particles and the length of the particle were
the important variables affecting the potency of such particles to
stimulate coagulation.

   His findings, coupled with platelet size, plus the work done by
Dr. Pool at Oxford at about the same time, led us to consider the
possibility that a prime function of the platelet is to make a quick
repair of a small lesion in the endothelium by being attracted to it
by the aberrant surface charge. This process would not be expected
to proceed to a platelet thrombus if it were "normal." The repair
process would then have a pathological outcome. Small wonder then
that while the idea was intriguing, we did not pursue it further.
We saw no mechanism for stopping the repair system.

Recently, however, I have had the opportunity in the course of
my ONR duties of observing the studies of Dr. Ramwell's laboratories
on the inhibition of platelet aggregation by prostaglandins. These
ubiquitous substances appear to be secreted by hard working or traumatized tissues. They have marked effects on vaso constriction. In
the kidney they are apparently secreted locally to control local
blood flow. Medullin 1 and 2 were their old names.

These recent findings on the prostaglandins, particularly as
regards platelet aggregation, open new areas for study of the role
and control of platelet function as regards endothelial integrity.
I do hope someone will be inspired to followup the implications of
these data.

DR. GRESHAM: The old notion of the thrombogenic theory was that
the thrombus, that is to say platelets and red cells and fibrin, became incorporated into the vessel wall and formed the atherosclerotic
lesion. More recently we have considered the view that platelet thrombi might damage the endothelium and can lead to the atherosclerotic
process.

DR. SCHWARTZ: I believe that one of the problems with relation
to the thrombogenic theory concerns the fact that many people be-   **RABBIT**
lieve, as Dr. French alluded to this afternoon, that the theories of
atherogenesis are mutually exclusive. We have looked at the organization of autologous artifically produced platelet rich thrombi in
rabbits (Ardlie and Schwartz, 1968a; Ardlie and Schwartz, 1968b and
Casley-Smith and Ardlie, et al., 1967) as have Chandler (Hand and
Chandler, 1962) and Still (Still, 1966) as well as a number of other
people. The organization of pulmonary thromboemboli in the normocholesterolemic rabbit results in a series of changes ultimately producing a fibro-fatty plaque. Mononuclear cells early in the organization of such a thromboembolus become foamy, swollen, and vacuolated,
pari-passu with the phagocytosis of platelet material.

At a later stage the lesion shows a dense fibro-elastic cap with
foam cells and fatty cysts centrally. One may also see cholesterol
clefts and calcification. Some lesions closely resemple the atheromatous plaque, or fibro-fatty plaque of man.

The effects of cholesterol feeding in this series of experiments
was to enhance the amount of lipid present, to increase the extent
and frequency of calcification of the fibro-fatty plaques, and finally
to slow down the rate of thrombolysis. In this sense an organizing
thrombus can result in a lesion that has some similarity to the human
lesion. I think it is still worth considering this as a mechanism
that may contribute to the growth of an atheromatous plaque.

DR. WERTHESSEN: May I make the suggestion here that you include
in your design an assay of the local lipid synthesis. I suggest this
because such assay permits analysis of the whole picture. It will be
helpful to know if local synthesis is increased or decreased under
these conditions.

DR. GRESHAM: How were the thrombi produced?

DR. SCHWARTZ: The thrombi were produced in the rotating Chandler
plastic loop using autologous platelet rich plasma or whole blood.
We used both. We obtained basically similar results whether red cells
were present or not. Cholesterol supplements in the diet were not
essential in the production of fibro-fatty plaques.

DR. GRESHAM: Isn't this what Harrison did years ago?

DR. SCHWARTZ: The difference between these studies and those of
Harrison (Harrison, 1948) relate to the fact that the thrombi we used
were platelet-rich. We used the head of the artificial thrombus. I
suspect that if one puts fibrin in, as a number of people have done,
one then finishes up with a lesion which is predominantly fibro-elastic; if you have many of the formed elements, particularly platelets
and leukocytes present, the resulting lesion is a fibro-fatty plaque.
It is possible that the platelets and perhaps also the polymorpho-
nuclear leukocytes may contribute to the lipid composition of these
lesions, together with, of course, the plasma lipid. The relative
contributions of each to the quantitative and qualitative lipid composition of organizing thrombi have yet to be determined.

DR. GRESHAM: Maybe so, but I think basically what you have done
is to injure the intima.

DR. SCHWARTZ: The thromboemboli almost certainly induce endothelial and arterial injury. There is also a spontaneous counter-
part of these lesions, for instance in people who have recurrent small
pulmonary emboli. In examining the lungs of such cases one can in
fact find lesions quite similar to those we have produced experimentally.

DR. GRESHAM: You can also produce the same thing with lycopodium
spores in the pulmonary artery of rabbits.

DR. SCHWARTZ: Yes.

DR. GRESHAM: Does the amount of lipid in the lesions depend on
the level of lipid in the blood?

DR. SCHWARTZ: Yes, except that lipid is prominent in these lesions in the absence of hyperlipidemia.

DR. FRIEDMAN: I must disagree with Dr. Schwartz. We have repeatedly produced thrombi in the aorta of the rabbit, and if that   **RABBIT**
rabbit isn't made hyperlipemic, and if new vessels have not been
brought in from the adventitia to introduce lipid, we find no increase in cholesterol in the thrombotic lesions. Furthermore, after
the entire thrombus has become a plaque, if we then produce another
thrombus on top of or in the plaque itself without feeding cholesterol, in two months there is no lipid accumulation.

CHAIRMAN FRENCH: May I just remind Dr. Friedman, and ask him
for his comment on Crawford's experiments in inducing rather large   **PIG**
mural thrombi in the aorta of pigs. His illustrations, as I recall
them, show a considerable amount of sudanophilic material in the lesions and appear remarkably similar to the so-called simple spontaneous atherosclerotic lesions in man.

DR. FRIEDMAN: I have an idea that the pig cholesterol value is
slightly higher than the rat's. As soon as you add a little cholesterol to the diet of one of the rats, its blood cholesterol may not
go up at all. In other words, if you add to a rat's diet 50 to 75 mg
of cholesterol in the daily diet, the plasma cholesterol might not
rise but an area of thromboatherosclerosis will collect lipid deposits.

CHAIRMAN FRENCH: I think that it is probably clear to everybody
that the absence of lipid in the organized thrombus in the rabbit
probably does not apply to man, because it does not apply to the pig
and the cholesterol values in man are higher than they are in the
pig. We would therefore anticipate that the organized thrombus, whatever way it is produced, would contain lipid in man.

DR. SCHWARTZ: There is one feature of the atherosclerotic plaque
which I believe is present in many lesions, which hasn't been mentioned, namely, the laminated nature of the plaque. This lamination is
present in most coronary plaques, and certainly can be seen in aortic
plaques as well. It can be easily seen with various staining procedures, particularly the elastic and trichrome stains and is a characteristic which led a number of people to suggest that the plaques
are at least in part laid down from the surface in an episodic manner.
I'd like Dr. Constantinides to comment
Explanation of   on the significance of the laminated
lamination in an   component.
atherosclerotic plaque

DR. GRESHAM: Also, I'd like
Dr. Constantinides to speculate as to whether the lamination is built
up in layers from on top downwards or from below upwards.

DR. CONSTANTINIDES: I might say that this lamination is not an
ccident. If all atheromata started as mural thrombi, then you would
xpect that the earliest lesions of atherosclerosis would be thrombi

in various stages of organization (half clotted blood and half collagen), and even more importantly, that they should all be sitting on
top of a normal muscular wall, which they are not. Most of us have
seen that the thrombi always sit on top of a fibrotic and thickened
arterial wall, so while the thrombus undoubtedly adds to the substance
of the atheroma it does not seem to initiate it. It is like a house
with a concrete foundation and a wooden superstructure. It starts as
an injury and repair focus and the thrombus is added on top.

DR. HAUST: Dr. Constantinides questions the role of mural thrombi as the initial lesions of atherosclerosis, because allegedly, no
thrombi can be observed on normal intima. To dispel this notion I
should like to show you some examples of small mural thrombi (microthrombi) composed variably of either fibrin, platelets or both, that
may be observed on normal intima of coronary arteries and the aorta.
Beyond infancy, most of the arteries with microthrombi show diffuse
intimal thickening; as discussed yesterday, the latter is a normal
feature. Moreover, many microthrombi may be found in various stages
of organization.

DR. WISSLER: I would like to propose another mechanism by which
fibrin gets into the plaque. Along with our fluorescent studies of
lipoproteins, albumin and globulins in the artery wall, we also used
pure antibody to fibrin. The only two consistently staining deposits
we would find in all ages of plaques were fibrin and the low density
lipoprotein. This has all been published (Kao and Wissler, 1965).
The fibrin that is there appears to be in the interstitium of the
artery wall. Since then a graduate student of mine, by the name of
Gordon Stoltzner, has carried this one step further, looking for
platelet antigens in the artery wall (Stoltzner, 1968). Dr. Stoltzner,
working with Dr. Dzoga in our laboratory, has produced a very pure
platelet membrane antigen which doesn't cross-react with any of the
other blood elements. They have found platelet antigen in the artery
wall, frequently superimposed on the areas where we find the fibrin
by fluorescence microscopy. At the time of the Chicago symposium Drs.
Levy and Day, from the University of Louisville, presented what I
thought was a very stimulating paper in which they indicated that the
surface properties of both fibrinogen and low density lipoprotein
were quite unique from the surface properties of any of the other
serum proteins that they have studied (Levy and Day, 1970). They hypothesized that there might be a good reason why these two blood elements would be preferentially trapped in the inner wall of the artery.
Presumably it might help to explain some of the perifiber trapping
that Dr. Smith observed (Smith and Slater, 1970b). So I would like to
suggest in the overall development of the filtration theory, if one
wants to use that term, that fibrin may well get precipitated among
the preformed elements in the vessel wall and this may be a part of
the reason that fibrin accumulates with time in the vessel wall. I
don't call this thrombosis, really, as I think it is a different process. It is clotting the fibrin in the wall of the vessel.

CHAIRMAN FRENCH: You say this is an alternative explanation of fibrin being present in the plaque. I think I personally would accept that. This is an extension of the filtration hypothesis, but are you thus implying a rejection of the interstitium hypothesis as also a possible explanation.

DR. WISSLER: In my own experience, based on consecutive autopsy samples of blood vessels that we sampled in a peculiar way, I must admit, sampled so they would be standard, we have seen very little evidence of fibrin forming on the top of plaques except in very advanced lesions (Wissler and Moskowitz et al., 1958). We have seen rare microthrombi, so I think they do occur, but I am not sure how much they contribute to the atheromatous plaque.

CHAIRMAN FRENCH: You did say there were platelet antigens in those particles?

DR. WISSLER: Yes, although this is preliminary data. This part of the study is still in progress.

DR. LAKI: In connection with fibrin being present in sclerotic plaques, I would like to make a brief comment. There are different **RABBIT** ways nature knows how to form blood clots; one is to clot fibrinogen. There are two different ways to clot fibrinogen. The most familiar one is the clot generated from fibrinogen by the enzyme thrombin (Laki, 1965; Laki, 1968). A less well-known clotting process is when a transamidase clots fibrinogen (Lorand and Urayama et al., 1966; Tyler and Laki, 1967; Farrell and Laki, 1970). In lobster's blood, for example, transamidase (transglutaminase) is the clotting enzyme (Lorand and Urayama et al., 1966). In man and in vertebrates, a similar enzyme (transglutaminase) also operates. Its usual function is not to clot fibrinogen, but to connect fibrin molecules in the clot with chemical bonds (Laki and Lorand, 1948; Chen and Doolittle, 1970). Only such a "cross-bonded" fibrin can fulfill its role in hemostasis. If the cross-bonding does not take place, the animal is in danger of bleeding. In addition, the stabilized clot (cross-bonded clot) is also needed for proper wound healing (Duckert and Jung et al., 1961).

Before making some remarks on the possible role of the fibrin clot in atherosclerosis, I would like to say a few words about how thrombin and the transamidase operate.

Fibrinogen consists of three different peptide chains which, in the fibrinogen molecule, appear in duplicates. Thrombin is a very specific, proteolytic enzyme which splits off a portion of two of the peptide chains by hydrolyzing a peptide bond between arginine and glycine residues. Thus, when fibrinogen clots, not only fibrin forms, but also two peptides are liberated (Laki, 1968).

When we see fibrin in the sclerotic plaques, we must also wonder
what the liberated peptides might have done.

The transamidase normally does not clot fibrinogen (although it
can) but connects the fibrin molecules together in the clot produced
by thrombin. This enzyme, instead of splitting peptide bonds, forms
peptide bonds, usually between the γ-glutamyl group of one fibrin
molecule and an ε-amino group of another molecule (Chen and Doolittle,
1970; Matacic and Loewy, 1968; Pisano and Finlayson et al., 1968).

The starting point for our experiments which I would like to
cite came from the consideration that fibrin in the sclerotic plaques
may serve as it does in wound healing.

To ascertain whether plaques contain stabilized clots, we decided
to determine the transamidase content of the plaques. After cutting
out the experimentally-induced diseased portion of the artery of rabbits, we found that the diseased portion of the artery contained three
times as much transamidase as the healthy portion of the artery of the
control animals (Benkö and Laki, 1968). Since the transamidase of the
plasma strongly and specifically binds to fibrinogen (its substrate),
we concluded from these experiments that sclerotic plaques contain
stabilized fibrin. However, these findings do not necessarily tell
whether the stabilized fibrin forms in the plaques to "heal" an in-
cipient damage or a severe damage induces a bleeding. Further experiments will have to decide this question.

One more point I would like to make. When the stabilized clot
is formed, some of the carbohydrate moiety of fibrinogen also becomes
liberated (Bray and Laki, 1968). Thus, when we see a clot we should
keep in mind that we know very little about what the liberated peptides, or the small carbohydrate chains, might do. The peptides have
constrictor activity on the smooth muscle of rabbit arteries and also
potentiate the action of bradykinin (Gladner and Murtaugh et al.,
1963). These peptides may also alter the metabolism of the arterial
wall.

I am mentioning these details because the microscope of the
pathologist does not show them, yet we should keep these in mind any-
time we see a fibrin clot.

COMMENT: Shirley Johnson and associates have reported that platelets are normally capable of entering endothelial cells, becoming
incorporated as part of the structure of the cells and controlling
their permeability.

Chapter 7

ENDOTHELIAL INJURY IN THE PATHOGENESIS OF ARTERIOSCLEROSIS

Opening Address by P. Constantinides, M.D., Ph.D.

Professor of Pathology, University of British Columbia Medical

School, Vancouver, Canada

I would like to summarize the characteristics of atherosclerotic
lesions very briefly and use them as points of departure for focusing
on the forces behind structural changes.

The first problem we immediately face when we start a discussion
of atherosclerosis in man is the problem of the identity of the first
lesions. How do we know that any lesions we choose to describe represent the earliest stages of atherosclerosis?

I think that in the case of a slow disease process that stretches
over decades we must satisfy the following criteria in establishing
any structural changes as the earliest stages of the process: (1) the
alleged earliest lesions must prevail in the earliest layers of time,
(2) they must be generally absent from the later layers of time, and
(3) there must be transition forms between the earlier and the later
lesions. Keeping these points in mind, most pathologists have over
half a century agreed that the earliest lipid deposits appear in certain areas of the arterial wall that show unmistakable signs of injury
and repair (or destruction and reconstruction). Injury is manifest
by various degrees of elastic destruction and infiltration with plasma
proteins, glucoproteins and mononuclear cells, while repair is manifest by the proliferation and longitudinal reorientation of the relatively undifferentiated muscle cells that make up arterial walls along
with the production of new extracellular materials: at first mainly
elastin, later increasing amounts of collagen. The earliest visible
lipids generally make their first appearance in the basal regions of
these injury and repair foci, in three locations: (1) within the
elastic lamella, (2) in small extracellular pools, and (3) within the
cytoplasm of cells (foam cells) that apparently come from two sources:

some of them are local muscle cells while others are evidently immigrant phagocytes that have crept into the wall from the blood, as
shown by the work of Geer et al. (Geer and McGill et al., 1961),
Movat et al. (Movat and Haust et al., 1959) and others. Using fluorescent techniques, Wyllie and Haust (Wyllie and Haust, 1963),
Wissler and Kao (Wissler and Kao, 1962), and Walton and Williamson
(Walton and Williamson, 1968) were able to show that these lipids
include low density lipoproteins and that they are accompanied by
deposits of fibrinogen and fibrin. These first lipid-containing
lesions are what most of us call fatty streaks.

The next basic problem we face here is the question of what
causes what: Does injury cause deposition of lipids or do lipids
cause injury?

While we have accepted for some time the idea that injury favors
the deposition of lipids, there is now growing experimental evidence
that the reverse may be equally true, namely that under certain conditions lipids in turn can injure the arterial wall - whether they
act from outside or inside the wall.

The idea that injury comes first and lipids afterwards was based
on the fact that at first, in the arteries of the youngest persons,
we usually find foci of injury and repair containing little or no
lipid whereas later, in older age groups, we find similar foci containing appreciable and increasing amounts of lipid. This idea has
also received more direct support from animal experiments which I
will discuss in a moment and which have shown that injury - no matter
how produced - enormously facilitates the deposition of lipids in
the arteries of lipemic animals, and that the lesions produced in
this manner resemble human fatty streaks more closely than those produced by any other technique.

The next question we have to ask ourselves is what factor decides
where fatty streaks will occur in the vascular tree. The answer to
this question has long constituted one of the most intriguing phenomena in human pathology and at the same time has provided us with some
of the best clues we possess as to the nature of some atherogenic
forces. For, as we all know, the location of the lesions shows a
striking hemodynamic pattern, i.e. a definite relation to blood pressure and blood turbulence: They always develop in arteries - never
in veins; within the arteries they develop in the large proximal
trunks - never in the small arteriolar twigs; and within the large
trunks they initially appear at certain typical sites which are exposed to highly turbulent flow, as well as to the stress of pulsatile
systolic elongation that Dr. Fremont-Smith (Fremont-Smith, 1969) talked about yesterday, and to the remodeling which results from the much
slower elongation and dilatation of growth that Dr. Gillman (Gillman,
1959) has been talking about for a long time. These sites show signs

of injury and repair even before lipids deposit in them. Finally, the development of fatty streaks is markedly increased by systemic and local hypertension.

I must emphasize, however, that although at first the fatty streaks tend to develop at such hemodynamic stress sites, later they begin to develop in between the hemodynamic sites, in an apparent geographic, i.e. random pattern. In fact, if we just stop and think of it, the majority of all atherosclerotic lesions will eventually occupy the large areas between the relatively small hemodynamic stress sites.

Through what mechanisms do hemodynamic forces promote athero-sclerosis? We do not know yet for sure, but several possibilities have to be considered: Blood pressure could work theoretically (1) by stretching the wall and making it more "permeable" to plasma (Duncan's original idea), (2) by "pushing" the lipoprotein molecules into the wall, or (3) by injuring the wall. While we cannot exclude the first two hypotheses, I hope to present to you some experimental support for the last possibility before I am through. Blood turbu-lence could work theoretically (1) by injuring the arterial wall through a direct shearing effect, (2) by slinging the large lipopro-tein molecules against the wall, and (3) by smashing platelets and leukocytes against it and injuring it through the release of chemicals from the smashed cells (e.g. serotonin or proteolytic enzymes). The first possibility has been recognized for several decades by bio-physicists, the second has not yet been tested to my knowledge and the third possibility has been supported by the recent experimental work of Mustard (Mustard and Murphy et al., 1964) who found that platelets constantly shower down at turbulent sites in artificial circulation systems. Systolic elongation could add to the effects of pressure and turbulence by stretch-injuring those arterial seg-ments which are close to fixed points in the course of the arterial tubes. So much about the fatty streaks.

The next stage is commonly referred to as the "raised plaque." In this phase, the lesion begins to become polarized into two distinct layers: a basal one which represents a region of destruction of the arterial wall and of its gradual replacement by a lipid nest (a mass with at first great numbers of foam cells), and a superficial one which consists of regenerating muscle and elastic tissue, representing apparently nothing else but the creation of a new arterial wall on top of the disintegrating old one - just as new bone forms on top of dead bone in osteomyelitis. We call this superficial layer the cap of the plaque since it sits like a lid over the lipid nest. Up to this point we may say that regeneration has balanced destruction and that there are more living cells than dead materials in the lesion. Were the disease process to stop here we would have no problems.

Unfortunately, the next series of changes leads to the destruction of the arterial wall through three chains of events that take place (1) in the lipid nest, (2) in what's left of the original wall, and (3) in the cap, respectively.

In the lipid nest the foam cells disintegrate and release their lipid contents producing a large pool of extracellular lipid, part of which crystallizes, the so-called "gruel." As Abdulla et al. (Abdulla and Adams et al., 1967) have found, several materials in this pool, notably free cholesterol and certain free fatty acids are very cytotoxic and they apparently destroy the surrounding arterial wall, causing its replacement by scar tissue. Next, the media of the vessel is gradually consumed and replaced by the expanding gruel and scar tissue. When it is completely destroyed, the last barrier between the gruel and the adventitia disappears and the following two things happen: (a) the vasa vasorum can now invade the interior of the lesion, where they sometimes bleed, and (b) the lipids of the gruel finally come into broad contact with the body mesenchyme where they perhaps act as antigens and provoke a lymphocytic rejection reaction directly underneath the atheroma. Finally, the cap changes: its primitive muscle cells start producing increasing amounts of collagen and gradually turn it into dense scar (fibrous) tissue which becomes further stiffened by the deposition of cartilage-like ground substance and calcium. Eventually most of the cells in the cap die and disappear leaving empty spindle-shaped caves behind them so that the whole cap becomes a dead structure, a cemetery. We do not yet know what causes this necrosis. Perhaps the cap cells die because they are cut off from their oxygen supply by the very dense fibrous matrix in which they bury themselves or perhaps they become victims of a chemical or immunological attack - and hypoxia, chemicals or immune insults might also contribute to the necrosis of some of the underlying foam cells. At any rate, at this late phase atherosclerosis can transform the artery from a flexible musculoelastic tube into a rigid fibrous tube with lipid and calcium deposits in its wall, i.e. it can turn a rubber tube into something like uncooked maccaroni.

And it is at this final stage that the disastrous atheroma complications develop: ulceration with thrombosis, aneurysm, arterial blow-out and thrombosis without apparent ulceration. While ulceration, aneurysm and blow-out are easily explained by the necrosis and the structural weakening of the atherosclerotic wall, the pathogenesis of thrombosis had until recently remained obscure. We have had only two real anatomical clues to the nature of arterial thrombosis: the first one was that it occurs only in arteries with advanced fibrous atherosclerosis - practically never in normal vessels - as shown by Strong and McGill (Strong and McGill, 1962), and the second was that it is very frequently accompanied by hemorrhages in the underlying plaques, as shown by Paterson (Paterson, 1938). But the mechanism through which fibrous atherosclerosis promotes thrombosis and the role of the hemorrhages were both unknown.

Seven years ago, following certain clues obtained in animal experiments, we started a complete serial section study of twenty successive coronary thrombosis cases and ten cases of cerebral artery thrombosis and, after examining more than 50,000 sections we found that every thrombus was caused by cracks of the underlying atherosclerotic wall and that most of the accompanying hemorrhages had developed from the entry of blood into the wall through the same breaks (Constantinides, 1964a; Constantinides, 1964b; Constantinides, 1965; Constantinides, 1966; Constantinides, 1967). Most cracks were extremely small, which explains why they were missed in the previous histological studies. If we consider that all studies in the past were made on just a few random sections or at best on step-serial sections at large intervals we will understand that under these circumstances only the largest breaks would be detected - all the small ones would be missed. Similar findings, at least as far as coronaries are concerned, have since been reported by five other workers namely Dr. Sinapius (Sinapius, 1965), Dr. Chapman (Chapman, 1965), Dr. Friedman (Friedman and VanDenBovenkamp, 1966), Dr. Harland (Harland, 1969), and Dr. Schwartz (Schwartz, personal communication). We may therefore conclude that thrombosis in the atherosclerotic arteries of the human heart and brain is initiated by breaks of atheroma surfaces and that the thrombi represent nothing but hemostatic seals for these injuries.

The next big question is, of course, what causes such breaks? Theoretically, they could be initiated (1) by the action of various chemicals on the endothelium and its intercellular junctions, (2) by mechanical forces acting from inside or outside the vessel wall (e.g. the rhythmic kinking of the coronaries with every heart beat which might eventually break these arteries if they become sufficiently brittle) and (3) by spontaneous changes in the atheroma cap itself leading to its increased fragility or disintegration (e.g. the cell depopulation of the cap or the shrinkage and the increasing molecular cross-linkages of collagen with aging).

So much about my summary of the lesions in man. Let us now turn our attention to the mechanisms that create the lesions, the theories about them and the experimental evidence.

The first theory we have to examine is the lipid filtration theory which considers the atheroma as a foreign body reaction in the arterial wall against excessive lipid invasion from the bloodstream.

Traditionally, this concept is based on the assumption that there is a constant stream of plasma from the lumen through the wall into the adventitial lymphatics, supplying the arterial tissue with oxygen and fuel; and that when too many or too large lipoprotein molecules appear in the bloodstream, some of them don't make it a-

cross but get stuck and accumulate in the inner wall; similar results
would be obtained if the wall were to get too thick or too dense for
the passage of lipoproteins.

There are two main arguments in favor of the lipid filtration
concept:

The first one is an epidemiological argument and it essentially
states that populations with higher blood lipids develop more atherosclerosis than populations with lower blood lipid levels, whether we
compare different nations with each other, or different groups of
people within the same nation.

The second argument is an experimental one and it states that
if through some means we produce abnormally high lipid levels in a
great variety of mammals and birds, lipids will eventually deposit
in the arterial walls of these animals (not in their veins) and they
will initially follow a rough hemodynamic pattern, just as in human
atherosclerosis.

For decades two serious objections had been raised against the
validity of this experimental evidence: First it was pointed out
that the lesions caused by hyperlipemia in animals did not reproduce
the features and complications of the advanced human disease - there
was no fibrosis, gruel, capillarization, hemorrhage, ulceration or
thrombosis. Secondly, it was pointed out that, such as they were,
the animal lesions required enormously high lipemia levels for their
production, levels of a magnitude not usually encountered in man.

In recent years, both these objections have really evaporated
because it was shown in a number of species, (including the all important primates, since the work of Dr. Taylor (Taylor and Cox et al.,
1962), (1) that one can reproduce all features of the advanced human
disease if the animals live long enough to develop them, i.e. if the
lipemia is prolonged or intermittent, and (2) that one can produce
atheromata in animals with the help of only a slight lipemia, a lipemia entirely within the human magnitude range, provided their arteries are injured in any of a dozen ways. It has also been shown
that one can even produce thrombosis and wall hemorrhage in such
experimental atherosclerotic arteries if one induces breaks of their
plaque surfaces through various auxiliary procedures (Constantinides,
1965).

Let me elaborate a little further on the role of injury because
I think it is rapidly becoming a factor of key importance.

It has been known for more than half a century since the original Russian experiments of Anitschkow (Anitschkow, 1913), Solowjew
(Solowjew, 1932), Schmidtmann (Schmidtmann, 1929), and others, that

if we injure animal arteries and then expose them to lipemia, lesions
will develop at the sites of injury much faster and at much lower
lipid levels than in intact arteries.

For example, if we take a highly susceptible species such as the
rabbit, we find that while in normal animals it takes an average blood
cholesterol level of approximately 1000 mg% for two months before any
visible lipid deposits develop, in animals with injured arteries lipid
lesions will appear at an average blood cholesterol level of only 150
mg% and in only three weeks (Constantinides, 1965). And if we take
a highly resistant species such as the rat, we find that while in normal animals a cholesterol level of 1000 mg% for two months will accomplish absolutely nothing, injured arteries will develop lipid lesions
with as little as 150 mg% in as short a time as three weeks (Constantinides, 1965). The same thing has been shown for monkeys by Dr.
Taylor et al. (Taylor and Cox et al., 1954).

The whole phenomenon becomes even more fascinating if we look at
it with the electron microscope in more acute experiments. We found
that while after repeated intravenous egg yolk infusions for three
days not a single yolk particles had penetrated into the wall of intact rat arteries, when we injured the vessels of these animals yolk
particles penetrated deep into the wall within five minutes of a
single infusion, and miniature atheromata with groups of foam cells
developed within three hours – in one of the most resistant species
known (Constantinides, 1968).

How does injury accomplish this fantastic acceleration of lipid
deposition? Simply by opening the junctions between endothelial
cells, by creating gaps through which plasma, lipoproteins and even
whole cells pour into the arterial wall.

One of the most urgent problems we now have to solve is the problem of what causes endothelial injury. There is no longer any doubt
about the importance of endothelial damage for both atherogenesis and
thrombogenesis but, at the moment, we know practically nothing about
the factors that produce it. For this reason we have started a systematic electron microscope study of the effects of a great variety
of factors on the endothelium of animal arteries, and I would now
like to summarize some of the results obtained so far before showing
them to you.

Our main method consisted of infusing various solutions directly
into the lumen of a rat femoral artery for 20 min – 30 min, following
this up with a glutaraldehyde perfusion to fix the endothelium in-
stantly, and making transverse sections for electron microscopy. Variations included intraaortic infusion into the streaming blood with a
very thin, hair-like needle and free perfusion of the artery after
distal transsection.

So far, we have studied the effects of general perfusion conditions (such as pH, osmolarity, and anoxia) (Constantinides and Robinson, 1969a), various vasoactive amines (Constantinides and Robinson,
1969b), enzymes (Constantinides and Robinson, 1969c), immune insults
and lipids, among other things.

As far as a pH is concerned, we were quite surprised to find that
the endothelium resisted solutions of increasing acidity down to a pH
value of 4.2 and increasing alkalinity up to a value of 11.0 before
its junctions began to open and its plasma membranes began to break.

As far as anoxia is concerned, the endothelium resisted the lack
of oxygen caused by clamping of the artery for up to 8 hr, but by 16
hr its plasma membranes began to break and its junctions began to
open. KCN produced the same changes in only 30 min.

Of the amines we studied, the most interesting results were those
obtained with tyramine, serotonin, and angiotensin.

Tyramine broke the endothelial cell membranes at a concentration
of 100 µg/ml.

Serotonin caused fluid accumulations within the endothelial and
muscle cells at a concentration as low as 10 µg/ml and at higher dosages it destroyed the endothelium when administered locally, while
angiotensin primarily opened the endothelial junctions and also caused
some fluid accumulations at concentrations as low as 1 µg/ml - an action that may explain the edema of the arterial wall in both human
and experimental renal hypertension. Minimum effective dosages have
not yet been determined.

Of the enzymes we investigated, the proteolytic and some of the
carbohydrate degrading enzymes broke the cell membranes while the
lipolytic ones had no effect.

Of the immune insults we tested, hemocyanine infused into the
arteries of rats previously sensitized to this antigen destroyed the
endothelium within a few seconds.

Finally, of the lipids and lipid derivatives we studied, triglycerides, cholesterol, and lecithin had no effects under our present
experimental conditions, but certain free fatty acids, desoxycholate
and phosphatidylethanolamine caused definite structural changes at a
few times their normal plasma concentration: they loosened or opened
endothelial junctions and caused endothelial contraction or vacuolation
or broke plasma membranes (see FIGURES 1 - 8 for hitherto unpublished
findings from these experiments related to the effects of angiotensin,
immune insult (hemocyanine) and free fatty acids.) The marked stimulation of endothelial pinocytosis induced by free fatty acids (even

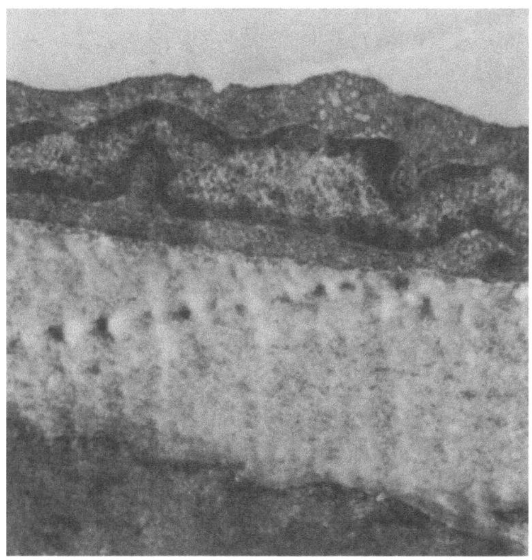

FIGURE 1. Normal endothelial cell of femoral artery attached to the
internal elastic lamina after control perfusion with tween-saline
solvent. The empty space at the top is the lumen of the artery
(x 7,300).

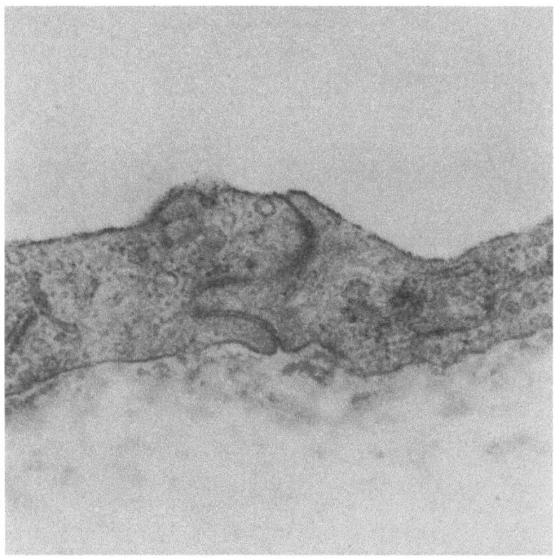

FIGURE 2. Normal (closed) interendothelial junction of femoral artery after control perfusion with tween-saline solvent (x 11,500).

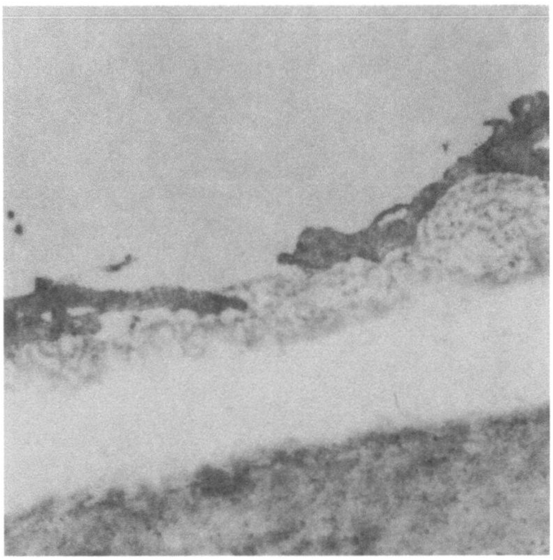

FIGURE 3. Opened interendothelial junction exposing subendothelial
collagen to the lumen after perfusion of palmitic acid, 4 mM/liter
in tween-saline. Note thinning of endothelial cytoplasm and development of a pseudopod (x 6,100).

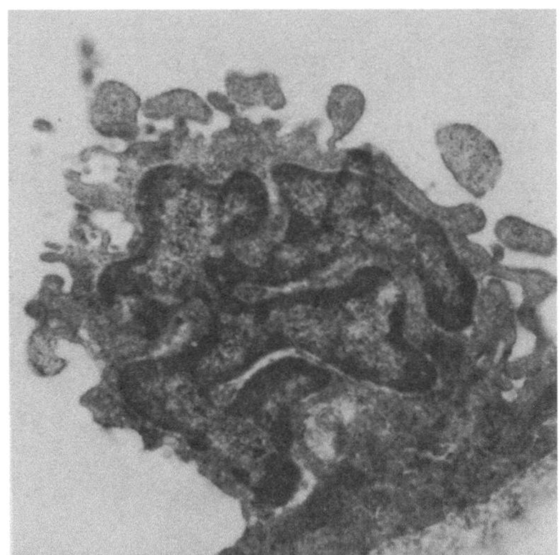

FIGURE 4. Marked contraction and multiple pseudopod formation in an
endothelial cell after perfusion with palmitic acid, 4 mM/liter in
tween-saline. Note the accordioning of the nucleus and the jutting
of the cell into the lumen (x 7,300).

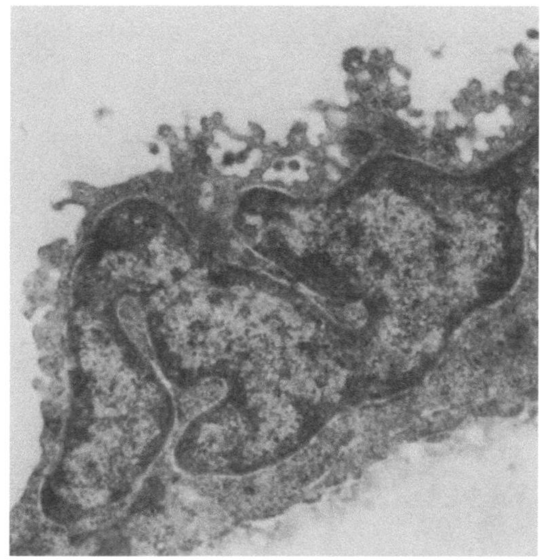

FIGURE 5. Marked pinocytotic activity with apparent confluence of
vesicles at the luminal side of an endothelial cell after palmitic
acid 4 mM/liter in tween-saline (x 7,300).

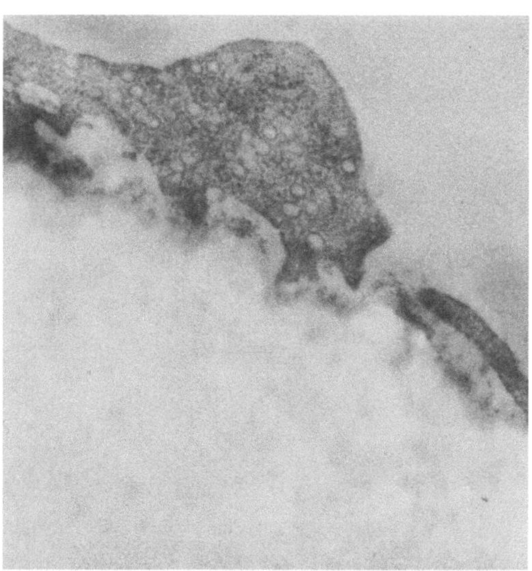

FIGURE 6. Opening of interendothelial junction after perfusion with
1 µg/ml angiotensin in saline (x 7,300).

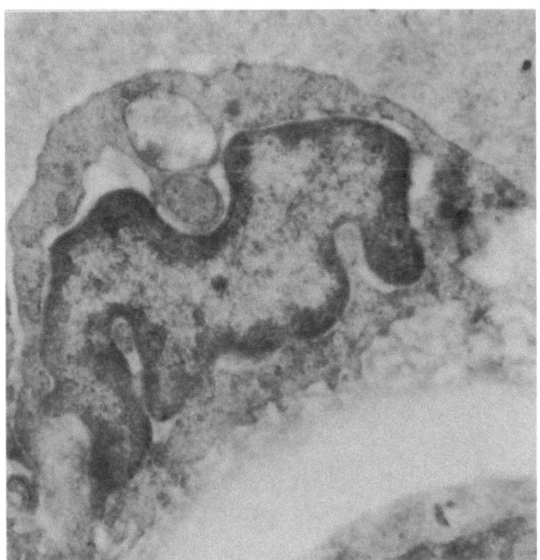

FIGURE 7. Fluid accumulation in the perinuclear space and development of a large cytoplasmic vacuole in an endothelial cell after infusion of a hemocyanine solution into the artery of a rat that was previously sensitized to this antigen through subcutaneous injections (x 7,300).

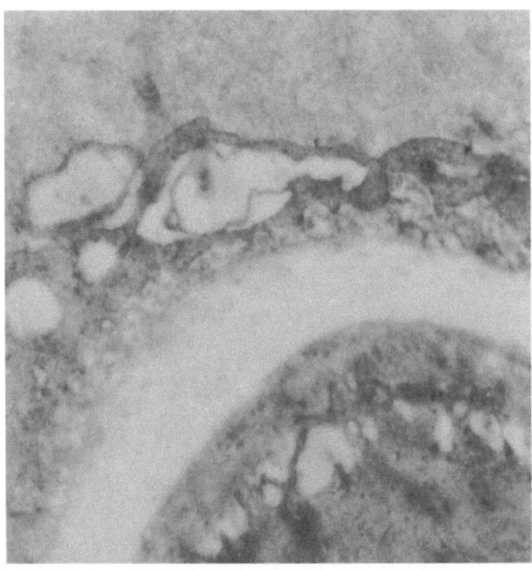

FIGURE 8. Vacuolar destruction and loosening of junction of endothelial cells and vacuolation of the periphery of underlying muscle cells after intra-arterial hemocyanine in a rat previously sensitized to this antigen (x 7,300).

in the presence of excess albumin) supports the hypothesis that the
latter normally cross the endothelium through vesicular transport
and invites further study.

How were the endothelial junctions opened by these various agents?
We don't know for sure yet, but it is likely that in some cases the
junctions opened because of a powerful contraction of the endothelial
cells, a contraction that forced them to pull away from each other,
while in other cases the treatments may have destroyed the "glue"
that binds cells together at the junctions.

I would like to finish the discussion of the lipid filtration
theory by proposing a modification of the traditional model associated
with this concept, a modification which is compatible with the ultrastructural evidence I just showed you, and is also, I think, supported by the recent kinetic studies of Adams et al. (Adams and Morgan et
al., 1970) and of Scott and Hurley (Scott and Hurley, 1970) on the
movements of labeled proteins and lipoproteins across arterial walls.

The old model which was put into a diagram by Page in 1954 assumed a constant percolation of lipoproteins across the normal arterial wall and postulated that when there are too many of them or when
the wall changes, they may get stuck there.

According to the new model we would postulate that under normal
conditions mostly the smaller molecules cross the endothelium by pinocytosis or by squeezing through the endothelial junctions. By smaller
molecules I mean O_2, water, electrolytes, glucose, free fatty acids
and perhaps a few of the smallest proteins and lipoproteins. Most of
the large proteins and lipoproteins and the chylomicrons will leave
the vascular tree the same way they enter it, i.e. by crossing the
very thin perforated walls of sinusoids to get to the liver, the
spleen, the intestine, and other tissues where they are consumed or
otherwise metabolized. When, however, an artery is injured, doors
are opened in its endothelium, allowing the entire plasma with most
of its content (small and big molecules) to pour into the arterial
wall much faster than normally and accumulate there. By "opened doors"
I mean either opened junctions, or gaps due to necrosis and sloughing
off of endothelial cells. Injury, as we have seen, can be caused by
many things, including sterols, anoxia, amines, enzymes, antigen-antibody complexes, certain lipids at high concentration and, as the
studies of Strong et al. (Strong and Richards et al., 1969) seem to
indicate, nicotine. I must emphasize that I regard the above concept
as merely a working hypothesis, to be confirmed or rejected by further research.

Having completed our discussion of lipid filtration and injury,
we may now turn our attention to the next major theory of pathogen-

esis, the thrombogenic theory. According to this concept, atheromata
are nothing else but organized mural thrombi that become incorporated
into the arterial wall. This idea is supported by the undeniable
facts that we sometimes catch mural thrombi in the process of organization, (particularly in the coronaries) and that we often encounter
plaques consisting of several layers, one on top of the other, as if
they had resulted from successive waves of mural thrombosis.

The main difficulty of the thrombogenic theory is the fact that
if it were valid we would expect all the early atherosclerotic lesions
to be mural thrombi in various stages of organization, sitting on top
of a normal arterial wall - which is not true. All the human arterial
thrombi I have seen have always been sitting on top of an atherosclerotic wall with a thick fibrous cap, or on top of a thickened fibrotic
wall, and this seems to be the overwhelming general experience.

Another difficulty of the thrombogenic theory is that it cannot
explain the development of massive lipid gruel in plaques without the
cooperation of hyperlipemia. Experimentally, whenever thrombi were
manufactured and stuck on the arterial wall they invariably turned
into simple fibrous thickenings with relatively tiny amounts of lipid
and at best a foam cell or two. Substantial amounts of lipid appeared in such fibrous thickenings only when the animals were made hyperlipemic - as was shown by the extensive studies of the Albany group
several years ago.

For these reasons we must conclude that mural thrombosis does
not usually initiate the atherogenic process, but that once plaques
are established by other factors, thrombosis most definitely adds to
their growth, often layer by layer. In fact, it seems likely that
as each layer of thrombus is transformed into scar tissue it is bound
to eventually crack and provoke a fresh layer of thrombus, which is
again turned into scar tissue, etc. In other words, we may regard
a thick multilayered plaque as a structure with two components, something like a house with a foundation built of concrete and the other
floors built of wood.

The last theory we have to look at is the lipid synthesis theory
which claims that the enormous amounts of lipids we find in atheromata
have been manufactured locally by smooth muscle or phagocytic cells
that have gone crazy metabolically. I am afraid that I haven't been
able to find any convincing support for this theory so far.

To start with, all data on local lipid synthesis that I know of
have been obtained in experiments where atherosclerosis was clearly
triggered by an exogenous factor, namely lipemia, so any lipid synthesis observed was a result and not a cause of atherosclerosis.

The interesting findings of McCandless and Zilversmit (McCandless and Zilversmit, 1956), Day (Day and Tume, 1969), Dayton (Dayton and Hashimoto, 1968), Vost (Vost, 1969) and others have shown us that the arterial wall replies to lipemic insults in an intelligent and rational manner. If you throw a lot of cholesterol at it, it will make fatty acids to esterify that cholesterol: if you throw a lot of fatty acids at it, it will make glycerol to esterify them; and in response to prolonged lipemia it will make phospholipid to manufacture the membranes it needs for new cells, new lysosomes, new phagosomes, new enzyme-charged surfaces, just like a healing wound or growing embryonic tissue.

Another argument against this theory is the fact that it has not yet been possible to produce atherosclerosis experimentally by any maneuver that would purely turn on local lipid synthesis, without at the same time producing hyperlipemia.

So we end up with the overall conclusion that the only pathogenic forces for which we have good evidence so far are hyperlipemia, injury, hemodynamic factors and thrombosis.

Summing Up
     In 1965 we summarized the main atherogenic forces – as manifest in human and experimental atherosclerosis – in the following crude formula:

$$A = \Sigma(L \times I \times h)t + \Sigma T$$

In this formula $\underline{A}$ stood for atherogenesis, $\underline{L}$ for lipemia, $\underline{I}$ for injury, $\underline{h}$ for hemodynamic forces, $\underline{t}$ for time and $\underline{T}$ for thrombosis.

Looking back at this summary five years later we see that (1) no new factors have appeared on the horizon since it was formulated, and (2) that we have gained some slight insight on the mechanisms of action of some of the already recognized factors. Let's quickly survey the present state of knowledge concerning each one of them in turn.

We know that we can get atherosclerosis with much lipemia (L) and little or no injury (I) as well as with little lipemia and much injury – hence the product relationship between L and I in the above summary.

What can cause arterial injury? Many things, such as calciferol (which could be a very real factor if the cholesterol of our food is turned into calciferol-like compounds by cooking, as Dr. Werthessen suggested), kidney disease, vasoactive amines or polypeptides (e.g. angiotensin, epinephrine), kinins, enzymes, nicotine, anoxia, radiation, and antigen-antibody complexes resulting from (1) vascular antigens (cf. rejection of transplant arteries) and (2) nonvascular antigens (cf. the arteritis of serum sickness and immune nephritis as well as the hemocyanine injury in sensitized rats).

Why does injury promote deposition of lipids in the arterial
wall? Apparently because the normal arterial endothelium represents
a barrier that allows only very few large lipoprotein molecules and
no chylomicrons to cross it. When the wall is injured, however, (1)
the endothelium becomes much more permeable, "doors are opened" in
that it allows large molecules and particles to cross it much faster
than normally, and (2) the wall becomes thickened by the plasma in-
sudation and the growth of repair tissue - which in turn makes it
harder for the immigrant lipoproteins to get out and also diminishes
(through hypoxia) the ability of the local cells to metabolize the
invading lipid.

What hemodynamic forces do we recognize? It seems that we have
to consider under this heading (1) blood pressure, causing a rhythmic
systolic dilation and elongation, and (2) blood turbulence, which has
shearing effects on and hurls particles against certain spots of the
arterial tree. The post-natal reconstruction of the arterial wall,
which is possibly due to post-natal pressure rise in the arterial
side of the circulation and to post-natal growth of arterial width
and length, seems to belong here, too.

The introduction of the factor time (t) in the above formula
indicates that the longer any atherogenic force lasts the more vascular change it produces, while the summation sign (Σ) indicates
that repeated atherogenic episodes cumulate. Finally, the addition
of a second thrombosis (T) term to the (L x I x h) term indicates
that repeated episodes of thrombosis can add to the mass of an atheroma, layer by layer.

One of the most intriguing phenomena about the above atherogenic
factors and one that is coming increasingly to the fore is that they
interact extensively. Thus, there are indications that lipemia itself can act as injury, and thus "open its own doors" into the wall -
as suggested by recent studies of the Albany group (Choi and Florentin
et al., 1969; Florentin and Nam et al., 1969a) and by our own fatty
acid data which were presented at this meeting. Similarly, hemodynamic forces can cause injury, injury can cause thrombosis and there
are data suggesting that thrombosis in turn (at least platelet microthrombi) may cause injury (Moore and Lough, 1970).

In closing, I have this to say: I think that we already know
the main atherogenic factors - at least the prime movers. I doubt
whether in the next ten years we are going to unearth any fantastic
new pathogenic factor. What we need to do now is to explore system-
atically the molecular mechanisms through which these factors work and
also to proceed from their general to their specific identification
so as to develop the most rational treatment possible. Then the ep-
idemiologists will be able to start evaluating the various treatments
in order to determine the most effective ones. Our physicians won't

have to wait for years, however, before they can start proven therapeutic action. On the basis of the evidence we already have it seems
highly probable that if they prevent or eliminate lipemia, hypertension and any known vasotoxic influence (e.g. nicotine) they will be
doing something real towards preventing or arresting arterial decay
in their patients.

Acknowledgement

The experimental findings presented at this meeting were the
result of work supported by the Medical Research Council of Canada
and the British Columbia Heart Foundation.

DISCUSSION

PARTICIPANTS: M. Anliker, P. Astrup, G.V.R. Born, P. Constantinides,
               G.A. Gresham, W.H. Hauss, A.L. Robertson, C.J. Schwartz,
               D. Sinapius, J. Stamler and C.B. Taylor

DR. ANLIKER: The patchy nature of atherosclerosis has been repeatedly related to hemodynamic phenomena, and various theories have
been advanced on the role of blood flow in the genesis of atheroma.
For example, it was hypothesized that atheroma develops preferentially
at those points of the arterial lumen where the hemodynamic stresses
are especially high (Rindfleisch, 1872). In support of this hypothesis it has recently been shown that rather severe endothelial damage can be produced by subjecting the endothelial wall to shearing
stresses of 350 to 450 dynes/cm^2 for periods of one hour or longer
(Fry, 1968). Even shearing stresses of lower magnitude may cause
substantial endothelial proliferation and damage in the chronic situation. It has also been postulated that those areas within the vessel lumen which are subjected to diminished lateral or static pressures are prone to atherosclerosis (Texon, 1957). Texon anticipates
the development of suction forces which tend to separate the endothelium from the vessel wall and which, if excessive, may produce
lesions. Such suction forces are envisioned as the result of a ven-
turi effect between the streaming blood and the extracellular fluid
in the vessel wall behind the endothelium. Finally, the most convincing arguments for a hemodynamic basis for the sites of predilec-
tion of atherosclerosis was given by an interdisciplinary research
team at the Physiological Flow Studies Unit of the Imperial College
in London (Caro and Fitz-Gerald et al., 1969). This team has performed extensive studies on human post-mortem material and also, under
the guidance of Professor M.J. Lighthill from Cambridge University,
on the mathematical analysis of blood flow in arteries. From their
studies they infer that early atheromatous lesions are localized primarily where the endothelial wall is subjected to low shear. The
shearing stresses along the wall due to the viscosity of the blood

are interpreted as having an inhibiting rather than a causative influence in the genesis of atheroma. They conclude that shear-dependent
mass transfer phenomena are ultimately responsible for the development of atheroma. Stated in simple language, the Imperial College
team suggests that there is an inflow into the wall as well as an out-
flow from the wall of cholesterol and other substances. Considering
the fact that the arterial wall is capable of synthesizing lipid, including cholesterol, from precursors, we may find an accumulation of
lipid and cholesterol in those regions where the shear stresses, and
thus the mass transfer rates, are low. By contrast, in those areas
where the shear stresses are high the mass transfer between the arterial wall and the blood is facilitated, and the lipid and cholesterol synthesized within the wall is more readily taken up by the
blood stream. Caro et al. find these propositions to be in substantial agreement with their own and others' published observations on
the location of early lesions and with qualitative identification of
regions of low shear on the basis of theoretical fluid-dynamic studies.
Yet there are additional aspects to be examined in the role of hemodynamics in the genesis of atheroma. Aside from the effects of shearing stresses acting on the endothelium taken into account by Fry and
Caro et al. and the possible influence of radial forces (considered
by Texon), we have to investigate what happens to the layer of endothelial cells as a result of the changes in the circumferential stress
(hoop stress) and axial stress produced by the pressure pulses generated by the heart and by the variations in the mean transmural pressure. Naturally occurring fluctuations in mean and pulse pressure
may give rise to wall stress fluctuations producing strains of as
much as 20 to 50%. With the endothelium subjected to such large
strains we can expect a corresponding variation in the separation of
the endothelial cells. It is quite conceivable that any increase in
cell separation may facilitate the passage of lipid and cholesterol
through the endothelium and that excessive separation might cause rupture of the endothelium and thereby produce a lesion. These possibilities suggest that areas of high and low strain in the endothelium
might also have a correlation with the sites of early atheroma. Sites
of excessive or very low strains may not only be defined by the hemodynamics but also by the tethering or anchoring of the vessels, by
non-uniformities in the vessel wall structure, by the anisotropy in
vessel wall material, and by the geometry, particularly at the branching sites.

In view of the complexity of every one of the phenomena and processes involved in the development of atheroma, including aspects of
hemodynamics and tissue elasticity, it is very difficult to arrive at
an incisive documentation of supporting evidence for any theory. We
are still far from a satisfactory understanding of hemodynamics and
have not yet acquired the ability to quantify such small changes in
the hemodynamic parameters as are needed for a meaningful assessment
of the validity of the various mathematical models which have been

postulated for blood flow. The pulsatile nature of the arterial flow,
the complicated geometry of the conduits and the vessel wall motion
due to the elasticity of the system invite approximations and over-
simplifications in the mathematical modeling of the mechanical behavior of the cardiovascular system. Accurate identification of local
variations in wall shear, pressure, wall stresses and strain calls
for more realistic mathematical models. The local variations of most
parameters are likely to be affected by secondary and second order
phenomena normally disregarded in the analysis.

DR. BORN: I would like to make the criticism that all the procedures to which Dr. Constantinides submitted the arterial endothelium
were so unphysiological that they permit no inferences about the behavior of endothelial cells and their junctions under physiological
or even under pathological conditions. For example, it is well established that a man will die if his arterial pH falls below 7.1 from
whatever cause. It seems pointless, therefore, to show that only
with solutions of pH 4.2 or less do endothelial cells and their junctions become morphologically abnormal. The same comments apply, muta-
tis mutandis, to his observations on the effects of osmolarity and of
respiratory inhibition by cyanide. Interestingly enough, there is
considerable evidence that hypoxia alters some permeability properties
of small blood vessels (Drinker, 1959); this would suggest that his
morphological method for demonstrating abnormalities is considerably
less sensitive than the physiological methods used by others.

Similar criticisms apply to his experiments with vasoactive substances including amines and angiotensin. Professor J.R. Vane and
his coworkers in my department are probably the foremost experts on
the concentrations at which these substances appear in the blood plasma under physiological and pathological conditions (Vane, 1969). Examples of the highest concentrations ever observed, even under pathological conditions, are as follows: angiotensin 1 - 2 ng/ml, i.e.
500-1000 times less than the lowest concentration mentioned in Dr.
Constantinides presentation; bradykinin 5 ng/ml; and adrenalin during
severest shock, 20 ng/ml. These values suggest to me that effects
demonstrable by concentrations at least a thousand times higher are
of little if any significance. Thus, choline acts cholinergically
just like acetylcholine, if the concentration is a thousand times
greater, but the natural transmitter at neuromuscular junctions is
acetylcholine not choline. It is axiomatic in pharmacology that high
enough concentrations make almost any agent toxic.

Concerning the effects of lipids, according to Bottcher and Woodford (Bottcher and Woodford, 1961), the concentration of total phospholipid in plasma is 250-300 mg/100 ml; phosphatidyl ethanolamine
constitutes 5-10% of that, i.e. at most 30 mg/100 ml. Therefore, Dr.
Constantinides' use of 300 mg/100 ml is 10 times more than the normal
concentration. The concentration of total free fatty acids in normal

plasma is about 10 mg/100 ml of which about 40% is palmitic. According to my calculation, that is about 25 times less than the concentration used by Dr. Constantinides. Even more important is the fact that phospholipids, including ethanolamine phosphatide, are almost wholly bound as lipoprotein, and the fatty acids are largely bound to albumin. It is not clear how Dr. Constantinides used the lipids, but the degree to which they are bound must affect – presumably diminish – any pharmacological activity they may have towards endothelial cells.

Dr. Constantinides remarks that structural endothelial damage depends not only on the concentration of the damaging agent but also on the time for which it acts is correct in principle but certainly not relevant under circumstances in which concentrations are many orders lower than those which are effective. It is not clear what "potentiating factors" may be.

My other criticism is that Professor Majno has provided sound experimental evidence for the view that the reversible appearance of gaps between endothelial cells is limited to venules and does not occur on the arterial side of the circulation; his evidence therefore supports my criticism that only extremely artefactual conditions will cause gaps to appear on the arterial side. (Recent experimental results of Professor Majno's show, indeed, that even on the venous side endothelial gaps occur only in certain organs and not in all. Gabbiani, Majno and Badonnel on p. 102 of the abstracts of the VI Conference of the European Society for Microcirculation, June, 1970.)

Please let me stress that these criticisms do not in the least detract from my admiration of the beautiful demonstration by Dr. Constantinides of the mechanism of occlusive thrombosis in human coronaries. That work is a most elegant and important contribution to our understanding of this terrible disease.

DR. CONSTANTINIDES: Concerning my findings that endothelial junctions open at pH 4.2 and 11, I certainly never for a moment believed that the streaming blood of a living person ever reaches such extreme values. The reasons I studied the effects of a whole range of pH values were (a) that this might tell us something about the nature of the hypothetical "glue" that was thought to fill the interendothelial clefts, and (b) that this was one of several necessary baseline studies. I had to know what the endothelial effects of certain non-specific parameters of solutions such as pH, osmolarity and temperature were before starting to perfuse arteries with various specific solutions. Most biologists I know would consider this a sound experimental procedure.

Next, my electron microscopic study of the arterial endothelium after various intervals of clamping-induced anoxia was never intended

to compete in sensitivity with physiological permeability studies,
but to complement them; I was searching for ultrastructural changes
that might accompany or help explain permeability changes - particularly in view of the fact that we had very little information on the ultrastructure of the acutely anoxic arterial endothelium before.

I accept Dr. Born's criticism that the concentrations of the vasoactive substances I used so far were unphysiologically high. I must
emphasize, however, that because of the considerable labor involved
I have not yet determined the minimum effective endothelium - damaging
concentrations of most of these agents. It is thus conceivable that
some of these substances may affect the endothelium at considerably
lower concentrations than the lowest I used. As if to confirm this
possibility, Professor Robertson has just informed me that he and his
coworkers at the Cleveland Clinic, using a variation of my perfusion
technique, have now obtained definite ultrastructural endothelial
effects with as little as 10 ng/ml angiotensin, i.e. a concentration
level that is 100 times less than the lowest I used and only 5 times
higher than the highest so far recorded in the blood.

And now we come to the criticisms of my recent lipid perfusions
which were (a) that according to Dr. Born's calculations I obtained
ultrastructural endothelial effects with 10 times normal phosphatidylethanolamine and with 25 times normal free palmitic acid concentrations, and (b) that perhaps some of these results might be due to the
form in which the lipids were perfused.

In the first place, rises of total plasma free fatty acid levels
approaching the order of magnitude I found effective have already
been recorded, e.g. in diabetes, where increments of up to 7 times
normal levels have been reported (Schatz and Williams, 1963). In
the second place, it is evident that anything that can cause structural changes at 10 - 25 times normal concentrations in 30 seconds
could be expected to be effective at much lower concentrations if it
were to act for 30 minutes, hours, days or weeks.

As for the free or bound state of my perfused lipids I could
add that ultrastructural endothelial changes were elicited not only
by free fatty acids but also by fatty acids in the presence of excess
albumin - although distinctly less intensely in the latter case.

Finally, the question of potentiating factors. I will quote
just two potentiating factors that were found to produce destructive
effects when combined with some of the vasoactive substances I studied and thus could, when present, induce these substances to exhibit
endothelium - damaging effects at lower concentrations than the lowest I used in my perfusions:

(1) Neither subcutaneous serotonin nor intravenous calcium glu-
conate have any structural effects on the skeletal muscle of the rat
when given alone, but they induce extensive necrosis of this tissue
when given together (Dieudonne, 1964). Calcium was also found to
sensitize tissues to other monoamines as well as its potentiating
effects were duplicated by vitamin D. The latter finding may have
very interesting implications if we consider the possibility that
we may turn a good deal of our dietary cholesterol into vitamin D -
like compounds by cooking.

(2) Tyramine from aged cheese has recently been found to cause
serious cerebrovascular accidents in persons who ingested it while at
the same time taking amine oxidase inhibitors.

I do not yet know what significance any of the above ultrastructural endothelial findings may have for human arterial pathology.
These studies merely represent initial explorations, to be extended
and, I hope, improved in sophistication with time. I reported them
because I had never seen unequivocal endothelial gaps in animal arteries before and because I thought that some of these results might
be useful to other investigators.

DR. STAMLER: I'd just like to remind the group of two old experiments. The first one was done decades ago by the father of experimental atherosclerosis, Anitschkow, who fed milk to rabbits over a
period of a year and a half. Although the elevation of serum cholesterol was minimal the procedure nevertheless produced atheromatous
lesions. I'm not here stating that injury plays no role. I'm merely
arguing that while injury may accelerate and intensify the process,
it is quite possible with so-called modest degrees of hyperlipidemia
at least in susceptible species or susceptible individuals to develop
atherosclerosis, including severe atherosclerosis. Now if we think
about human beings this is really the nub of the question, because
millions of people develop severe coronary atherosclerosis in the
middle decades of life without severe hyperlipemia. And the first
question is, can we make an experimental model of this, and the
second question is, must there be injury? I don't think there needs
to be injury. Katz and I fed chickens a diet containing 1¼% cholesterol. The birds' blood cholesterol levels increased only from
approximately 100 mg% to 150. Nevertheless in a matter of 9 to 18
months atheromatous lesions developed.

I also would like to defend Dr. Constantinides against the attack of the extremity of his methods, on philosophic grounds. For
years in this field, from Anitschkow on, up until ten or so years
ago, it was argued that all cholesterol feeding was irrelevant because a) it was extreme in the amounts of cholesterol fed, b) the
hyperlipemia was extreme, and c) for a considerable period it could
not be produced in another animal. But all of those problems have

since been solved and if Dr. Constantinides starts to research tissue
injury, intimal injury and its role with relative extremes, I don't
think he can be put down simply if he starts that way, to use an
American youth phrase.

DR. TAYLOR: I feel it should be pointed out that we observed a
proliferative "chemical-type" intimal reaction in monkeys to modest **MONKEY**
elevations of serum cholesterol levels (as low as 250 mg%), (Taylor
and Cox et al., 1962).

DR. ROBERTSON: In collaboration with Drs. R.G. Favaloro, D.B.
Effler, W.C. Sheldon and F.M. Sones we have just completed histochemical and ultrastructural evaluation of symptomatic segmental coronary
artery disease in patients that underwent direct coronary artery
surgery.

We believe that clinical use of selective cineangiography and
autologous vein replacement in the surgical treatment of segmental
coronary lesions provide a unique opportunity for anatomopathological
evaluation of symptomatic coronary disease during life.

Evaluation of specimens from over 150 patients have shown that a)
only 1/3 of the lesions fulfill histochemical and ultrastructural criteria of typical atheroma, b) proliferative inflammatory lesions of
intima and media were often found with small lymphocytes and plasma **HUMAN**
cells surrounding newly formed capillaries, c) prominent adventitial
non-myelinated nerve fibers and arterioles showing medial thickening
were common beneath stenosing intimal lesions, d) type and severity
of coronary artery lesions did not necessarily correlate with those
found in other arteries in the same patient, and e) bilateral ventricular biopsies in the presence of main coronary artery disease showed
that these arterial lesions may occur without involvement of small
intramuscular coronary arteries.

These findings suggest that clinically significant segmental
coronary artery disease may occur without diffuse atherosclerosis
and that surgical repair of main coronary artery lesions may be an
effective deterrent to further ischemic damage to the cardiac muscle.

DR. ASTRUP: Attention has for many years been focused on the
possible injurious effect of nicotine on the cardiovascular system
while the carbon monoxide in tobacco smoke was not considered to have
any pathogenetic importance. In animal experiments, however, it has
not been possible to prove an atherogenic effect of nicotine by itself (Thienes, 1960; Wenzel and Turner et al., 1959). The cholesterol
content of aorta in cholesterol-fed animals continuously exposed to
carbon monoxide for 10 weeks (15% carboxyhemoglobin for 8 weeks, 30%
the last 2 weeks) was at an average of 2.5 times higher than in the
control animals which had not been exposed to carbon monoxide, but

Intimal injury from carbon monoxide and hypoxia
also were fed cholesterol (Astrup and Kjeldsen et al., 1967). By intermittent exposure, 8 hours a day for 10 weeks, to a carbon monoxide gas mixture leading to 20% carboxyhemoglobin concentration, the experimental animals attained as much as 5 times higher aortic cholesterol concentrations than the control animals.

Also without giving the animals cholesterol, it was possible by carbon monoxide exposure to induce arterial lesions as endothelial hypertrophy and proliferation, splitting of the subintimal structure with a tendency to pronounced focal subintimal edema (Wanstrup and Kjeldsen et al., 1969).

Many experimental findings indicate that it is an increased permeability of the vessel walls which explain an enhancing effect of hypoxia and carbon monoxide exposure on the development of atheromatosis. Moderate carbon monoxide exposure (20% COHb) in the course of hours leads to a considerable increase of the vascular permeability for albumin in normal human individuals (Siggaard-Andersen and Petersen et al., 1968). It is known that acute exposure of animals and men to higher concentrations of carbon monoxide (30-40% COHb) leads to congestion of tissues, and a decrease in the plasma volume with increased hematocrit values (Asmussen and Knudsen, 1943). The same occurs in hypoxia, which is known from high altitude expeditions and especially from studies during the Chinese-Indian war (Singh and Khanna et al., 1969).

Studies on human individuals in a low pressure chamber at a simulated altitude of 4500 m, have demonstrated an increased vascular permeability to albumin, of the same degree as at exposure to carbon monoxide (20% COHb). An increased permeability of intimal cells to cholesterol was demonstrated by Robertson in experiments with absorption of radioactive cholesterol in intimal cells exposed to varying degrees of hypoxia (Robertson, 1968).

The binding of carbon monoxide to various enzymes is in competition with oxygen. It should be emphasized that in working cells the oxygen tension approaches zero while the carbon monoxide tension does not change from the arterial values, as no metabolism of carbon monoxide takes place. Under such circumstances the ratio between the carbon monoxide tension and the oxygen tension will therefore become high. This circumstance would be unfavorable for the function of enzymes that require oxygen. The carbon monoxide furthermore influences the oxyhemoglobin dissociation curve by displacing it to the left. Hereby the unloading oxygen tension of blood is decreased and the tissue oxygen tensions are reduced. This has been demonstrated by human experiments as well as by animal experiments and occurs also at low carboxyhemoglobin concentrations (Campbell, 1929; Klausen and Rasmussen et al., 1968).

The well documented increased risk of smokers for getting obliterating arterial diseases should be reevaluated by estimating, in prospective studies if possible, the relation between carboxyhemoglobin levels and the incidence of arterial disease.

A proven atherogenic effect of carbon monoxide exposure in man will be of interest for arteriosclerosis research and may influence the views on etiology and pathogenesis of the disease, especially concerning a relationship between vessel permeability and filtration of lipoproteins into the arterial walls.

TABLE I contains data on cholesterol accumulation in the aortas of rabbits following tissue injury by carbon monoxide and hypoxia. **RABBIT** The protective effect of hyperoxia is also shown.

TABLE I

MEAN OF TOTAL CHOLESTEROL CONTENT OF AORTIC TISSUE

(mg/100g WET WEIGHT)

	1	2	3
Experimental group (n=12)	1774	1399	303
Control group (n=12)	703	412	596
Significance	$p < 0.001$	$p < 0.001$	$p < 0.001$

1. Cholesterol feeding and moderate carbon monoxide exposure for 10 weeks.
2. Cholesterol feeding and hypoxia (10% O_2 in N_2)
3. Cholesterol feeding and hyperoxia (28% O_2 in N_2)

DR. GRESHAM: Many of us who have worked in this experimental field have come to recognize fatty streaks as the earliest stage in the development of atherosclerosis. May I ask Colin Schwartz to propound a view which he and Mitchell put forward that this was not so on the grounds that the distribution of fatty streaks was different from the distribution of more advanced lesions in the human arterial tree. Can the belief that fatty streaks are the initial lesion be reconciled with the theory that endothelial injury is primary?

DR. SCHWARTZ: I'm not sure that one can answer this question with certainty. There are, however, certain features of the distribution and behavior of fatty streaks which should be considered. In looking at pediatric aortas one of

the most striking features is the early and almost universal development of fatty streaks within the first year of life (Schwartz and
Ardlie et al., 1967). This fatty streaking first appears in the
aortic sinus of Valsalva region, and subsequently in other areas of
the thoracic arch. (Schwartz and Ardlie et al., 1967). In the aortic
valve ring region the extent of fatty streaking shows little progression with age, and the subsequent development of fibrous plaques is
minimal. In other words, the early development of fatty streaking
is not necessarily associated with the early or late development of
fibrous plaques.

There are other characteristic differences. In children and
young adults the areas immediately below the intercostal ostia are
usually free of fatty streaking, although these sites characteristi-
cally develop fibrous plaques (Schwartz and Mitchell, 1962). Moreover, we have found, for both the aorta and coronary arteries (Mitchell
and Schwartz et al., 1964; Schwartz and Stenhouse et al., 1965) that
the extent of arterial surface covered by fatty streaking was un-
related statistically to age, or diastolic blood pressure levels,
whereas the extent of raised lesions (fibrous plaques) did show a significant positive correlation with these variates. Thus, on the basis
of differences in topography and subsequent lesion development, and
also on the basis of differences in behavior in relationship to age
and blood pressure levels, I would tentatively conclude that fatty
streaking is not necessarily the precursor of the fibrous plaques,
or alternatively that not all fatty streaks need evolve into fibrous
plaques. It is quite possible the factors responsible for the development of and subsequent evolution of fatty streaks may be different.

MONKEY DR. TAYLOR: I think that one of the best experimental studies
providing evidence that foam cell lesions can regress is the study
of Armstrong, Warner and Connor (Armstrong and Warner et al., 1970).
Significant coronary atheromatosis was induced by feeding Rhesus
monkeys a high-fat, high-cholesterol diet for 17 months. Much smaller
fibrotic lesions (average cross-sectional area of lumen was 80% greater) were observed in regression in animals which had been subsequently fed a cholesterol-free diet for 40 months. It would appear that
uncomplicated (principally foam cell) atheromata can regress in the
presence of low normal serum cholesterol levels.

DR. SINAPIUS: We have not yet had an answer to the question of
Dr. Gresham whether fatty streaks constitute the earliest lesion of
atherosclerosis.

DR. GRESHAM: I think we've done remarkably well really, and I
think the conclusion we might have reached is that one needs to look
at the premorphological state, that is to say the biochemical processes that precede the appearance of a lesion.

DR. HAUSS: I do not believe that a biochemical change is the
beginning of atherosclerosis. The first step is injury and I think
the best experiments were related by Dr. Constantinides. He couldn't
make atherosclerosis with only a high level of lipids in the blood.
But with an injury, a mesenchymal reaction in the wall, he produced
atherosclerosis. Not alone the fat but this mesenchymal reaction
is required.

DR. SCHWARTZ: I would like to suggest that injury can cover a
very wide range of changes in the vessel wall from gross endothelial
disruption down to subtle changes in membranes, and in the intracellular organelles. When we consider certain characteristics of
atheroma, in particular its consistent pattern of localization, we
should seriously consider the possibility that we are dealing with
a process of subtle and continuous endothelial injury, perhaps relating to and mediated by the pattern of blood flow in arteries. In
this context I should like to refer briefly to some experiments that
we have been doing in young pigs on a normal diet. These animals
weigh about 30 lbs, and are only some 6-8 weeks of age. The protein-
binding azo dye Evans Blue was used to identify areas of increased
accumulation of protein in the arterial wall. This model was first
described by Mustard and Packham (Packham and Rowsell et al., 1967).
They showed that with this technique, one can define focal areas of
blue accumulation which correlate with areas of I^{135} albumin accumulation in the aorta. We have used this approach to study the uptake
of isotopically labeled ($^{3}HevC^{14}$) cholesterol in the aorta of the
pig. Three hours after the intravenous injection of Evans Blue, a
characteristic and focal accumulation of this dye in the aorta can
be seen. These zones of blueing are the zones which subsequently
become areas where lipid accumulates either spontaneously or experimentally in older animals. Blue and white aortic segments were removed, extracted, and the cholesterol activity in the blue and white
areas expressed as dpm/100 mg dry weight (Schwartz and Nishizawa
et al., 1968). We observed that the white zones have significantly
less activity than the blue zones. Using the Evans Blue technique
to define focal areas of aortic uptake accumulation of arterial cholesterol in normocholesteremic pigs that have been subjected to no
dietary or other manipulation, the difference between blue and white
areas is apparent histologically. In other words, in normal untreated
animals one can identify focal areas of high cholesterol uptake, and
in these areas there are already some structural changes present within the aortic endothelium and intima. These changes have also been
studied with the electron microscope and again there are subtle but
definite differences in the endothelial structure of these blue zones.
We believe that the cholesterol uptake in both blue and white areas
is due to transport from serum lipoprotein, and I think that we should
address ourselves to the problems of how is the cholesterol transport-
ed; which, if any, are the specific lipoproteins that donate cholesterol to these areas? How does cholesterol or lipoprotein get across

cellular membranes and into cells? What happens to it once it gets
there, and then perhaps how does thrombosis influence this process?
We know that in these blue zones, from the work of Mustard (Packham
and Rowsell et al., 1967) there is indeed a high frequency, of endothelial platelet microthrombi in these blue areas. The possibility
that at least part of the endothelial damage may have been mediated
through the release of platelet constituents at these points has to
be carefully looked at.

Chapter 8

THE PROLIFERATIVE NATURE OF ATHEROSCLEROSIS:

ADAPTIVE AND REPARATIVE

PARTICIPANTS: P. Alaupovic, C. Cavallero, P. Constantinides,
               J. French, T.E. Gillman, G.A. Gresham, C.G. Gunn,
               W.H. Hauss, A.N. Howard, G. Junge-Hulsing, K.T. Lee,
               R.M. O'Neal, A.L. Robertson, D.D. Rutstein, J.
               Stamler, C.B. Taylor, K. vonBerlepsch, N.T. Werthessen
               and R.W. Wissler

The concept of a preliminary proliferative phase of the process
of atherosclerosis not necessarily dependent on injury was discussed
by Dr. Junge-Hülsing and Dr. O'Neal.

DR. JUNGE-HULSING: In Chapter 5 we discussed available evidence
of lipid synthesis in the arterial wall. In considering the process
of atherosclerosis it would probably be more pertinent to ask about
the synthesis of mesenchymal substances (for example, mucopolysaccharides, collagen, glycoproteins). These are of great importance for
atherosclerosis and for the aging process of the vessel wall as well.
I would therefore like to call your attention to the changes of connective tissue cell metabolism in aging and atherosclerosis.

In the process of age, you can find some typical changes with a
decrease of sulfated mucopolysaccharide metabolism (FIG. 1), of protein metabolism or in collagen metabolism and activity of the enzyme
PAPS. On the other hand, in the case of atherosclerosis, you can find
a reactive increase of mesenchymal metabolism in the aorta. These results have been confirmed by Dr. Lindner and Dr. Hilz in Hamburg and
Dr. Sanwald of the group of Professor Schettler in Heidelberg (Sanwald
and Ritz et al., 1968).

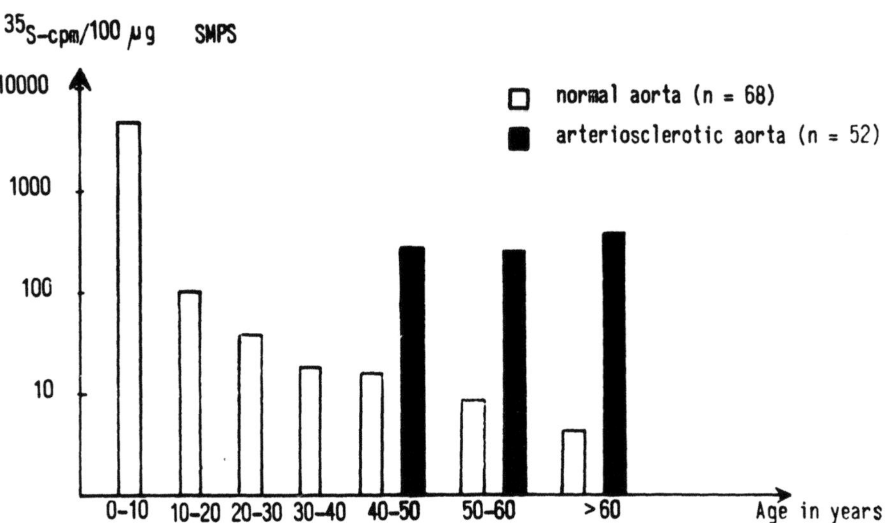

FIGURE 1.   Incorporation of ^{35}S-sulfate into the SMPS of ground substance in human aortas (incubation assays). There is a distinct decrease in incorporation rates with age and a distinct acceleration
of the mesenchymal metabolism in arteriosclerotic aortas.

     Moreover, Dr. Lindner and his group have shown that in the early
stage of atherosclerosis, in the areas with hyaline swelling, the
metabolism of connective tissue is markedly increased; whereas in
areas with severe atherosclerosis with fat and calcium deposition,
there is only a very small activity of mesenchymal metabolism. So
we can conclude that early stages of atherosclerosis are combined
with a typical increase of metabolism of connective tissue and that
this metabolic disturbance is the 'pace maker' of morphological
changes, with increased amounts of mesenchymal compounds in the mesenchymal membranes and the condition for later and secondary fat-
and calcium-deposition, and, as a secondary phenomenon, thrombosis
on the disturbed vessel wall.

     In Dr. Constantinides' excellent address he asks what is the
first step in atherogenesis, and he answered on the basis of his histological methods that endothelial cell injury followed by fat deposition is the first step, the second is repair by connective tissue
and the third step is rupture of vessel wall. Concerning the first
step, we have to consider that aortic walls have a content of more
than 90% of connective tissue, that - as has been demonstrated by
biochemical methods - this connective tissue has a very high metabolic

turnover rate, that connective tissue is a very sensitive reactive
tissue (and not only a tissue of repair), and that in this meaning
the first step of atherogenesis is a primary alteration (i.e. metabolic injury) of connective tissue with a consequent disturbance
in membrane function, and secondarily a deposition of fat, calcium,
and so on. So the question as to the first step of atherogenesis is
not to be answered by histological methods. We have to keep in mind
and look by chemical and biochemical methods to the premorphological
step, to primary reactive injury of connective tissue, and we have
to notice that fat deposition is a secondary step. FIGURE 2 shows
the effect of acute experimental hypertension on connective tissue
metabolism in the aortic wall.

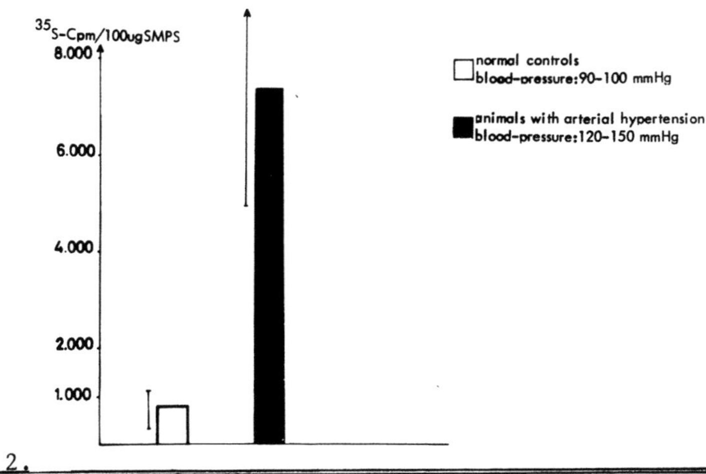

FIGURE 2.

During the first hour of acute hypertension the biosynthesis
of mucopolysaccharides is increased up to sevenfold in the aortic
wall. Up to the fourth hour of hypertension, when connective tissue
metabolism is decreasing, there is no change in the cholesterol content of the vessel wall. Only after 8 and 24 hours can you see increasing cholesterol concentration in the aortic wall.

DR. HAUSS: The structural alterations in the arterial wall are
not only a consequence of increased formation of extracellular substances by the arterial wall cells
Early hyperplastic   but also of cellular proliferation.
changes in arterial   We measured the multiplication rates
wall antedating   of the cells in the arterial wall by
lipid deposition   labeling with ^{3}H-thymidine before
                              and after stimulation. We counted
the numbers of labeled cells in 150 microscope fields in sections
of aortas from normotensive rats. TABLE I shows that multiplication
rate of the aortic wall cells was considerably increased by acute and
chronic hypertension. It is remarkable that this increased cell di-

vision started within 1 hour after the beginning of the arterial pressure elevation (Schmitt and Knoche et al., 1970).

TABLE I

	A Controls	B Acute Hypertension (1 hour)	C Chronic Hypertension (weeks)
Intima	3	14	59
Media	12	136	235
Adventitia	4	218	255

TABLE I. Number of marked cells in 150 microscopic fields in the
aortic wall of normotensive, acute hypertensive and chronic hypertensive rats (^{3}H-thymidine post-labeling method).

After some weeks of arterial hypertension we always found a
broadening of the subendothelial zone due to deposition of newly-
formed ground substance and collagen fibers (FIGS. 3A and B). Moreover in many places there were cells which resembled smooth muscle
cells. We postulate that these new born "multifunctional cells" are
the producers of the newly-formed ground substance and the fibers
surrounding them. Another consequence of the disturbed mesenchymal
metabolism is the malformation of the elastic fibers which became
thin and fragmented (Hauss, 1971).

While the resulting tissue proliferation with increased amounts
of ground substance and collagen fibers is often reversible, beyond
a certain point there is destruction of elastic fibers with permanent
structural consequences. Our work suggests that this proliferative
mesenchymal reaction is the first step in atherosclerosis.

COMMENT

The rapidly developing arterial lesions in steel head trout as
they swim from salt to fresh water to spawn, and the complete reversal
of the process in those that are able to regain their sea water hab-
itat, may be relevant to this discussion of reversibility (VanCitters
and Watson, 1968).

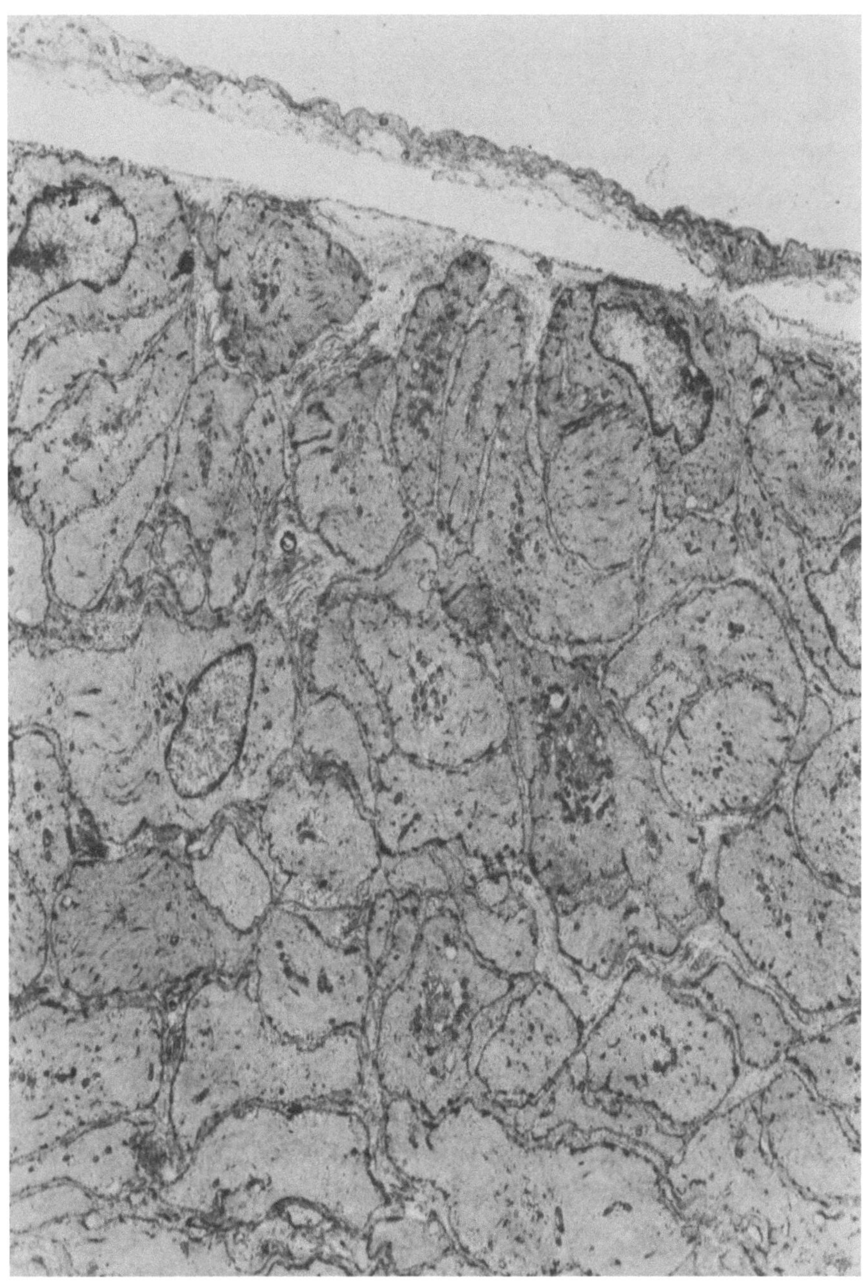

FIGURE 3A. Electron microscopic picture of the coronary artery of
a normotensive rabbit (x 4,550).

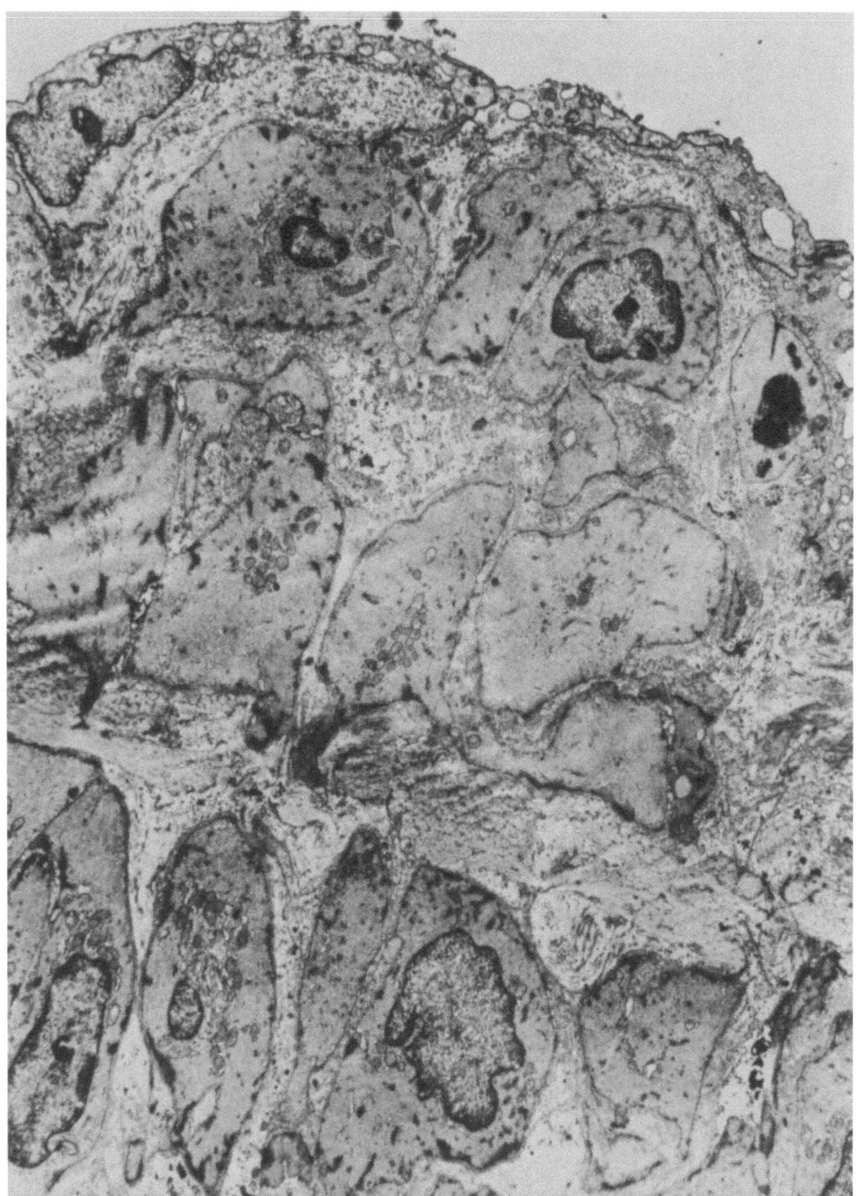

FIGURE 3B. Coronary artery wall of a rabbit, suffering from renal hypertension for 2 months: Many cells, a great amount of ground substance and many collagen fibers are to be seen in the subendothelial area of the intima. The elastica interna is considerably fragmented (x 6,500).

DR. O'NEAL: Whenever "the early lesion" is mentioned, controversy arises. Before we leave this subject I would like to present **SWINE**
some of the recent work of our group in Albany. The cellular proliferation which leads to the formation of the lesion has been so
far largely ignored in our discussions. On the basis of this recent
study, it appears that beginning proliferation, as evidenced by increased mitotic activity, can be detected in swine aorta after only
three days of cholesterol feeding (Florentin and Nam et al., 1969b).
We have studied 92 of these early mitoses in swine aorta by electron
microscopy and find that they are essentially all within cells that
can be classified as smooth muscle cells (Imai and Lee et al., 1970).
Normal young adult swine aortas contain considerable number of mitoses
but the number is doubled within 3 days after institution of cholesterol feeding. I submit that, at least morphologically, this
evidence of proliferation is truly "the early lesion."

DR. LEE: In the past we have demonstrated an increased rate of
[3]H-thymidine incorporation into the aorta of swine fed a hypercholesterolemic diet for one month, suggesting that an increased rate of
cell division takes place long before the development of gross lesions
(Thomas and Florentin et al., 1968). More recently we have studied
the rates of ^{3}H-thymidine incorporation and mitosis in the aorta of
swine as early as 3 days after the initiation of the diet and found
both parameters to be increased as compared to controls (Florentin
and Nam et al., 1969b).

I would like to present briefly some of the results obtained
from these studies. TABLE II shows the composition of the basic **SWINE**
stock diet, and either 8 or 20 g of cholesterol was added for the
hypercholesterolemic diet.

TABLE III shows the results of ^{3}H-thymidine radioautography of
an en face preparation of the abdominal aorta of swine fed the hypercholesterolemic diet for one and three days.

TABLE II

COMPOSITION OF BASIC DIET CONSUMED PER DAY

Ingredients	gms
Peanut Oil	38
Butter	38
Cholesterol	0
Choline Chloride	1
Casein	100
Salt Mix (Wesson)	22
Vitamin Mix (less choline)	11
Sucrose	155
Cellulose	35
Total in gms	400

Total Calories	1704
Fat	40%
Protein	24%
Carbohydrate	36%

TABLE III

^{3}H-THYMIDINE RADIOAUTOGRAPHY
OF EN FACE PREPARATIONS OF ENDOTHELIUM
OF SWINE ABDOMINAL AORTA

AVERAGES

DAYS ON DIET	CHOLESTEROL GROUPS			CONTROL GROUPS		
	NO OF ANIMALS	LABELED CELLS / TOTAL CELLS	% LABELED	NO OF ANIMALS	LABELED CELLS / TOTAL CELLS	% LABELED
1 Day (20 g)	5	393/69,520	0.57	5	242/42,206	0.57
3 Day (20 g)	5	430/39,010	1.10	5	214/41,707	0.51
3 Day (8 g)	4	516/33,078	1.55	3	196/37,308	0.53

In this experiment two different amounts of cholesterol, 8 and
20 g, were given. After one day no difference was observed between
the cholesterol and control groups. By three days significant differences were observed between the two groups regardless of the
amounts of cholesterol used.

However, these increased rates of ^{3}H-thymidine incorporation
cannot be regarded as absolute evidence for increased cell division
(Florentin and Choi et al., 1969). For this reason mitotic activity
was determined after colchicine injection in the aorta of swine fed
the diets for three days.

The results of mitotic counts of the aortic trifurcation region
of swine fed cholesterol for 3 days are shown in TABLE IV. Twelve
swine were used for both the cholesterol and the control groups.
Mitotic counts were carried out in the inner media, subendothelial
intima, and endothelium, and recorded as number of mitoses per 10^4
cells per hour. The cholesterol group had significantly higher values than the control group in all three layers of the aorta studied.

TABLE IV

Mitotic Counts of Aortic Trifurcation Region
of Swine Fed Cholesterol for 3 Days

	Cholesterol (12 swine)		Control (12 swine)		
	Mitoses/Total cells counted	Mitoses/10^4 cells/hr.	Mitoses/Total cells counted	Mitoses/10^4 cells/hr.	P
Inner Media	457/233,492	4.0	253/248,766	1.9	< 0.01
Subendo-thelial Intima	179/104,979	3.2	76/102,741	1.5	< 0.01
Endothe-lium	195/148,432	2.3	82/138,142	1.1	< 0.01

In another experiment we compared the effect of serum from hypercholesterolemic swine and serum from control swine on the DNA synthesis and cell division of primary cultures of aortic intima and media
cells. The cholesterol level used in this experiment was 700 mg% for
the hypercholesterolemic (H) serum and 76mg% for the stock (N) serum.

Two-mm^2 intima-media strips taken from the aortic arch of cholesterol-fed and control swine were sandwiched between two coverslips
and placed in Leighton tubes to which were added a mixture of Eagle's
basal medium and either H or N serum in various proportions: 20,
40 and 80% serum. When daily inspection by phase-contrast microscopy
revealed that new cell growth in most cultures exceeded twice the
area of the original explant, the latter was removed, leaving only
new cells. These cells grew in monolayers. In this experiment,
cells derived from the cholesterol-fed swine (Ht) were grown in the
H serum (Hs) and cells from the control swine (Nt) in the N serum
(Ns).

The results of the radioautography studies of ^{3}H-thymidine incorporation are presented in TABLE V and the mitotic indices in
TABLE VI.

TABLE V

DATA ON CELLS GROWING IN 20, 40 OR 80%
SERUM LABELED WITH ^{3}H- THYMIDINE

Days After Explant	Group	No. of Cells Labeled / Total No. of Cells Counted	% Labeled
8	Nt – Ns 20	671/3,054	22.0
	Ht – Hs 20	629/2,192	28.7
8 (1)	Nt – Ns 40	268/1,741	15.4
	Ht – Hs 40	1,039/3,928	26.5
8 (1)	Nt – Ns 80	537/2,811	19.1
	Ht – Hs 80	499/2,562	19.5

Significance of Selected Comparisons By Chi Square

Ht – Hs 20 > Nt – Ns 20   P < 0.001

Ht – Hs 80 VS Nt – Ns 80   N.S.

Ht – Hs 20 > Ht – Hs 80   P < 0.0001

Nt – Ns 20 > Nt – Ns 80   P < 0.05

On the 8th day the cells from cholesterol-fed swine grown in
20 and 40% H sera showed a significantly higher percentage of labeled
cells than cells from stock diet-fed swine grown in similar concentrations of N sera. Cells grown in 80% H or N serum showed no difference in the percentage of labeled cells.

TABLE VI

DATA ON MITOSES OF CELLS GROWING IN
20, 40 OR 80% SERUM

Days After Explant	Group	No. In Mitosis / Total No. of Cells Counted	% Mitosis
8	Nt - Ns 20	163/9,703	1.7
	Ht - Hs 20	260/7,844	3.3
8 (1)	Nt - Ns 40	125/5,257	2.4
	Ht - Hs 40	119/3,928	3.0
8 (1)	Nt - Ns 80	174/9,110	1.9
	Ht - Hs 80	59/5,139	1.2

Significance of Selected Comparisons By Chi Square

Ht - Hs 20 > Nt - Ns 20 $P < 0.001$

Ht - Hs 80 < Nt - Ns 80 $P < 0.001$

Ht - Hs 20 > Ht - Hs 80 $P < 0.001$

Nt - Ns 20 VS Nt - Ns 80   N.S.

Mitotic indices were greater in cells grown in the H serum than those grown in the N serum with serum concentrations of either 20 or 40%. However, with the serum concentration of 80% the mitotic indices in cells grown in the H serum were significantly less than in those grown in the N serum. Many of the cells exposed to 80% of the H serum were degenerate or dead, whereas those exposed to 80% of the N serum were indistinguishable from those in 20% serum.

These results suggest to us that H serum contains some element that under appropriate circumstances helps to trigger DNA synthesis and cell division in primary cultures of aortic tissue. The proposed substance could be cholesterol per se (which was the only dietary constituent that was different between H and N groups) or an entirely different molecule produced in response to the hypercholesterolemic diet.

As I mentioned in the earlier part of this presentation, in the preproliferative period, prior to the appearance of gross lesions, there was an increase in the rate of entry of aortic smooth muscle cells (SMC) into mitosis. In order to obtain information on the effects of hypercholesterolemic diet on the generation cycle of aortic SMC that might account for the increased mitotic rates prior to the development of gross atherosclerotic lesions, the following study was carried out (Nam and Florentin et al., to be published). The approach chosen was to pulse-label swine aortic cells with ^{3}H-thymidine and carry out grain counts of labeled cells at the out-

set of the experiment (baseline) and after 30 days on either hypercholesterolemic or stock diet. Since with each division of a labeled cell half of the ^{3}H-thymidine would be expected to go into each
daughter cell, a comparison of the grain counts of the baseline
group with those of the two 30-day dietary groups would provide the
number of divisions that had taken place in the two dietary groups.

Eighteen male Yorkshire swine of similar age and weight were
given 0.5 mc of ^{3}H-thymidine per kg body weight intravenously at
the outset of the experiment. Six were sacrificed 2 hours after
injection (baseline group), six were fed a stock diet for 30 days
and then sacrificed (stock group), the remaining six were fed a hypercholesterolemic diet for 30 days and then sacrificed (cholesterol
group). The hypercholesterolemic diet is the same as the stock diet
except that 8 g of cholesterol was added daily. Aortic tissue was
obtained from the trifurcation region of the abdominal aorta and
cross-section histological slides were prepared and processed for
radioautography.

The number of grains per labeled cell in the inner media was
counted by a single observer. The mean grain counts for each swine
in the baseline group were 47, 44, 44, 42, 51, 47; in the cholesterol
group 11, 12, 8, 9, 11; in the stock group 19, 14, 15, 18, 22 (TABLE
VII). The frequency distribution curves of the grain counts for each
group are shown in FIG. 4. The following factors may contribute to
the shape of the curves at 30 days (1) generation time of labeled
cells in the continuously dividing population, (2) drop out rate of
labeled cells from the dividing population into the non-dividing population, that is, labeled cells that remain viable but do not divide
and so retain the same number of grains for the remainder of the experimental period, (3) degree of synchrony maintained by the labeled
population over the 30-day period, (4) death of labeled cells, (5)
migration of labeled cells, (6) rate of re-entry of labeled dropouts
into the dividing population, and (7) reutilization of tritium from
dead cells.

The mean grain counts in the three groups (baseline, 46; cholesterol, 11; stock, 17) strongly suggest that more divisions took
place in the cholesterol group than in the stock group. However, the
means do not permit quantitative assessment of the difference, especially since they are biased by "losses" due to cells that have divided until their grain numbers are below the threshold of count-
ability.

With the help of Dr. John Reiner of our department, who is a
mathematical biologist, a new mathematical approach was developed
for analyzing the grain count distribution data. The aim of the
mathematical analysis is to predict the grain count distribution at
any time after initiation of the experiment, given the initial dis-

TABLE VII

MEAN GRAIN COUNTS PER LABELED CELL IN INNER MEDIA

OF AORTIC TRIFURCATION

	0 DAY	30 DAYS	
Animal No.	Baseline Group	Stock Group	Cholesterol Group
1	47	19	12
2	44	14	11
3	44	15	12
4	47	22	8
5	42	15	9
6	51	18	11
Mean	46	17	10

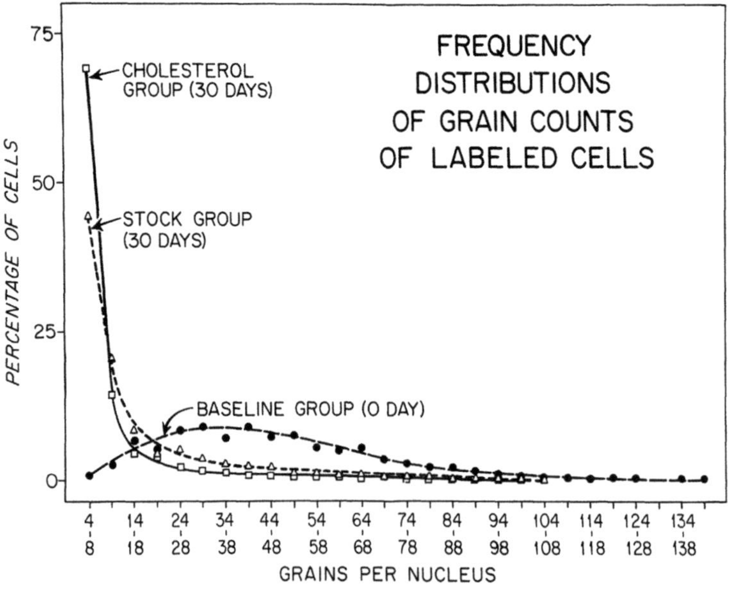

tribution (baseline group), in terms of such parameters as number of generations elapsed, dropout rate, death rate, and so forth. The first two of these parameters proved to be sufficient to fit the data, strongly suggesting that the death rate, at least during the period of this experiment, is negligible, and that re-entry from the dropout population also is either small or absent. Support for the first of these suppositions is given by measurements of ^{3}H-thymidine activity in the aortas of half of the animals at 0 and 30 days; no significant decrease was obtained.

The following is the basic equation to calculate the fraction of dropouts per generation and maximum generation time.

$$N^i_g(\text{obs.}) = 2^i(1-f)^i C^g_i + \sum_{j=0}^{i-1} 2^j f(1-f)^j C^g_j$$

No. of cells   No. of fertile cells   No. of dropout
with g-grains   cells accumulated
at i-generation

The results of the mathematical analysis suggest that hypercholesterolemic diets (1) shortened generation time of the aortic SMC and (2) decreased the rate of dropout from the dividing to the non-dividing population.

DR. CAVALLERO: I would like to show you the results we have obtained in some studies concerning the cellular kinetics of the arterial wall during experimental atherogenesis. Our experiments have been carried out on cholesterol-fed rabbits by using colchicine as a mitosis blocking agent and tritium labeled thymidine as an index of DNA synthesis. Radioautographic visualization of DNA synthesis and mitotic arrest by colchicine afford two relatively simple approaches to the study of this aspect of the problem.

Rabbits fed a cholesterol enriched diet for various periods of time and rabbits fed cholesterol for two months and then returned to a normal diet were used as experimental material. Labeled thymidine was injected one hour before sacrifice intravenously 1 mC per kg body weight and colchicine subcutaneously 1 mg per kg body weight nine hours before sacrifice.

In normal conditions the cellular constituents of the rabbit arteries represent a rather stable population. In animals fed a normal standard diet no colchicine mitoses were seen in several sections of the aortic and pulmonary wall; only exceptionally labeled nuclei were observed in the media after thymidine administration.

Conversely, in the aorta, pulmonary artery and coronary vessels of the cholesterol-fed rabbits colchicine mitoses (FIGS. 5 and 6) and tritium labeled nuclei (FIGS. 7 and 8) were regularly found in

Enhanced mitotic   plaques as well as in the smooth
activity in the   muscle cells of the media. In the
artery of choles-   plaques they were mainly located
terol fed rabbits   in the innermost layers. Colchicine
                                mitoses and labeled nuclei were some-
times found in smooth muscle cells halfway between intima and media.

As to the cellular site of proliferation, it was rather difficult
to establish in conventional histological sections and in radioautographs whether the endothelial cells enter mitosis. In any case, the
labeling of the superficial lining of the plaques was generally low.
Conversely, high numbers of labeled nuclei were seen within the
plaques; the dividing cells were in part spindle shaped cells of un-
determined type, probably myointimal cells; and partly foamy, vacuolated cells and true foam cells.

As to the cell type(s) involved the question arises whether they
are modified muscle cells or macrophages migrated from the blood.
The preferential localization of the label in the most superficial
parts of the plaques might be consistent with the view that they are
mainly macrophages. But we can also suggest that the higher proliferation in this area should be due exclusively to a better trophism
of the cells more directly accessible to the nutrients from the bloodstream. On the other hand, the finding of mitotic activity in the
deeper parts of the plaques, the dividing cells mid located between
intima and media, and the higher numbers of DNA synthesizing nuclei
in the inner media, clearly indicate that also muscle cells are
actively proliferating.

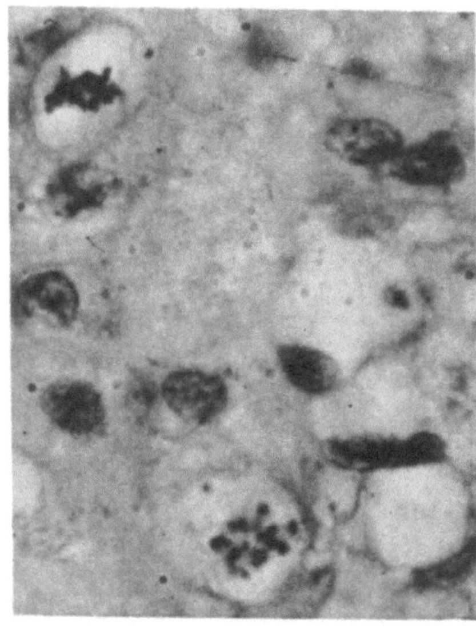

FIGURE 5.

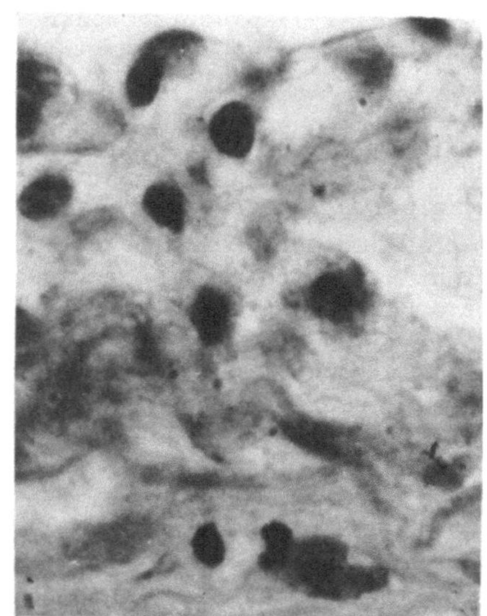

FIGURE 6.

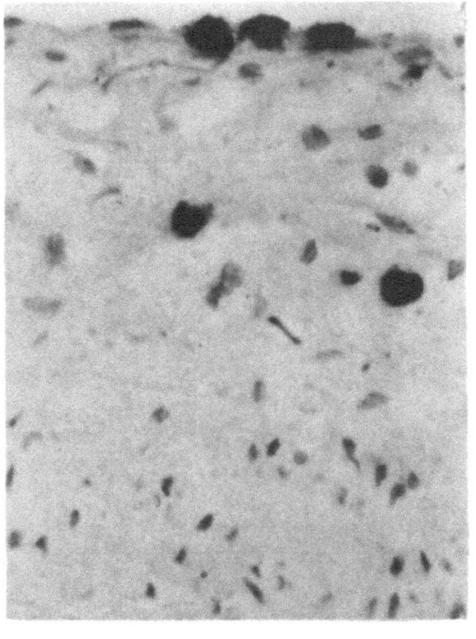 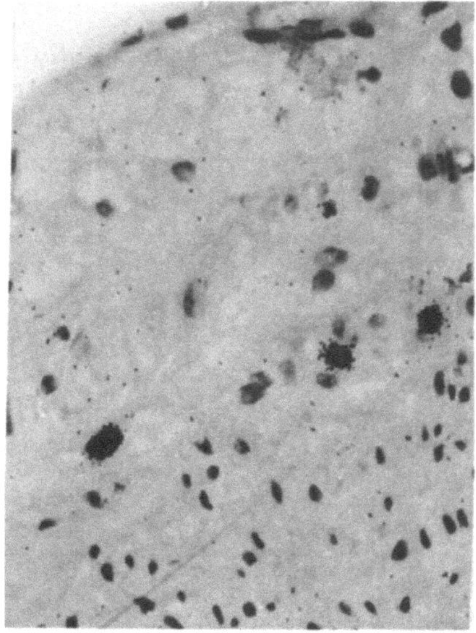

FIGURE 7.   FIGURE 8.

In this connection, we have performed parallel radioautographic
and enzyme histochemical studies of 1μ thick sections of aortic
plaques and we have seen that the
Proliferation   labeled cells were partly esterase-
of muscle cells   positive like macrophages, and partly ATPase-positive like smooth muscle.

In the media colchicine mitoses and labeled nuclei were frequently seen in smooth muscle, but only in those medial regions corresponding to the intimal plaques.

The frequency of the label and of the mitotic index was found
to be closely related to the morphological type of the plaque (TABLE
VIII and IX). Moreover, even after discontinuance of treatment proliferation was still present both in plaques and in the underlying
·media. Active nuclei were found, but evidently in lower number, even
five months after withdrawal of treatment. It is noteworthy that at
this stage plasma cholesterol was returned to normal levels.

From the results obtained it may be concluded that 1) the proliferative changes are a prominent feature of the atherosclerotic
process; 2) that during atherogenesis proliferation seems to occur
both in smooth muscle and in macrophages; 3) that foam cells also
are mitotically active and 4) that the smooth muscle of the medial
coat seems to play a prominent role in the initiation and the evolution of the arterial disease.

TABLE VIII

MEAN NUMBER OF COLCHICINE MITOSES IN VARIOUS MORPHOLOGICAL

TYPES OF AORTIC PLAQUES

Type of plaque	No. of mitoses per mm^2 plaque
Cellular (4 plaques)	24.53 ± 4.70 Range 20.5 - 30.0
Fatty (8 plaques)	6.86 ± 4.88 Range 2.4 - 17.1
Fibrous (5 plaques)	1.85 ± 1.01 Range 0.9 - 3.5

TABLE IX

MEAN TRITIUM-THYMIDINE INDEX IN VARIOUS MORPHOLOGICAL TYPES

OF AORTIC PLAQUES

Type of plaque	Tritium-thymidine index $^o/oo$ cells labeled
Cellular (5 plaques)	20.4 ± 10.9 Range 28.9 - 12.1
Fatty (4 plaques)	13.6 ± 8.8 Range 26.7 - 7.8
Fibrous (5 plaques)	5.9 ± 3.9 Range 10.7 - 0.5

The results here outlined fully agree with those obtained by
others (Spraragen and Bond et al., 1962; Stary, 1967; Stary and
McMillan, 1970; Florentin and Nam, 1968; Florentin and Nam et al.,
1969b) in their studies on rabbit and pig atherosclerosis. Proliferation of medial smooth muscle has been observed by us in other
experimental models too; in short-term experiments in which an anoxic
aortic medial necrosis was induced in rabbits by means of several
orthostatic shocks, we (Cavallero and Turolla et al., 1969) have

found as early as 24 hours after the acute lesion high numbers of colchicine-blocked mitoses in smooth muscle cells of the undamaged media beneath the necrotic foci. Similarly, high numbers of colchicine mitoses were seen in the tied carotid arteries of rats as well as in the aorta of epinephrine treated rabbits in which not only anoxic factors but also hemodynamic changes were operating (unpublished observations). Thus we can assume that the proliferation of medial smooth muscle might take a fundamental part in several pathological processes of the arterial wall.

DR. ROBERTSON: Using the already described tissue-organ culture techniques to isolate arterial cells, we recently studied the effects of similar concentration of several pooled homologous lipoprotein fractions (some of the serum fractions were prepared in the laboratory of Dr. L. Lewis, Cleveland Clinic). Both mitotic index and tritiated thymidine incorporation rates by human and baboon (baboon aorta specimens used for this investigation were part of a combined study with Dr. A. Howard, University of Cambridge, England) intimal and medial cells were compared with those of two fast growing human cell lines, prostatic adenoma MA 160, (supplied by Mr. M. Vincent, Microbiological Associates, Bethesda, Md.) and fetal smooth muscle cells (TABLE X).

TABLE X

EFFECTS OF LDL AND VLDL FRACTIONS ON MITOTIC INDEX

AND TRITIATED THYMIDINE INCORPORATION

	Intimal Cells		MA160	HEM
	Human	Baboon		
NS 10%	1.4%/15/6	1.2%/12.8	16.4%/68.2	9.8%/38.2
NS 10%+ 0.5 Chol.	1.2%/14.6	1.4%/16.4*	9.4%/29.6	----
+LDL-S 10%	2.6%/32.8	2.8%/31.2	10.2%/33.2	12.6%/38.7
LDL F. 10%	3.5%/31.2	3.4%/33.2	8.2%/26.7	7.2%/28.7
VLDL F. 10%	1.6%/14.2	2.1%/12.6	9.4%/29.3	6.8%/18.6*

* Insufficient samples

As shown in TABLE X, although the established cell lines had
a higher growth rate than the arterial cells in media containing 10%
homologous normal sera, they were considerably inhibited by addition
of homologous low density fractions (LDL) that significantly increased
mitotic indexes and thymidine incorporation rates of both baboon and
human intimal arterial cells. All cells were inhibited, on the other
hand, by addition of similar concentrations of baboon or human high
density lipoproteins (HDL) or cholesterol emulsions in homologous
normolipemic sera.

These findings suggest that primate arterial intimal cells are
growth stimulated specifically by LDL fractions and that cholesterol
alone, although a major component of LDL, cannot account for such
stimulation. Furthermore, the factor or factors involved do not
seem to relate to increased metabolic requirements of cells in culture since both tumor and fetal cells were inhibited by LDL. Finally,
they indicate that specific increases on serum LDL concentrations in
some types of hyperlipoproteinemias (type II) may be a factor on the
initiation of early stages of arterial intima proliferation that precede overt atheroma.

COMMENT

In the course of further discussion, there gradually emerged
the concept that the adaptation of arteries to ordinary wear and tear,
and to the strain imposed by the blood within the vessels and the
cardiovascular dynamics, as well as to specific injuries, involves
intimal hyperplasia, with consequently increased connective tissue
metabolism and an increased demand for fuel, mainly in the form of
fat. Most of the participants agreed that somehow, either because
of a discrepancy in supply and demand, or because of changes in the
permeability of the endothelium, or both, there results an accumulation of lipid and collagen with a degree of thickness of the wall
that, in the absence of vascularity, leads to impaired nutrition,
impaired tissue cell renewal and repair, and ultimately necrosis.

Among specific injuries that elicit proliferative responses in
the arterial wall, immunological mechanisms were discussed by Dr.
Wissler, referring to the work of Beaumont.

DR. WISSLER: I would like to make a very brief remark. I am
really sorry that Dr. Beaumont isn't here from Paris because he
spoke so eloquently about the role
of immunological mechanisms in the
development of atherosclerosis in
Chicago. I can't really summarize
his talk but would recommend you
read it in the proceedings (Beaumont, 1970). I would also like to
mention two groups in New York with whom I am familiar who are both

Cellular proliferation
related to immunological
mechanisms

working along the same lines. They use a model of serum sickness in
the cholesterol fed rabbit. They find that much more severe atherosclerosis will develop in the animal with arteritis induced with
heterologous serum than in the normal rabbit (Hirsch and Kellner;
Minick and Murphy et al., 1966).

DR. ROBERTSON: The role of vascular injury and subsequent repair in the development of diet-induced or spontaneous atherogenesis
is receiving increasing attention.

Experimental and clinical evidence have suggested for some time
that one of the commonest complications of long-term vascular transplants in hyperlipemic recipients was the development of localized
atherosclerotic lesions in the newly formed pseudointima of both
homografts or man-made arterial prosthesis.

We found extensive sudanophilic deposits immediately above the **HUMAN**
fibers of a Dacron prosthesis implanted for 14½ months in a hypercholesterolemic patient.

We have recently applied a technique originally developed for
the gradual dissection of the vascular intima in vitro (Robertson
and Insull, 1967) using segmental irrigation of proteolytic enzyme
solutions, to the removal of arterial intima in vascular segments
in vivo.

When we irrigated the isolated femoral artery in a dog in the **DOG**
manner described with enzyme mixtures combined with mechanical removal of intimal cells, using conical plastic brushes, we were able
to demonstrate preservation of the internal elastic lamina. A well
organized pseudointima was present 305 days following intimectomy
of normolipemic animals.

TABLE XI summarizes the effects of mechanical intimal injury in
the abdominal aorta of normolipemic
Cellular proliferation   dogs. Although intimal proliferation
following mechanical   and increased ^{3}H-thymidine incorpo-
injury   ration was the rule in the early
                                stages of organization and repair
(up to 30 days) intimal fibroplasia without lipid deposits was present
in all animals studied for longer periods.

If the recipient was hypercholesterolemic, on the other hand,
extensive intimal proliferative and lipid rich deposits developed
in areas of vascular repair. These changes closely resembled those
shown on the next illustration as part of chronic arterial homograft
repair showing extensive involvement with typical atheroma in the
transplanted arterial segment but not in the recipient artery.

TABLE XI

MECHANICAL INTIMAL INJURY
ABDOMINAL AORTA-NORMOLIPEMIC DOGS
IN VIVO-BRUSH-ENZYMATIC INTIMECTOMY

DOG #	TIME P.O.	RESULTS
1) 307K	5 hours	Exposed IEM-Scattered Fibrin & Platelet Aggregates. No Lipids.
2) 255K	15 days	Patchy Endothelial Lining-↑ Mitosis Adherent Thrombus at Arteriotomy. No Lipids.
3) 351K	15 days	Patchy Endothelial Lining-↑Mitosis Scattered Platelet Aggregates. No Lipids.
4) 195K	27 days	Organizing Pseudointima-Few Mitosis No Lipids.
5) 170K	30 days	Organizing Pseudointima-Few Mitosis No Lipids.
6) 436K	8½ months	Organized Pseudointima-Extensive Collagen Deposits-No Mitosis or Lipids.
7) 353K	9½ months	Organized Hyperplastic Pseudointima-Extensive Collagen Deposits. No Mitosis or Lipids. Delivered 4 Puppies.
8) 805J	10 months	Organized Hyperplastic Pseudointima Above Intact IEM. No Mitosis or Lipids.

RABBIT

Earlier work from our laboratory (Gutstein and Robertson et al., 1963) have shown that local "arterial irritability" following pin-pointed selective intimal injury of the abdominal aorta in rabbits resulted in abnormalities in the balance of the repair process that induced elastodynamic and hemodynamic changes tending to enlarge and propagate the intimal arterial wall defect.

In order to determine if other more diffuse types of arterial injury may also induce accelerated athero-arteriosclerotic changes, periodic immunization with heterologous sera was used in rabbits as shown in TABLE XII. Pooled horse serum was injected intravenously with a schedule similar to that described by Minick, Murphy and Campbell (Minick and Murphy et al., 1966). Other groups of animals received similar doses of pooled calf serum or bovine serum albumin. All animals were injected after the first dose of serum with a de-sensitizing injection every 16-21 days.

As shown in TABLE XIII, rabbits were divided in 3 groups: A, receiving a cholesterol supplemented semi-synthetic diet containing 17% fat as hydrogenated coconut oil (Mälmros and Sternby, 1968); group B receiving the same diet without cholesterol added and group C maintained on standard rabbit chow. Serum injections were initiated

either preceding, simultaneously or following initiation of the diet.
The results were that all animals in the semi-synthetic diet, with or
without cholesterol supplement, devel-
Effects of   oped arterial fatty lesions. The le-
immunization   sions were more severe and proliferative when immunization and diet were
started at the same time (S.T.). Short term immunization alone induced endothelial proliferation and intimal fibroplasia. Diet alone
induced the less severe vascular changes.

Aortic lesions were characterized by intimal proliferation with
abundant lipid deposits extending both in the thoracic and abdominal
aortas with both intra- and extracellular lipid deposits.

Intimal changes were characterized by increased ^{3}H-thymidine incorporation followed by cell proliferation (endothelial and smooth
muscle cells) in 2-3 weeks similar to those shown by Stary and McMillan
(Stary and McMillan, 1970). Positive immunofluorescence for anti-
rabbit gamma globulin Ab was localized in areas of intimal proliferation. These findings do not distinguish whether this deposition occurred due to increased vascular permeability or specific immunological injury.

TABLE XII

IMMUNIZATION SCHEDULE TO INDUCE ACCELERATED

ATHEROGENESIS IN HYPERCHOLESTEROLEMIC RABBITS

(HS) Pooled horse serum (TC) 10cc x kg*

(CS) Pooled calf serum (TC) 10cc x kg

(BSA) Bovine serum albumin (A) 0.25cc x kg

Administered by _slow_ intravenous injection
every 16-21 days

All animals received a desensitizing dose of 1cc
of serum 24-36 hours preceding immunization.

---

*(Minick and Murphy et al., 1966)

Evaluation of renal changes in hyperlipemic animals receiving
multiple doses of heterologous sera failed to show the typical renal
changes of serum sickness. This may be explained as suggested by

Dixon (Dixon, personal communication) because the anamnestic response elicited after the first injection is so early and so strong that the excess antigen Ag is rapidly eliminated and (Ag-Ab) antigen-antibody complexes are in circulation only for very brief periods.

The experimental findings described both in dogs and rabbits emphasize the significance of hyperlipemia when combined with intimal injury.

TABLE XIII

ACCELERATED ATHEROGENESIS IN RABBITS

Diet	Average Total Cholesterol (mgs %)	Diet Before Ag (days)	Diet After Ag (days)	Ag	Total time (days)	Severity & Extent Vascular Lesions
A	97/2600	22	----	HS	35/123	2-3 (Fatty)
A	1860	----	51	CS	165	3-4 (Fatty)
A	1435	S.T.	S.T.	BSA	276	4-5 (Fatty)
A	2200	----	----	----	270	Aorta 0-1 (Fatty) Pulmonary 1-2
B	1600	S.T.	S.T.	BSA	109	2-3 (Fatty)
B	290	8	----	BSA	130	2-3 (Fatty)
C	82	----	----	CS	12/30	1-2 (Fibroelastic)

Diet A - Mälmros diet + 5% cholesterol
    B - Mälmros diet without added cholesterol
    C - Standard laboratory rabbit chow (0.5% cholesterol by weight)

The observations may also extend to vascular changes in allograft rejection. As shown on the slide, typical obliterative arteritis is often found as part of chronic renal transplant rejection. Intimal proliferation with extensive intra- and extracellular lipid deposits is not unusual.

Accelerated athero-arteriosclerosis may also occur in coronary branches in cardiac allografts. FIGURE 9 A, B and C shows intimal proliferation and typical foam cells (atherocytes) (arrows) in a coronary artery of a heart obtained from a young female donor (21 years old) without previous history of coronary artery disease that was transplanted by Dr. R. Favaloro and had excellent functional results for 15½ months in a 46 year-old recipient without previous history of serum lipid abnormalities, diabetes or hypertension. Typical diffuse coronary atherosclerosis was present at autopsy in all major branches, although the atrial portion of the donor heart showed no evidence of vascular disease. Tissue immunity and rejection phenomena Furthermore, the recipient's own heart had no histological evidence of coronary artery disease after removal and the cause of his intractable cardiac failure proved to be subendocar-

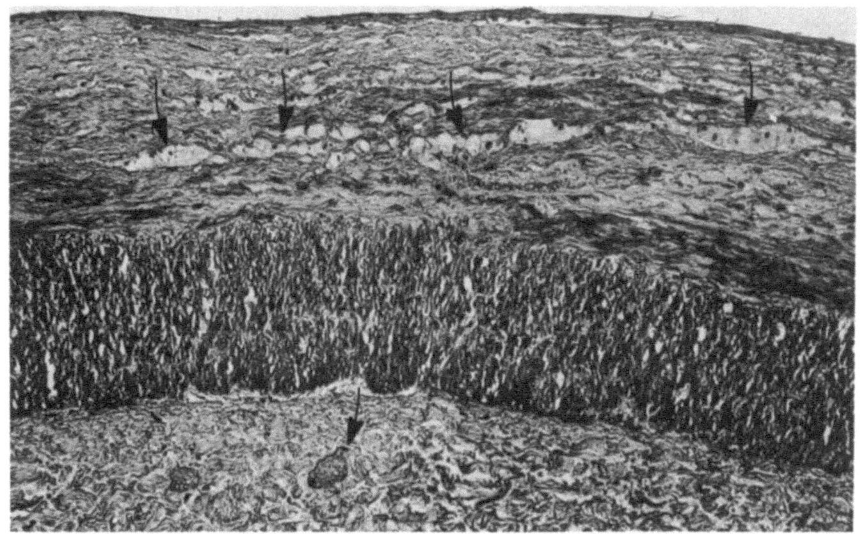

FIGURE 9 A. Atherosclerotic changes in coronary artery of cardiac allografts. Arrows show foam cells in thickened intima with minimal medial changes as well as congested adventitial arterioles (15½ month transplant). Masson Trichrome Staining (470 x).

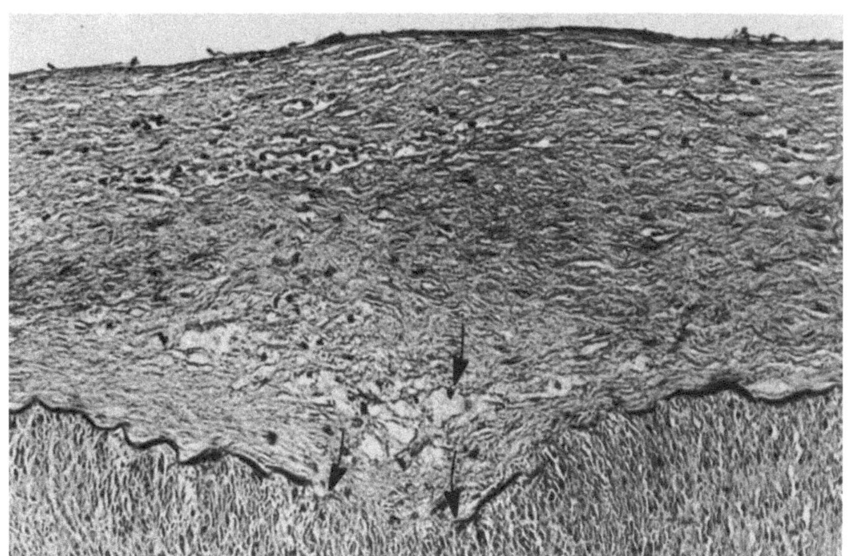

FIGURE 9 B. Atherosclerotic changes in coronary artery of cardiac allografts. Foam cells invading media in areas of fracture of internal elastic lamina (arrows) (15½ month transplant). Verhoeff Staining (520 x).

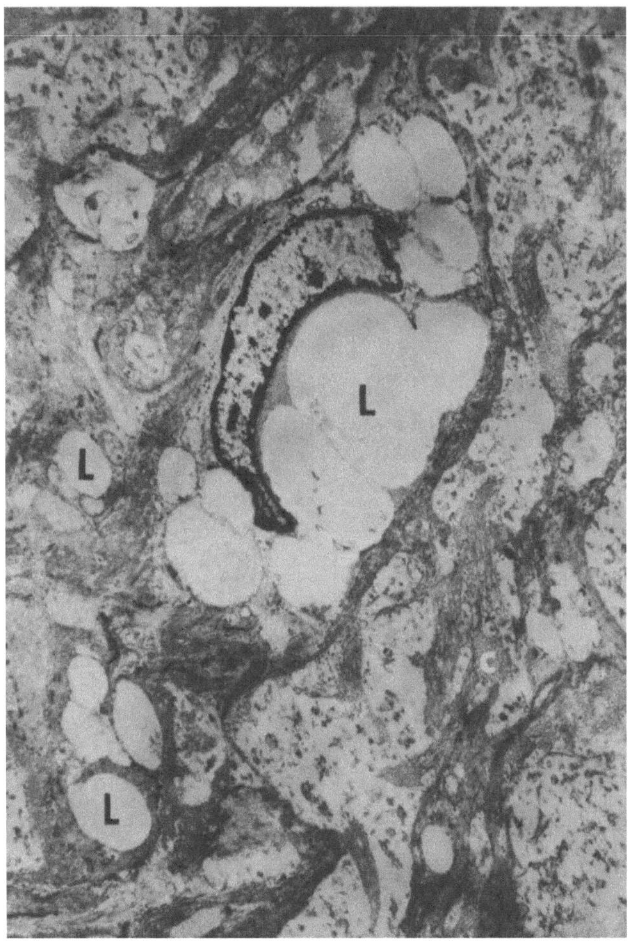

FIGURE 9 C. Atherosclerotic changes in coronary artery of cardiac
allografts. Ultrastructural changes showing typical lipid laden (L)
intimal smooth muscle cell (atherocyte) in collagen matrix (c) (15½
month transplant). Uranyl Acetate - Lead Citrate Staining (10,600 x).

dial fibroelastosis. That these vascular changes may occur early
during rejection is also illustrated in FIGURE 9 D showing severe
intimal fibroplasia with intracellular lipid deposits in a cardiac
allograft transplanted in a 22 year-old male for only 30 days.

As recently reported by Thomson (Thomson, 1969) on the series
of transplants studied at Capetown, South Africa, accelerated atherogenesis may be a serious and common complication of cardiac allograft

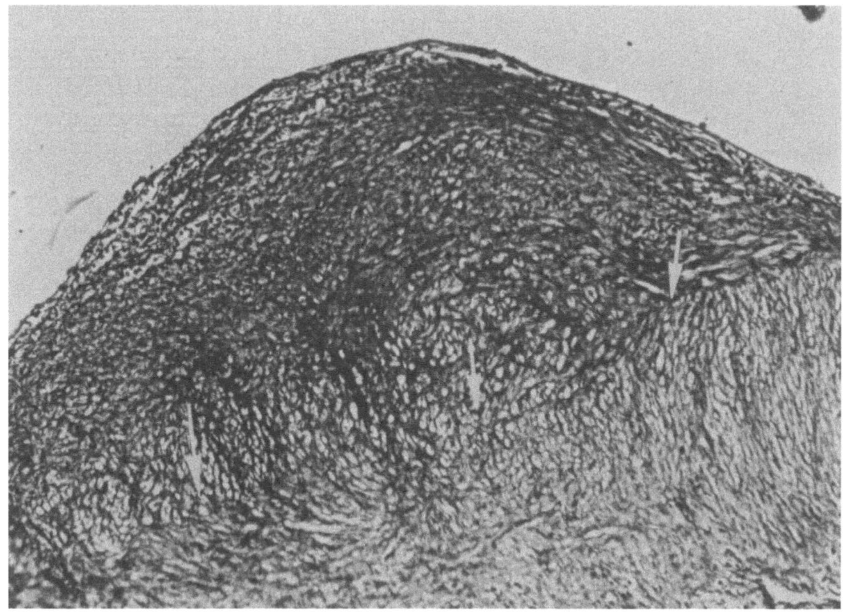

FIGURE 9 D. Atherosclerotic changes in coronary artery of cardiac
allografts. Area of intimal fibroplasia with foam cells (arrows) in
coronary artery (30 day transplant) in a 22-year-old male recipient.
PAS - Alcian Blue Staining (200 x).

rejection, particularly in recipients showing serum lipid abnormalities.

Athero-arteriosclerosis may be initiated as an inflammatory response of the arterial wall to injury, variable in its intensity and
in the metabolic changes induced, depending on the duration and severity of the injury and on the
Effects of   reparative processes elicited.
inflammation
Chronic allograft rejection ful-
fill all requirements to induce accelerated atherosclerosis particularly in recipients with serum lipid abnormalities. A very careful
screening and effective treatment of hyperlipidemics preceding graft-
ing seems to be warranted in order to prolong survival rates of clinical renal and cardiac transplants.

DR. RUTSTEIN: I am very much interested in the accelerated
atherosclerosis in the transplanted heart. This same phenomenon has
been reported many times in transplanted abdominal aortas. Do we
really have evidence that the mechanism is an immunological one?

In the case of the abdominal aorta, it would appear that the active
process of atherosclerosis, which destroyed the original abdominal
aorta occurs at a more rapid rate in the transplanted segment. I
assume that Dr. Blaiberg had serious
The coronary arteries   atherosclerotic disease which was
after heart   the reason for the heart transplan-
transplantation   tation operation. One will have to
distinguish between the mere con-
tinuation in the transplanted heart of the underlying atherosclerotic
process, or the development of a new mechanism based on immunological
response.

DR. GRESHAM: May I say about the Blaiberg heart in response
to Dr. Rutstein, that the donor was a young Cape colored man and that
Blaiberg's cholesterol was in the 350 range. The heart had been
transplanted for not more than two years anyway, and yet the degree
of coronary atherosclerosis was very severe. I cannot believe that
the elevated blood cholesterol was the only factor here. The second
point is that we know from the work of Porter and others that the
rejection of the renal transplants is largely accompanied by massive
platelet accumulations on the intima in renal vessels. We know that
platelets clump because of many factors, including antibody complexes
within them or upon them. I think that another atherogenic factor
may be that of an immunological effect on platelets.

QUESTION: Dr. Gresham, do you have any evidence, or does anyone
on the panel have any evidence, that patients who have a history of
allergy of any sort or who have various kinds of history of being
sensitive to their own tissues have more atherosclerosis than people
who do not?

DR. GRESHAM: No, I do not have any evidence.

DR. ROBERTSON: As Dr. Gresham pointed out, Blaiberg had severe
hypercholesterolemia and advanced coronary artery disease that induced
terminal cardiac failure. As far as I know, the case I just reported
is the first one of cardiac allograft with diffuse atherosclerosis
in which there was no evidence of coronary artery disease in the recipient's heart. The second point to be made is that immunological
injury may provide local arterial changes that will make possible the
accelerated deposition of lipids. Although in itself a nonspecific
phenomena, antigen-antibody complexing on the endothelial surface may
provide enough changes in permeability of the wall, in direct local
tissue hypoxia (Robertson, 1968) and in synthesis of lipids therein
that will accelerate atheroma.

DR. STAMLER: Does anybody know whether the denervated heart (of
course, the transplants are all denervated hearts) is more susceptible? Has anyone done any experiments on that question? This would
shed important light on the hypothesis that it may relate to denervation.

DR. ROBERTSON: Although denervation may play a role, it should be pointed out that inverted autologous transplants, although also denervated, do not seem, in the absence of rejection phenomena, to be more susceptible to atherosclerosis than the host artery.

Effect of dener-
vation vs. tissue
rejection

DR. WERTHESSEN: We have already shown denervated blood vessels increasing their rate of lipid synthesis (Chapter 2).

DR. GUNN: The development of severe generalized atherosclerosis, after a 19 month interval, in the coronaries and aorta of a heart from a 24 year old man, into Dr. Blaiberg was attributed to the elevated serum cholesterol (300 mgm), and an immune rejection phenomena in the 58-year-old recipient (Thomson, 1969). Transplanted hearts and their vasculature are also denervated and are presumably subject to the same metabolic alterations as the experimental arteries which have lost the modulating benefits of neural stimulation. It is interesting that the donor's proximal aorta was also described as newly atheromatous except that section of suture line nearest to the recipients distal aorta (Thomson, 1969). If an immune reaction were operating, would not this area of donor-recipient interface be the most susceptible? Perhaps this junction is reinnervated, or maybe vascularized from the recipient aorta, allowing increased norepinephrine transfer from an innervated aorta to a denervated one.

Another cardiac transplantation team has been unable to correlate either the degree of chronic rejection phenomenon or serum cholesterol levels to the vascular pathology (Bieber and Stinson et al., 1970). HUMAN While discussing atheromata in the transplanted hearts, Kosek and Bieber (Kosek and Bieber, 1970) mention the similarity of the intimal and medial lesions in both spontaneous atherosclerosis and in visceral grafts, which they termed, "graft arteriosclerosis."

Perhaps another etiological mechanism, i.e., the loss of neural innervation, should be considered as a contributor to occlusive vascular pathology in organ transplants.

One of the phenomena of tissue rejection may be the rejection of neural elements growing from the recipient to the donor organ. This would continue to deny the presence of local catechol release, suppressing the activation of adenyl cyclase, decreasing cyclic AMP function, thus inhibiting lipase activation and lipid mobilization. Even more fundamental to transplant atherosclerosis may be the absence of the catechol system serving as a naturally occurring brake on lipid synthesis.

Although it is attractive to postulate a neurogenic integrative influence on local arterial metabolism, based on preliminary observations, further data is essential and we hope forthcoming.

RABBIT

BABOON

DR. HOWARD: We have been doing work in baboons (Howard and Patelski et al., 1970) similar to Dr. Robertson's experiments, and those of Levy (Levy, 1967; VanWinkle and Levy, 1968) and Minick and Murphy and their coworkers (Minick and Murphy et al., 1966; Minick, 1966) in rabbits. The design of our experiment is shown in TABLE XIV: two groups were receiving hypercholesterolemic diets and two control diets. Two of the groups received 5 injections at 16 day intervals of 250 mg/kg bovine serum albumin (BSA) intravenously during the last 2 months of a 6 month experimental period. Two days beforehand 25 mg/kg BSA was given to prevent anaphylactic shock. As expected the plasma cholesterol with the hypercholesterolemic diet was elevated $2\frac{1}{2}$ - 3 fold, but only the group receiving the BSA showed aortic atherosclerosis. With a much longer period of feeding the diet alone, it is, of course, possible to produce the disease. The value of these experiments is to show that it is precipitated more rapidly. Histologically the lesion resembled the early human fatty streak (FIGS. 10 and 11) having both lipid, collagen and elastin, and also is similar to the spontaneous lesion in older baboons (Gresham and Howard et al., 1965).

Humeral immunity

TABLE XIV

PLASMA LIPIDS AND AORTIC ATHEROSCLEROSIS (mean ± s.e.m.) IN BABOONS GIVEN

HYPERCHOLESTEROLEMIC DIETS AND INJECTED WITH BOVINE SERUM ALBUMIN

Group	No. examined	Diet	BSA	Plasma Cholesterol mg %	Plasma Phospholipids mg %	Cholesterol / Phospholipid	Aortic atherosclerosis % area
1	8	H	+	245 ± 15.6	281 ± 11.3	0.96 ± 0.09	46.3 ± 12.5
2	5	H	-	286 ± 17.3	272 ± 23.4	1.08 ± 0.10	0
3	5	C	+	118 ± 13.1	125 ± 20.9	1.08 ± 0.26	0
4	5	C	-	116 ± 7.5	119 ± 9.8	1.00 ± 0.09	0

H = hypercholesterolaemic   C = control

BSA = bovine serum albumin
(5 x 250 mg/kg at 16 day intervals)

One can speculate on the cause of the immunological damage and Dr. Robertson has already given his ideas on this. It may be that the antigen antibody complex is affecting platelet aggregation which Dr. Gresham has already drawn attention to in causing vascular injury. Also, the antigen and antibody reaction will affect permeability. This will mean that there will be an increased influx of macromolecules, particularly lipoproteins, into the injured area. Either of these two mechanisms may operate. Certainly we have no further light to throw at this moment on what may be the injury factor. There is

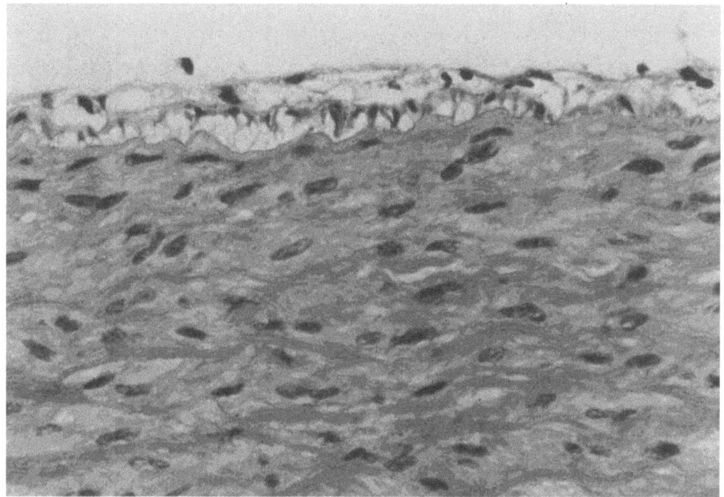

FIGURE 10. Aortic intimal thickening containing vacuolated cells. (H & E; 750 x)

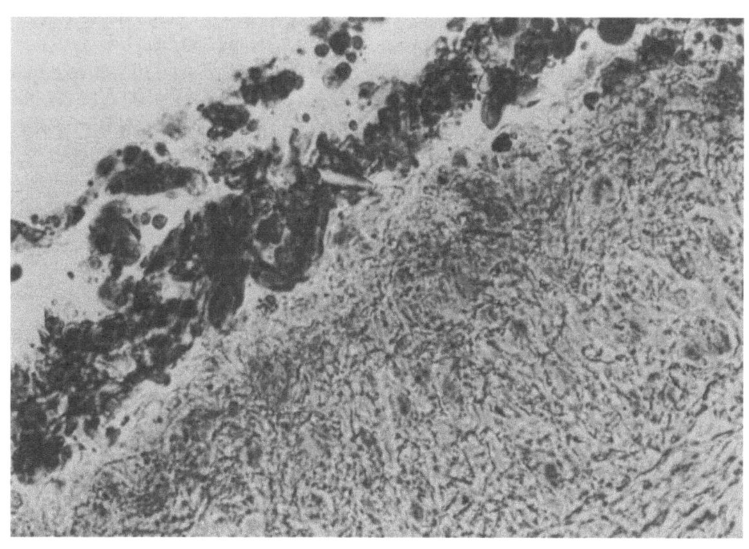

FIGURE 11. Sudanophil lipid in aortic intima. (Sudan III/IV; 750 x).

no measurable decrease in platelets on injecting the bovine serum
albumin over a short period.

DR. TAYLOR: In connection with Dr. Robertson's theories on
arterial lesions in transplanted hearts, I would like to bring out
the fact that in any transplanted artery, excepting an autologous
artery, there is death of many of its medial cells and quite a bit
of intimal proliferation. Therefore any transplanted artery would
be expected to be forming reparative intimal scars and have a greater propensity to accumulate lipids.

Proliferation in re-
newal of dead tissue

Dr. Robertson in his cardiac
transplantation study has also provided corroborative support to our
reported studies showing that arterial
scars healing in the presence of normal circulating lipids are quite
immune to the subsequent development of atheromata (Taylor and Trueheart et al., 1963).

DR. WERTHESSEN: May I take it as your view then, that this immunological idea is fundamentally another method of injury?

DR. TAYLOR: No, he may have a rejection phenomenon in this
heart but he also has arteries that are not terribly responsive to
immune mechanisms. The major factor may be that the artery didn't
survive. Any repairing arterial structure has a greater propensity
for accumulating lipids.

DR. CONSTANTINIDES: There is not the slightest doubt that immune injury against the arterial wall constitutes one of the most
powerful injury-inducing mechanisms that we know of in animals. I
will never forget a tremendous immune damage to the internal elastic
lamina of coronaries. It was shattered to pieces and a thick muscular-
elastic hyperplasia was induced up above it in rabbits that Charles
Cochrane had made nephritic with antikidney serum. There was an
antigen-antibody reaction in the kidneys and as a byproduct of this

RABBIT the coronary showed a classical injury syndrome. So the possibility
that this may happen in man is a very important and very serious one.

Absence of immuno-
globulins in
fatty streaks

We tried to operate on this hypothesis
and I asked a graduate student of
mine (Mr. Reynold Orchard) to look
for the IGG and IGM antibodies and
the beta 1C component of complement
in the earliest microscopic lesions of atherosclerosis in man (in
about a dozen fatty streaks) but the results were very disappointing.
We didn't find a single trace of immune globulin or complement in the
early fatty streaks, which may mean one of two things: either this
does not operate in man as dramatically as in animal experiments, or
else if some fatty streaks are initiated by immune injury, the antibody globulins are washed out of them very quickly without leaving a

trace; in other words we can't catch the culprit. While this may be
useful to some of the members here who might want to follow this up,
it is interesting that you, Dr. Wissler, several years ago, although
you found fibrinogen and fibrin in human atheromata, you never did
find gammaglobulin. Now, in essence I have been confirming what you
found, in a more elaborate way. I didn't find IGG, IGM or beta 1C
and neither did Walton and Williamson find any gammaglobulin. This
is a very important and very interesting problem we will have to
followup.

DR. ROBERTSON: I think a point can be made in what Dr.
Constantinides just said, that perhaps the antigen-antibody complex
has a very short life and once the endothelium is damaged it will
disappear. But the damage is already there.

DR. TAYLOR: We decided to test the old question about the effect on lipoprotein during filtration through the arterial wall as
discussed by Page in 1954. Dr. Constantinides pointed out earlier
today that atheromata secondary to endothelial injury are accelerated
and enhanced in the presence of hypercholesterolemia. We therefore
produced a lesion in the monkey by **MONKEY**
Lack of lipid freezing the arterial wall. Athero-
deposition in sclerosis developed within three weeks
scar tissue if the blood cholesterol was over 350.
When we produced a lesion in the pres-
ence of a blood cholesterol of only 154, however, let it heal for six
or eight weeks and then challenged the animal with high cholesterol
feeding we found that the scar was immune to the deposition of lipids.
Florid atherosclerosis was evident on either side of the scar but none
in the scar itself. I hope that you vascular immunologists can explain that to me.

DR. GILLMAN: One of the phenomena which is not generally appre-
ciated about scar tissue is the much more rapid rate of turnover of
at least some of the components of the scar than in the neighboring
healthy tissue - a matter badly in need of further critical study.
Dr. Taylor didn't quite give us the time of onset or age of the scarring. Would you mind repeating it again?

DR. TAYLOR: It was a minimum of six, eight and twelve weeks.

DR. GILLMAN: Could you perhaps answer the question yourself by
giving your animals labeled proline
The high metabolic and seeing how quickly the proline
activity of scar will be taken up by the collagen in
tissue the scar during its formation as
opposed to other neighboring tissue
normal collagen and how quickly it (proline in collagen) will disappear from that scar tissue? If there is a quick turnover of tissue

elements (and it may well be and this is purely a suggestion), then you may perhaps get an uptake of lipid followed by a rapid removal as part of the overall connective tissue turnover. The collagen and other components may be turning over more rapidly in the scar.

DR. TAYLOR: After the scar is all fully developed and it has laid down its collagen, is it then still a more active tissue?

DR. GILLMAN: Can I simply tell you this. In the "old days" when scurvy was rife among sailors all the doctors and ship surgeons reported that when you exposed mariners to scorbutic conditions the very first tissues to undergo scorbutic degeneration were in old scars, even twenty year old scars. So we may be quite wrong in believing scars to be "dead tissue" that are rigidly "fixed." Recently, at Hopkins, a very much greater content and turnover of vitamin C was found in scar tissue as compared to healthy tissue, the vitamin C content of scars being 64%, or much greater than in neighboring collagen. So I don't think that we should look at scars as rigidly fixed structures but should consider the possibility that their vitamin C needs and collagen turnover may be considerable.

DR. VON BERLEPSCH: It appears to me that the nature of the connective tissue components may determine the degree to which macromolecules are filtered through the artery wall. If filtration determines whether or not a blood vessel is to harbor fatty deposits, susceptibility to spontaneous sclerosis may depend upon the chemical composition of the ground substance. The macromolecular composition of the ground substance differs widely from one species to the other and may determine susceptibility to atheromatous change. We made more than 10,000 single analyses in six different species. The fact is that in these six animal species the composition of all the different mucopolysaccharides i.e. hyaluronic acid, the chondroitin sulphates, and so on are very, very different. You find species with almost none of one of the components and others with almost none of the others. In other words, at the present time it is not possible to see any direct relationship between the composition of mucopolysaccharides of an arterial wall and the susceptibility of that type of blood vessel to spontaneous atherosclerosis.

The variable composition of connective tissue among different species

DR. ALAUPOVIC: A similar comment applies also to plasma lipoproteins. There is a great difference in the distribution of plasma lipoprotein density of electrophoretic classes between various species (Campbell, 1963). Just to mention one example: Whereas dog, horse or deer contain almost exclusively high-density or α-lipoproteins, the guinea pig lipoprotein spectrum is characterized by the absence of high-density lipoproteins. It would be interesting to explore whether susceptibility of certain animal species to atherosclerotic process could be correlated with a specific plasma lipoprotein class and a specific carbo-
hydrate composition of the ground
substance. There is an urgent need
for a more thorough characterization

Species differences
in lipoprotein
of lipoprotein families of the most frequently used animal species
such as rabbit, rat and primates.

DR. WISSLER: I think we can all agree that heightened metabolism
and cellular proliferation takes place in the arterial wall prior to
lipid deposition in the process of atherosclerosis. This does not in-
validate the filtration theory as long as we understand the sequence
of events and if it is clearly understood that whatever is filtered
may be modified by the metabolism of the artery wall. This is the
major direction in which new evidence, some of it not so new, is
leading us. We get the kinds of depositions that we do in the artery
wall because we are dealing with cells that have the ability to metabolize and to alter, to deesterify, to reesterify cholesterol esters,
to probably manufacture phospholipids and do many other things that
require modification of the old simple interpretation of the filtration theory.

DR. FRENCH: I suggest that the various hypotheses of the atherogenic process are not mutually exclusive. Rather than concluding that
an hypothesis is not valid if it won't answer some point, we should
ask how each one may contribute to the lesion. I agree with Dr.
Wissler that it is not necessary to explain everything in one hypothesis. The very fact that there are different hypotheses indicates
that there is some sense in all of them.

Chapter 9

ATTEMPTS AT SYNTHESIS

PARTICIPANTS: P. Constantinides, E. Erdos, M. Friedman, T. Gillman,
               W.H. Hauss, M.D. Haust, N.T. Werthessen, R.W. Wissler
               and S. Wolf

CHAIRMAN WOLF: This Conference has provided a gratifying example of free discussion and dispute, without hostility. We have
clearly generated more light than heat. In very large measure this
is due to the wonderful atmosphere that has been created here, and
the superb hospitality of our German friends, Professor and Mrs.
Schettler and Dr. Schlierf.

We have witnessed the usual conclusion of controversy, namely
that everyone turns out to be partly right. If the participants
leave here with a new perspective on the problem, the meeting has
been successful. If they go home and design new approaches, incor-
porating ideas or methods from other disciplines, then the Conference
has been extremely successful. Finally if interdisciplinary or even
international collaborative activities develop from this meeting,
then it will have been successful beyond the wildest dreams of the
organizers. In this last session of the Conference we have attempted
a synthesis.

DR. WERTHESSEN: On Tuesday, we attained agreement in this room
on the point that at the site of the lesion, the metabolism of the
artery is different from that which one finds in the adjacent normal
tissue. It should be noted that such agreement was applicable only
to the general term, metabolism. To me this meant, as I trust it did
to the Conference, that if one examined the mode of behavior of the

carbohydrates, proteins and lipids within the lesion area and in the normal tissue in the same aorta, that one would be able to delineate a long series of differences. In some, the biochemical evidence would substantiate what the histological, cytological and electron microscope had proven to those who use those methods of looking at things. It was also found that the evidence at hand was sufficient to induce no argument on the point that the substances found in excess within the lesion can be derived from either the plasma or from the cells within the abnormal tissue or normal tissue. We had agreement on that point as long as no attempt was made to delineate the extent of the contribution from either of these sources. And the reason for that careful delineation came out later when we found that as of now nobody can calculate in quantitative terms how much the local synthesis produces, so we have to assume that most of the lipid comes from the rich source in the plasma. No matter from where the material under discussion is derived, we seem to have agreed that cells of the lesion probably dispose of it or metabolize it in a quite different fashion than do the cells in the normal portion of the vessel. There is no certainty, obviously, as to what all these differences are. Our enzymologists haven't run up the list long enough and quantitatively enough, but that there is a difference I don't think we'll argue.

Now, let's turn to a more anatomical point, if I can call it that. First of all, no one objects to the idea that the nurture of the cells in a vessel is in major part due to the passage of plasma components, and please note what I said "plasma components," through the vessel wall. Where the wall is too thick for this to be efficacious, evolution has provided a back circulation in the form of the vasa vasorum and the nature, the extent and the beautiful construction of that was well illustrated at the Conference. Now to me it follows, from this anatomical fact, that the cells of the inner intimal surface of an artery function in a plasma, which is rich in oxygen, low in CO_2, rich in nutrient and low in waste products from the cells. I'm talking about the top surface, the intima. The farther below the surface the cell happens to lie, the less it has available to it in the way of the nutrients and the more it is surrounded by the debris and waste products of the cells above it and, in a sense, it has to cope with those waste products. The anatomical facts about the vessel indicate to us that there are limits within which the lower cells can function. When those limits are exceeded in the larger vessels, the vasa come in from the bottom and rectify matters. So, obviously, here we have a gradient down from the surface in which the biochemists could talk about the varying situation in which a cell would metabolize.

The point that came up at the meeting which startled me, is the demonstration of the rapidity of the response in an artery at the biosynthetic level. It was demonstrated that at the end of an

hour of induced hypertension one can see a tremendous increase in the
synthesis of the ground substance and connective tissue. I had never
realized that proliferation could occur that fast. This point is
important to the development of my thesis. It can only be taken to
mean that we must regard the artery as an organ continuously under
load. When this load changes with the interior pressure, the arteries' metabolism undergoes change. Obviously, to achieve an increase, more plasma components must pass through the channels provided for them within the artery walls. The increased pressure,
which has increased the load, is also able to drive the needed ex-
tra fluid through. In sum then, we can take the viewpoint fortified
by this high speed biosynthetic performance, and picture a normal
artery as one which is nurtured by the fluid which it carries.
This has been obvious for a long while, but I am just saying it
slightly differently. To conduct the fluid it must work. When the
pressure goes up, it must work harder and, I might add, this is not
a low level of effort.

It has long been a private hunch of mine, that we have been
misled by the amount of connective tissue there is in an artery's
wall. We've looked at the sections of an artery, noted their strength
when we pull on the artery when we're doing surgery, and calmly assumed that this organ accomplished the load imposed upon it in the
same way that a brass pipe does. But the connective tissue is not
able to function when inert and dead like a metal pipe. By these
experiments it is proven to be in the need of constant repair. Obviously, when you increase the load the repair needs increase.

I think what happened to me the other day was that I had to
change my hidden working hypothesis. That hidden working hypothesis
was, and I think a number of us have had the same idea, that the
physiology of the nutrition of the blood vessel wall ran something
like this: Once built, a connective tissue net and an artery carried
most of the artery's load imposed upon it by the blood pressure.
That since no pipe, composed of cells and connective tissue, can be
other than a semipermeable membrane, there had to be a leakage of
plasma components through the wall. This leakage is presumably ultimately collected by the lymph system on the outside of the artery.
This was what, I for one, maybe all of you, assumed was adequate
and sufficient to nurture the tissue. But what has bothered me for
a long time in thinking about this problem, is the amount of glucose
that our perfused arteries consumed. It seemed extraordinarily high
for the red cells that were present in the perfusate and we used it
primarily as an index that there were no bacteria growing in the
perfusion. I never could understand this high utilization, but now
if we start to think about the artery as hard working then high glucose comsumption becomes rational.

Things then begin to fall into place, particularly with regard to
atheromatous development. First of all, this new viewpoint obviates

the need to look at lipid penetration into the artery wall as something bad. Lipids have to penetrate the wall and they are needed
by the cells in the arterial wall for nutrition, just as they are
needed everywhere else. This is particularly true when the workload
goes up and metabolic activity increases but, and I believe this is
critical, we have no reason to assume that the normal arterial wall
is any less selective in what it permits to penetrate through it than
is the infinitely less thick capillary wall. Not, that is, unless
there has been an injury.

It is here I think, where I took a major step forward on Tuesday. From where I stood, it became apparent that once there had
been insult to the wall then all things changed. Several kinds of
insult were presented, among them were immune reactions and anoxemia
and, of course, the feeding of cholesterol, and I emphasize now the
simultaneous feeding of its oxidation products. When I say cholesterol and its oxidation products, the latter is what people leave
out when they say they feed cholesterol, because unless they make
a terrific attempt to purify and maintain the purity of the cholesterol, they're feeding the oxidation products too, up to ten to
fifteen percent of the cholesterol they say they administer. Now,
once the artery wall has been traumatized by one of these agents,
then it appears that one could expect to see a lesion develop. Indeed, unless I am grossly mistaken, the sentiment of the Conference
appeared to be that once you could manage to induce a trauma these
sequela were pretty much the same except as to later development
and some specific items of detail.

Species differences, too, were important. But out of the mass
of evidence, one point stood clearly: "Injure the wall and trouble
ensues." If there is even a mild hyperlipemia the injured site contains excess lipid.

In summary, then, one could take these data and package them
into the concept that the primary phases of lesion development are
specialized responses in the arterial wall and/or what one could
call a healing process. This concept gained support from the discussion on the early fatty streak. This stage of atherogenesis is
now regarded by many as one which can regress. Indeed, several of
our members regard the real problem today to be that of determining
what it is that induces a benign fatty streak which can regress to
go forward and become the full blown lesion. If we could stop atherogenesis at this point, then we could expect to stop the occur-
rence of all the rest of it.

We run into a difficulty at this point, however, because a
number of use have already presented adequate evidence that at the
fatty streak stage of development, the metabolism within the fatty
streak is already different from that of adjacent normal tissue.

To get around this difficulty, I had to back up somewhat and
consider some data presented only in part at this Conference. The
data to which I refer is that which demonstrates, (a) that the artery's metabolism can respond to physical force changes, (b) that
the artery's metabolism is susceptible to alteration by hormones
and is dependent on vitamins, (c) that arterial metabolism is subject to neural control. Mind you, I said metabolism not function.

At this point we have to make the first assumption that I found
necessary in developing this thesis. That assumption is that whatever it is that leads to the fatty streak involves a specific manipulation of the control systems that normally organize the arterial wall metabolism. If we don't so assume, then the fatty streak
is an abnormal state and can not be expected to regress. The only
other way out would be to assume that unless a second event occurs
a fatty streak and the cells in it have a limited life, sort of like
the red cell that is expected to die at the end of 100 days. At
this stage, I don't know how to decide between these two possibilities.

But, as I think I have mentioned once before I was trained primarily as a reproductive physiologist and, as a result, I had to
know what goes on in an ovary. Therefore, I submit to you that the
change that goes on in a follicle when it is under the influence of
FSH and pops open and converts to a corpus luteum is of the same
order of magnitude, if not greater, than when a normal arterial
wall cell converts to a fatty streak. Now the critical point here
is that when the stimulus of corpus luteum maintenance ceases, the
corpus luteum regresses and dies. So I can't see any need to get
bothered by assuming that if the ovary can do this, the endometrial
wall can do it and the cells of the lacunae in the mammary glands
can do it, under appropriate stimulus, that it would be irrational
to expect the cells in another organ to do it. The only difficulty
at the moment is that we don't know all the controls that regulate
the function of the arterial wall tissue.

If you're going to have a good thesis you've got to not only
cover the facts, but use them. And one of the facts that particularly suits this thesis is that it has been demonstrated that there
is a genetically determined susceptibility to recognized atherogenic
stimuli. Now in those days when one measured hormones, not chemically but by bioassay procedures, one of the things you had to do
was to use inbred stock carefully selected as to age and weight;
otherwise, you got a mess for data! Now what this means conversely
is that if you are looking for something that is to be regulated by
a hormone, you should expect to see differences genetically determined in the quantitative response to a specific set of hormones.
(You're just flipping the thing around and looking at it the other
way.) Therefore, I am delighted to know--I noted some time back on
this one--that two strains of pigeons showed differences in susceptibility to an atherogenic stimulus. I was particularly pleased at

this Conference, when it was shown that cross-breeding demonstrates
the difference to be gene dependent and, of course, I am further delighted to find that now in all probability, we are going to see the
same kind of thing in a species of monkey. It has already been shown
long ago in rabbits.

Now let's move to something else we have to cover. We were
shown here that cells derived from normal and abnormal tissue from
the same human vessel retain a differential response when exposed
to similar lipid challenges. Secondly, we were shown that cells
obtained from the intima of experimental animals, challenged by
cholesterol feeding, were, within a few days after the feeding began,
grossly different as to thymidine incorporation and as to dropout
rate from the population. What is critical here, is that in each
instance cells are being delineated as different from the normal
population from which they were derived. Criteria of molecular biology were required to demonstrate that difference, cytological criteria not being sufficient to do so.

Now we come to the end, almost. What do all these data seem
to drive us to? I think it's the following: (1) When a blood vessel wall receives an insult or injury from an atherogenic stimulus,
such as those discussed, its responses can be considered two-fold;
(a) the insult permits an excessive influx of plasma born material,
(b) the insult induces the development of new cell-types from the
local population. (2) The repair process proceeds under a control
system not yet delineated and is distinguishable in its maximal normal stage as the fatty streak. (3) If the insult continues, the
cell transformations are maintained. (4) Because the regeneration
time and dropout rate of the cells that are newly formed to produce
the repair job are 10 days and 0.3 respectively, as compared to 15
days and 0.5 for the preexisting cells, it follows that these new
cells must cause an increase in thickness of the intima. We can call
on Dr. Lee if need be, to explain that. I'll just say it for the
moment.

If successful repair occurs, this process can cease and we observe regression of the fatty streak. But if the injury is too
severe for repair to be rapidly accomplished or, secondly, if the
insult continues, and I think this is a major contribution if my
thinking was anything worthwhile, then this very repair process leads
to further trouble. It does this because it interferes with the nutrition of the subjacent tissue by inhibiting the filtration of plasma
nutrients through the surface and down to the lower layers. Anoxemia
and pH changes occur, the lipids that could have been nutrients are
now inappropriate. Ground substance and smooth muscle maintenance
is inadequate and we end up with what the pathologists describe as
an early lesion. There isn't time, and/or the need for this audience
to develop all phases of this thesis. The only point I need to make

is to repeat the item about the "fed cholesterol." It's not pure
cholesterol--it has a lot of oxidation products in it and these can
be nasty. I can give you the data on that.

Again, I apologize for not citing names in this performance
but I learned long ago that there's only one thing worse than not
citing names and that's to ascribe to A what B did and my notes were
insufficient to prevent me from doing it. Thank you for the cathar-
sis you have permitted me to take.

DR. WOLF: Thank you very much Dr. Werthessen. I can tell you
that his thinking didn't just start on Tuesday. It was Dr. Werthessen
who provided the original idea for this Conference.

DR. WISSLER: I am intrigued by Dr. Werthessen's fear of con-
tamination of cholesterol with oxidation products. I'm not clear as
to whether he is talking about cholesterol as we buy it when we include it in our diets or cholesterol as it occurs in egg yoke, meats,
milk products and so forth. Is it something that happens during
the preparation of food?

DR. WERTHESSEN: There are two points to make. I believe it
was Wintersteiner who showed that cholesterol is so labile that all
you need to do to obtain a good yield of oxidation products is to
bubble air through a suspension or solution in liquid. The second
point is that Dr. Altschule who did the studies on nicotinic acid
and atherosclerosis happened to be a friend of my collaborator and
sterol chemist Dr. Erwin Schwenk.

Altschule began to use a better grade of cholesterol in his
studies and his rabbits began to show a poor grade of atherosclerosis. He wrote a letter of complaint to Schwenk.

Schwenk then advised him to thoroughly mix the cholesterol in
the meal, then bake it and feed it to the rabbits. Altschule was
delighted at the hyperlipemia and atheromatosis that resulted. Need-
less to say I was delighted to hear Paris elaborate on the potency
of calciferol as an atherogenic agent. It can be made by oxidizing
cholesterol.

To me, the inability to feed cholesterol without also feeding
oxidation products explains the differences in atherogenicity of a
hypercholesterolemia induced endogenously by hormonal manipulation
and that induced by feeding cholesterol. Had Schwenk isolated the
factors in Altschule's well baked diet that induced the excellent
results, I believe we would now be using a variety of agents like
calciferol instead of cholesterol in our experimental diets. But
in the late forties we were all more interested in cholesterol biosynthesis than in oxidation. It seemed then to be far more important.

DR. ERDOS: I should like to emphasize the complexities of the situation that may follow injury to endothelial lining. This may lead to the activation of Factor XII (Hageman factor). Active Factor XII can trigger three simultaneous processes: clotting of the blood, the release of plasma kinins and the activation of the complement system. The factors liberated in turn may aggravate the existing conditions and cause further injury to the endothelial surface.

DR. GILLMAN: On the first day of this meeting I referred to a number of basic processes that are involved in maintaining the integrity and continuity of both healthy and diseased tissues, including arteries - apart from the now generally conceded "wear and tear" turnover of various molecular species comprising "resting" arterial (and other) tissues. Among these basic processes are growth, with attendant remodeling of tissues and the healing, by either regeneration and/or repair, of any injured tissues.

These terms have so often been misused that I would like to propose here simple, potentially useful brief definitions. Thus, growth is taken to mean an increase in the size of any organ (or tissue(s) in accordance with genetic and environmental requirements and, for arteries, involves increments in wall thickness together with the inevitably associated simultaneously occurring increases in both arterial length and caliber. The latter, most probably occur together with increasing size of the body or heart (or for that matter of any other growing organs and tissues e.g. pregnant uterus). Such simultaneous increases in all the parameters of arteries, anywhere, - whether in conformity with genetically and/or environmentally determined healthy growth, or due to hyperplasia and/or hypertrophy in disease, or as an adaptation to increased work load must surely be achieved not only by increases in tissue mass but also by the inevitably associated remodeling and attendant changes in component tissues including arteries.

We were astonished when, about 15 years ago, we found, almost accidentally, that the susceptibility of the rat's aorta to the experimental production of dissecting aortic aneurysms seemed to be directly related to the rate of daily postnatal increments in aortic length. Later we found that this held, but much more so, during the period of maximal intra-uterine embryonic aortic elastic membrane (and also, at least, of collagen and mucopolysaccharide) synthesis. This we have previously shown characterizes the last 3-4 days of the mouse's intra-uterine life (Fyfe and Gillman et al., 1968). Indeed, severe aortic lesions, including aneurysms (with or without ruptures), can be produced in almost 80% of a litter, and within 2 to 3 days at that, by treating the mother with toxic nitriles only on days 17 to 21 of her pregnancy (Pyorala and Punsar et al., 1957; Gillman and Hathorn, 1958; Gillman and Hathorn, 1959; Fyfe and Gillman et al., 1968).

It has also been shown that the extent and severity of myocardial, coronary and vascular lesions in general, are far more severe and extensive in baby rabbits fed cholesterol during their rapid post-weaning growth phase than in full grown rabbits fed the same dose of cholesterol for only a single period of about 100 days, and then placed onto a standard non-atherogenic diet for the subsequent 4-6 years of their lives (Gillman, 1968 and more recent confirmatory unpublished data).

So, it would seem that arteries - including the coronaries - may be much more susceptible to serious injuries induced by various endogenous and/or exogenous metabolic agents - when they are growing rapidly and hence probably remodeling.

This has also been shown to apply to those arteries known to grow rapidly postnatally, - especially if such growth is episodic and even more so if soon followed by an even more speedy episode of "degrowth" or what is generally called "involution." Thus, the uterine arteries of multiparous women have been clearly demonstrated to become so grossly pathological between pregnancies and at the menopause as to resemble premature arteriosclerotic degenerative diseases, even in African women who are otherwise relatively "immune" to death-dealing progressive lesions in coronary arteries, even more so than African men (FIGURE 1, A-H). The same has been shown to hold for the uterine (and for the ovarian and mammary) arteries of sows, goats and sheep after multiple pregnancies (FIGURE 2, I-T) (Gillman, 1964; Gillman, 1967; Gillman, 1968).

The above remarks and demonstrations of the apparently increased susceptibility of rapidly growing and remodeling arteries to endogenously and/or exogenously determined growth and metabolic changes and to "nocuous agents" are by no means the only remodeling to occur in arteries. For, we have now clearly shown, for example, that incisional scars in the skin and the entire dermis of autografts grow rapidly and in pace with the increase in body surface and hence the animal's cutaneous dimensions - a phenomenon seen so strikingly in piglets wounded and/or grafted at birth as they grow rapidly in size during the first 3-6 postnatal months.

The same perhaps occurs in intramural arterial scars during growth and aging. Moreover, there is some evidence that the rate of collagen and ground substance turnover in cutaneous scars, and possibly therefore also in arterial scars, may be considerably more rapid than in healthy neighboring dermal (or arterial) tissues. Certainly the far greater susceptibility of very old scars to scurvy, recorded in mariners of yore, and confirmed for the guinea pig only 20 years ago (Pirani and Levenson, 1953) provides strong ancillary evidence for this view. The atonishingly high vitamin C content of burn scars, compared with neighboring unscarred tissue in man also supports this view (Abt and von Schuching et al., 1959a and b). We

are presently checking this possibility for cutaneous and arterial
scars made in healthy guinea pigs who were then fed scorbutic diets
6-8 months later.

It would seem desirable to examine these processes in other
species than pigs, rats and guinea pigs and perhaps particularly
to study closely the dynamic biological processes of the normal
growth and remodeling of arteries (and of their intramural scars)
postnatally, after active episodic growth, however promoted, in
man, as during pregnancy and in trained athletes. This applies perhaps especially when such periodic growth is shortly followed by
periods of sudden "degrowth" as exemplified by the involuting uterus, and perhaps also by the "involuting" athlete's heart after he
stops training and "goes to seed." For that matter, similar dynamic
tissue remodeling and/or turnover studies would also seem to be
desirable on human arterial thrombi and intramural scars, and even
in the hearts and arteries of non-athletes as their tissues involute
(as in brown atrophy) during aging which follows, slowly or rapidly,
the speedy growth inevitable in the previously physically highly active adolescent.

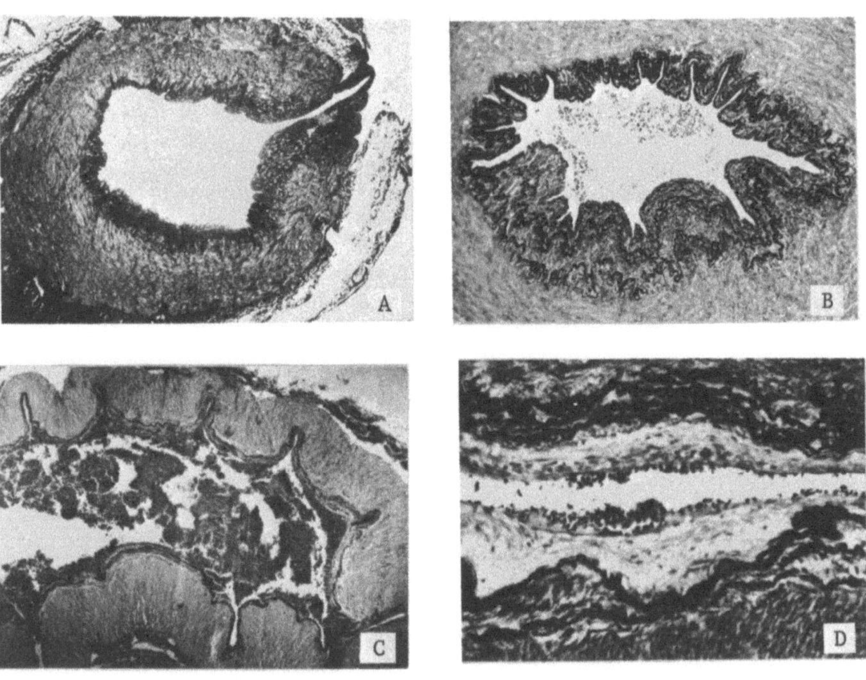

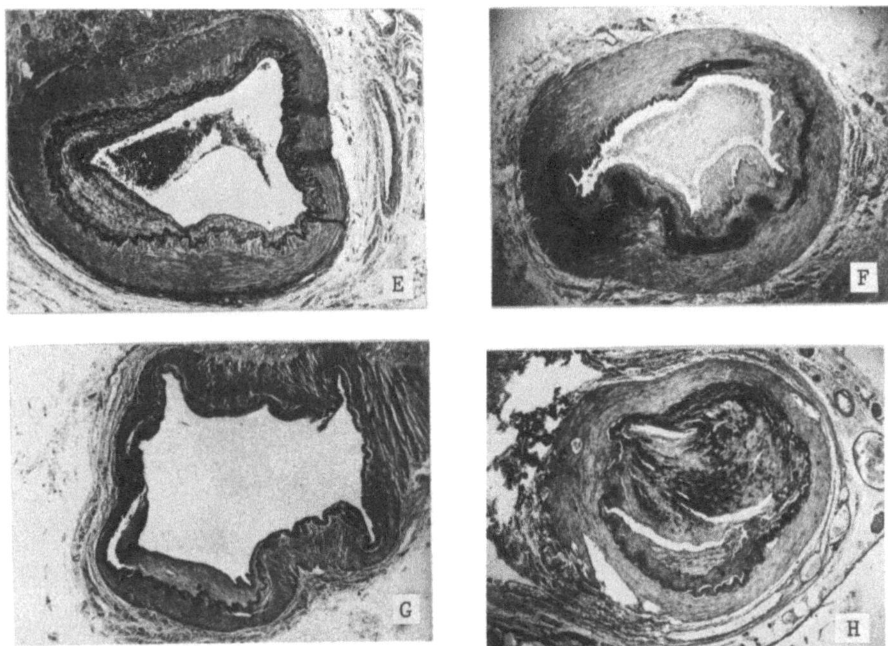

FIGURE 1 A - H. All these are photomicrographs of human uterine arteries (main para-uterine trunks) in women of differing parity at the
end of pregnancy (by caesarian sections - A & B), between pregnancies
and at the menopause. Note that, at the end of pregnancy and regardless of parity, in both A and B (para. 5 & 2 respectively) the lumen
of the arteries are widely dilated and the intima is laden with mucopolysaccharides (dark staining material in A) and usually shows markedly "reduplicated" elastic (pseudoelastic) laminae (B) i.e. presumably remodeled with growth during pregnancy. However, after multiple
pregnancies, the lumen of the main arteries become markedly sacculated
probably due to longitudinal contraction (C), and almost invariably
show intimal fibrosis (D), varying degrees of intimal thrombotic
fibrosis (E & G) and, later in life, medial calcification as well,
with luminal thrombus organization amounting to frank occlusion shortly after the menopause (F & H). Thus, the main trunks of uterine arteries, in young African women, notably "resistant" to degenerative
diseases in other arteries, almost invariably show marked "degenerative changes" following repeated growth (pregnancy) followed by active (involutionary) degrowth (post partum) e.g. FIG. 1 D from a 35
year old para 8 woman. This series of figures suggests that if growth
and remodeling, accompanying great functional activity, is followed
by degenerative-like and even thrombotic changes during subsequent
(involutionary) degrowth this may well happen in other arteries
e.g.? coronaries.

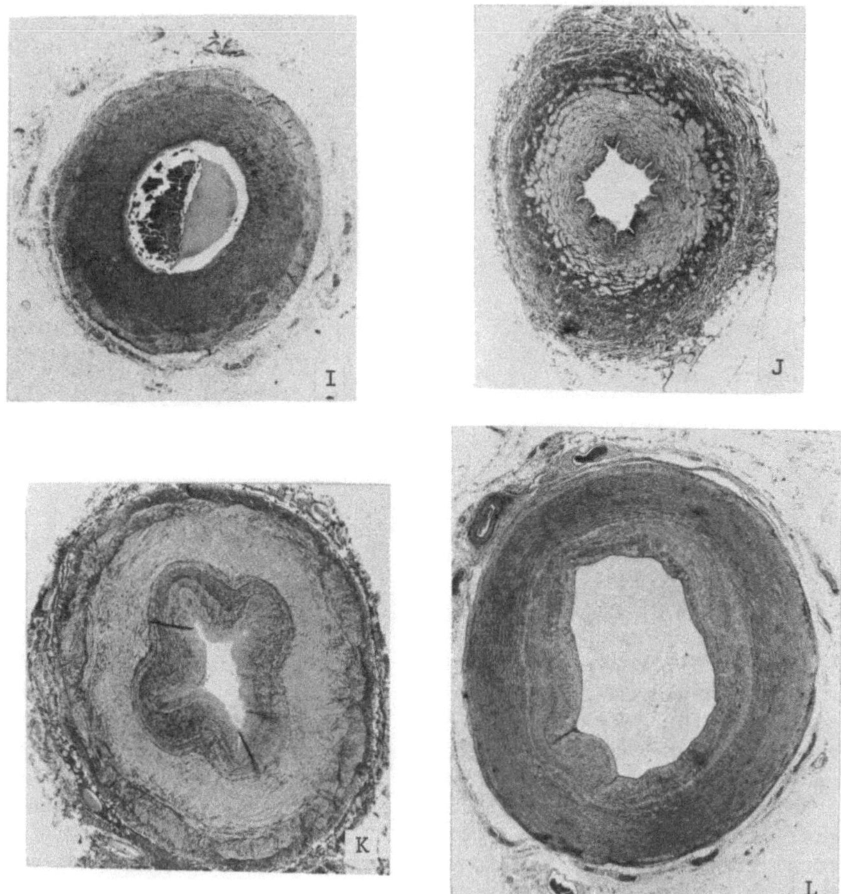

FIGURE 2 I - T. Figures I to R (inclusive) are photomicrographs of
the main trunks of the uterine arteries of sows of different parities.
Thus, Figs. I (x 12) and O (x 45) are from a sow on the last day of
its first pregnancy; Fig. J, 41 days after the first pregnancy; K and
P at 50 days after the 6th pregnancy; L and Q in the middle (day 65)
of the 7th pregnancy; M at 32 days after ninth pregnancy; N at 8
months after second pregnancy and R at 95 days after pregnancy 10.
Note, in Figs. I, K, L (all x 12), P and R (x 45), how the intima,
in particular, undergoes progressive thickening with increasing numbers of pregnancies due to accumulations of reticulin, collagen,
smooth muscle and mucopolysaccharides. Fig. J shows involution (compared with I) at 41 days after first pregnancy (x 12). Figs. L
(x 12) and Q (x 45) (when compared with K and P at same magnifications)
demonstrate the capacity for resorption of the markedly increased
intimal components (after pregnancy 6) by the middle of the next,

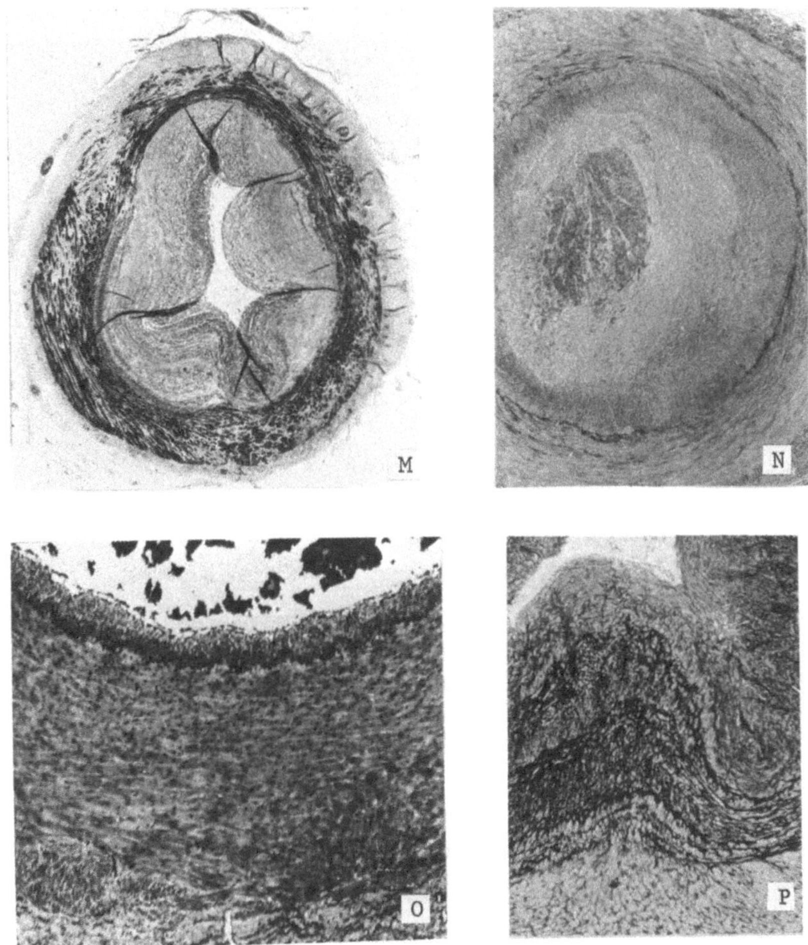

seventh pregnancy. On the other hand Fig. N (x 45) shows true thrombotic occlusion with irregular intimal sclerosis in a para 2 sow
allowed to remain "empty" for 8 months. Thus, pregnancy profoundly
influences the structure of the uterine arteries but such structural
changes are partially reversible during a new pregnancy, thus indicating the capacity of this artery, at least, for dynamic changes
attendant on functional state - especially rapid growth followed by
rapid "degrowth" (involution). The occlusion of the artery in a
sow left empty for 8 months (N) demonstrates that the arteries,
altered by previous pregnancies, are liable to thrombotic occlusion
if allowed to involute progressively, whereas arteries kept "active"
(Figs. L, M, R) will remain patent despite marked intimal fibrosis/
hyperplasia.

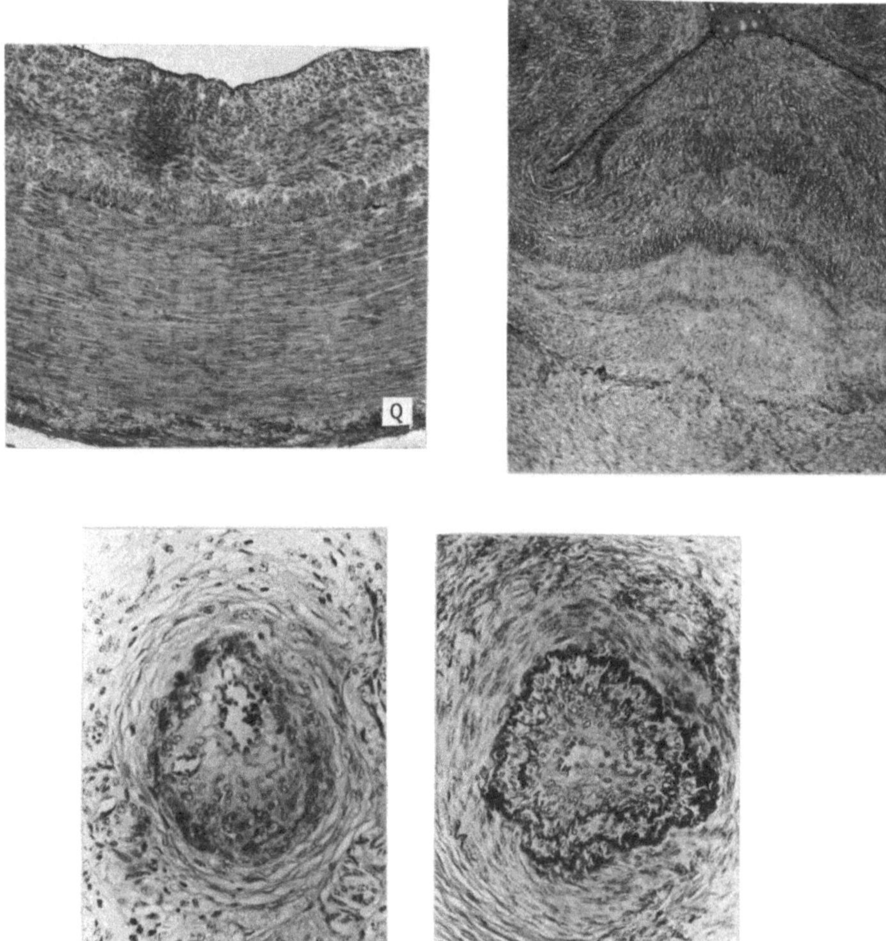

Figs. S & T (x 100) show the intimal and medial degenerative
changes tending to arterial occlusion (S) with reduplication of
internal elastic laminae (T) in the main artery supplying the involuting corpus lutum in a sheep's ovary - again demonstrating occlusive changes when very "active" arteries are allowed to become
"inactive", i.e. to grow and subsequently "degrow" rapidly.

DR. WISSLER: First I'd like to present a diagram which was
originally modified from a figure that Gofman and Young produced
in Sandler and Barnes very stimulating book on Atherosclerosis and
its Origin, published in 1963 (Gofman and Young, 1963). We made some
modifications in it when we used it at the time at the International
Symposium on the Comparative Pathology of Atherosclerosis which was
held in October 1964 (Wissler, 1965). I presented this modification
at the International Symposium at Chicago in November of 1969 (Wissler,
1970b), (FIGURE 3). Now I'd like to indicate where I think it needs
to be modified further in the light of this Conference that we've had
here. I have found this meeting very useful as I'm sure the rest of
you have, in terms of redefining goals and identifying areas which
need further work. To begin with, I believe the factors in the lumen
of the artery have to be thought of a little more broadly. The next
time this chart is modified, it should really include the two major
factories or production centers that we have to consider in relation
to low density or very low density lipoproteins, namely the liver
and the intestines. As is so frequently the case, some of the major
contributions of a Conference like this take place in the halls and
around the table at mealtime. This one has been no exception, and
the conversation the other day between Ted Gillman and Larry Pottinger,
our student who has been attending this Conference, indicated to me
that we really probably should be thinking at the hepatic or gastro-
intestinal tract level, depending on where one thinks the major part
of the lipoproteins that are dangerous are produced. This may be
another place where the major modifications can be made that will
prevent the disease in the artery. I think this Conference has, if
anything, reinforced my view that the critical factor that is probably most easily altered and has the most to do with the epidemiological aspects of the disease, is really what is circulating in
the lumen. Then we have to think of the overlay of this in terms
of genetics. One comes up against the important question - Are
genetic factors exerting their greatest effect on circulating lipoproteins as Frederickson's work emphasizes? Certainly, we've had
abundant evidence at this Conference that genetic factors are important. Nevertheless, I submit that the evidence still supports
the concept that environmentally induced epidemiological factors
are predominant. After listening and participating for five days
here it appears to me that we are frequently faced with cases in
which we really can't explain the variations of disease by any measurement we know of so far of what is circulating. We have to admit
that there must be some cases in which genetics may be primarily
involved with the cells, either the endothelial population of cells
or the smooth muscle cells in the media of the vessel, so that as
we try to dissect this disease further, I think we're going to have
to document the importance of genetics at the artery cell level.

Now, as a pathologist, I want to emphasize two points I found
that impressed me very greatly here and which will certainly lead

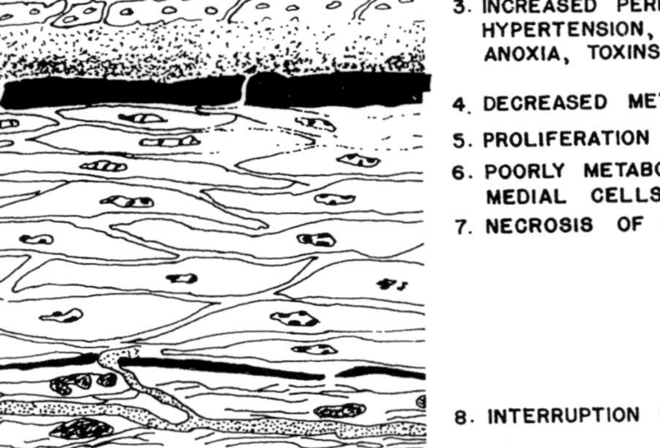

FIGURE 3.   Factors in the cellular pathogenesis of atherosclerosis.

to some modifications in the chart. You notice how amorphorus we
made the area between the endothelium and the internal elastic membrane in FIGURE 3. I have been impressed by the evidence presented by a number of colleagues here that we must think more about the
function of this subendothelial area -- the area that was so beautifully demonstrated in some of Ted Gillman's slides. The acid-
mucopolysaccharides and other ground substance materials in general,
while probably a product of the medial cells, must be thought of in
relation to what they may do to help bind or trap certain of the
lipoproteins from the plasma. We may have the beginnings of knowledge that will help us in understanding that there could be a vicious
cycle here. In other words, factors coming in from the blood stream
affect the metabolism of the medial cell. This, in turn, leads to
modification of the quantities of products it makes, i.e. collagen,
elastin and ground substance. When these accumulate they may lead to
a greater trapping of lipoproteins and in turn to further modification of cell metabolism. This then becomes a vicious cycle center-
ed, if you will, right on the amorphorus area that I have really
never filled-in in the diagram and which wasn't filled-in in its
original form. So the first major point that I am suggesting is
that there should be a modification of the diagram and our thinking
in relation to the effect of certain lumen derived substances which
we will call "x" substances at the present time. They may be part
of the lipoprotein molecule or, as Nick Werthessen has suggested,
they may be cholesterol oxidation products. These stimulate the
myointimal cells to proliferation and to abnormal metabolism, with
greater output and perhaps production of abnormal forms of acid mucopolysaccharides, collagen and elastin.

The second remodeling of my own thinking has been in what's happening in the adventitia. On the basis of the work of a number of
people, those who transplant segments of vessels or produce experimental injury to the outside of the vessel, and in certain disease
processes, such as luetic aortitis, I think it's been apparent for
some time that one has to think of the interruption of lymphatic
drainage and interruption of vasa vasorum as being important in the
development of the disease. Here, we've heard a number of the ways
that inflammatory changes in the adventitia, whether from neurogenic
origin or other origins, may also be correlated with the development
of the disease in the inner portion of the vessel. I would simply
like to mention in passing that it was no accident that in one of
the slides that I showed of the coconut oil lesions in the monkey
there was an active inflammatory change in the adventitia. In fact,
we have noted this in almost every animal that we've ever studied
that was fed coconut oil. There is almost always an inflammatory
area of lymphocytic cells on the outside of the artery just opposite
each plaque. Does this mean that whatever is coming through this
artery wall that stimulates the intimal proliferation also makes
its way through the vessel wall and incites an inflammatory response?

I don't know whether this concept is correct or not but I'm interested in the fact that others, by entirely different means, are now
observing inflammatory cells, principally lymphocytes, in the adventitia of arteries at points that appear to be particularly susceptible
to the development of atherosclerosis.

DR. HOWARD: As we know in atherosclerosis, this is an intimal
disease in which the smooth muscle cells and so on accumulate in
the intima. And I was wondering whether Dr. Wissler would be prepared to accept some modification to his diagram. We know from the
work of Wilbur Thomas that the medial cells migrate through gaps in
the internal elastic lamina and this may explain why they accumulate
in the intima. On the basis of the discussion we've just heard, we
have had no explanation as to why atherosclerosis is an intimal
disease.

DR. WISSLER: I think we first have to establish that atherosclerosis is really primarily an intimal disease. In the rabbit it
is usually an intimal disease and most of the proliferation occurs
inside a rather prominent internal elastic membrane. In the primates
in general, including man, the lesion that I see appears to consist
of a small, frequently very slight, proliferation of subendothelial
cells that can be considered a part of the intima. The cells that
show the first evidence of cell damage that will progress to a necrotic center are in the inner media. I think that this area is
particularly at risk in the sense that Dr. Werthessen was describing
the cells being at risk in the artery wall. The necrotizing reaction really occurs in the inner media and this means that we can't
think of this as purely an intimal disease. I don't ignore the
intima at all. I think the fibrous cap which is the proliferative
product of cells that were in the media primarily does ultimately
show up in the intima. But the media can't be ignored and many
much wiser and more experienced pathologists than myself have thought
of this as a disease involving the inner part of the media. I believe that one really shouldn't try to label the disease as intimal
or medial. I think both are involved and they're both important.

DR. FRIEDMAN: I have no objection whatsoever to the statement
that the medial cell may be the preponderant cell in the well developed human atherosclerotic plaque. But in our animal studies,
specifically those concerned with the cholesterol-fed rabbit, the
very beginning arterial plaque is composed of foam cells that originally were endothelial cells. We are certain of the identity of
these cells for the following reasons. First, we were able to prepare in vivo arterial plaques which consisted only of endothelial
cells (Friedman and Byers et al., 1966). Such plaques lack a
specific framework of elastic fibers and the foam cells which are
polygonal in form, are piled upon each other in a quasi-palisade
manner (FIGURE 4). Thus this lesion is exactly like the lesion
seen occurring spontaneously in the aorta of the cholesterol-fed

rabbit. Secondly, we also have been able to prepare an in vivo arterial preparation containing a plaque composed solely of hyperplastic medial cells (Friedman and Byers, 1965). These cells as
one might expect are spindle shaped and even when they are engorged
with lipid-cholesterol they still resemble in their earliest stage,
spindle cells. More important, such medial cell hyperplasia is accompanied by a laying down of new elastic tissue in a relatively
regular fashion (FIGURE 5), - a phenomenon never seen in the early
developing spontaneous plaque of the cholesterol-fed rabbit. Thus
when one induces a true hyperplasia of the media, one gets not only
cells whose morphology but also whose functional capacity (i.e. the
laying down of regular patterns of elastic fibers) differs totally
from those cells found in the early stages of a spontaneous plaque
in the cholesterol-fed rabbit. Thirdly, we have been able to produce an in vivo arterial plaque consisting of only fibroblasts
Friedman, 1969) and this plaque (FIGURE 6) differs in its structure
from that of the endothelial or medial cell plaque. What I am saying is that the various cells comprising the arterial coat are each
capable of producing a plaque. Such cells when they eventually ab-
sorb enough lipid/cholesterol all become "foam cells." Finally, it
should be emphasized that any cell in contact with excess cholesterol
not only may become hyperplastic, but may become metaplastic. In
this latter event the electron microscope cannot identify its original
provenance. One cannot easily describe the roots of a tree by the
first appearance of its buds.

DR. WISSLER: Well, I didn't want to rehash this really but I
must emphasize that I did have the endothelial cell in the diagram and
I think that it is extremely important in the development of atherosclerosis. I'm not, however, convinced that the proliferation in the
rabbit lesion is endothelial cell proliferation. In general, I believe the evidence indicates that these cells are either coming from
the bloodstream in the rabbit disease or they are coming from the
media. I know that endothelial cells can proliferate but I've not
seen the proof that they ever make up a very large part of the lesion.
I have seen tracer evidence and ultrastructural evidence of various
kinds indicating that the rabbit lesion, at least with time, becomes
a smooth muscle lesion and that early on it is a macrophage lesion
(Imai and Lee et al., 1966). I just don't know how to be sure that
you're right about the endothelial cell proliferation being the
principal part of the foam cell lesion in the rabbit, but don't assume for a moment that I don't think the endothelium is extremely
important in the development of atherosclerosis. I'm tremendously
impressed by Mustard's work (Mustard, 1967) and the possibilities
that the opening up of the endothelium to greater permeability may
be produced by a number of products and conditions in the lumen of
the vessel-particularly agglutinated platelets liberating vasoactive
amines.

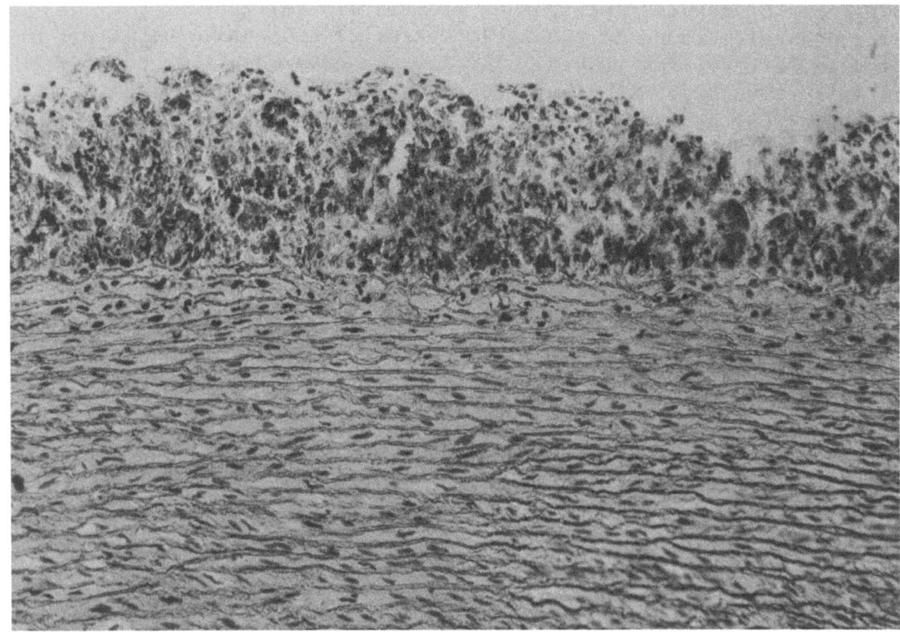

FIGURE 4. Photomicrograph (Weigert's resorcin-fuchsin x 160) of a
spontaneous lesion in the ascending aorta of a cholesterol-fed rabbit. Note the irregular proliferation and palisade-type of growth
of these cells. Note also the total absence of a regular pattern
of elastic fibers.

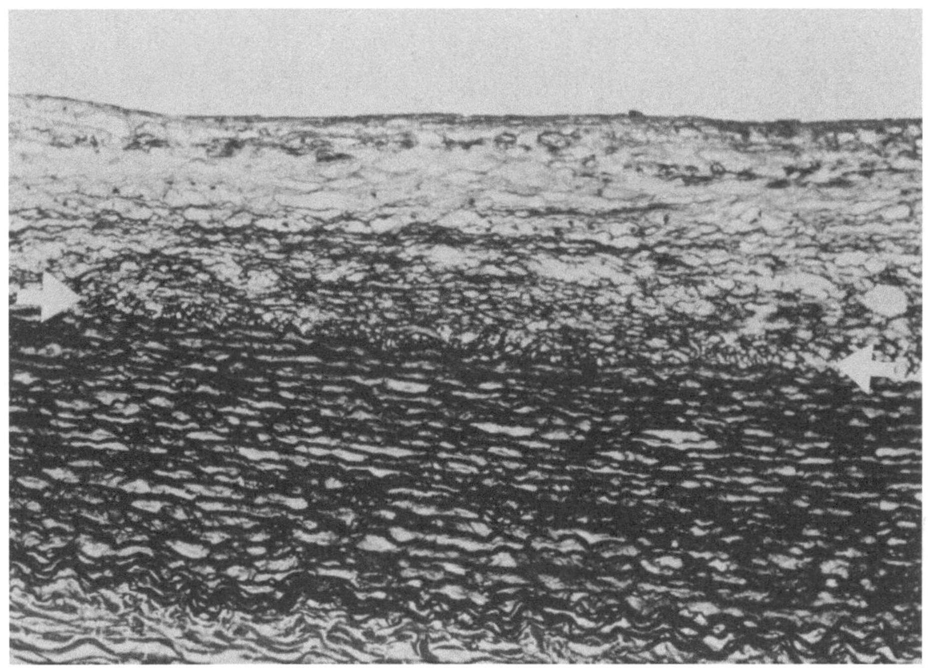

FIGURE 5. Photomicrograph (Weigert's resorcin-fuchsin x 160) of a
segment of induced medial cell hyperplasia in the abdominal aorta
of the same cholesterol-fed rabbit described in FIGURE 4. Note the
regular, smooth growth of the hyperplastic medial cells (above arrows) and the rich deposit of new elastic fibrils present in the
new growth. The morphological differences between this type of
hyperplasia and that depicted in FIGURE 5 are quite obvious.

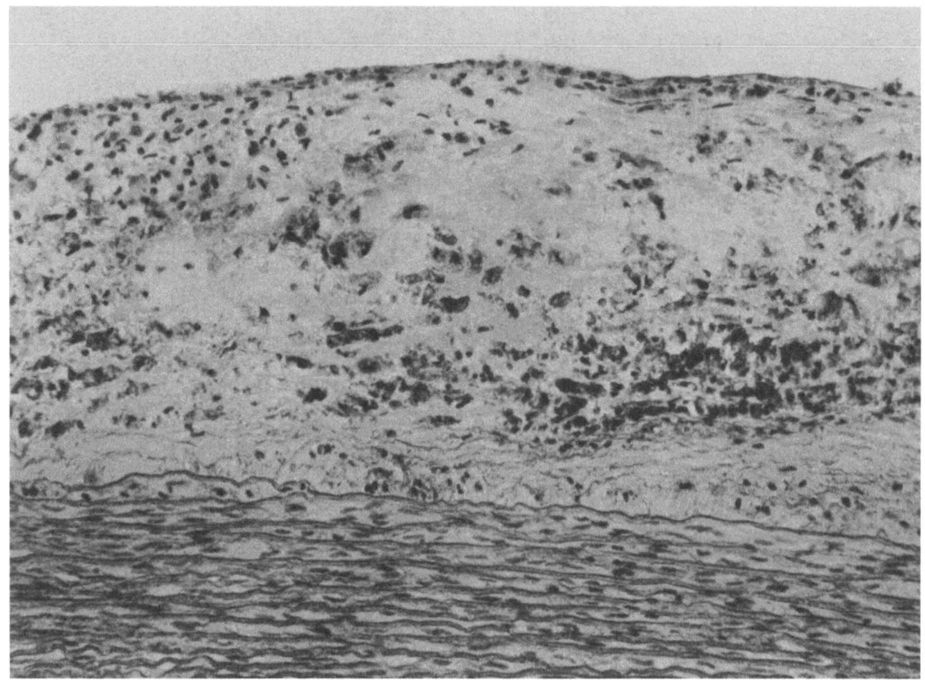

FIGURE 6. Photomicrograph (Weigert's resorcin fuchsin x 160) of a
segment of thrombo-atherosclerotic plaque (induced by insertion of
an aluminum-magnesium alloy) lying in the abdominal aorta of the
same cholesterol-fed rabbit shown in FIGURES 4 and 5. Note its
fibrous, rather irregular growth and the absence of any regular pattern of elastic fibrils within the plaque tissue.

DR. HAUSS: I would only like to give a brief general remark
about our theory of sclerogenesis based on our clinical and experimental research since 1959:

1.   Cells which produce ground substance and fibers and their
stem cells are denoted mesenchymal cells.

2.   Mesenchymal cells have an active metabolism and a most sensitive reactivity and numerous factors induce an acceleration of mesenchymal metabolism ("nonspecific mesenchymal reaction").

3.   The nonspecific mesenchymal reaction in the arterial wall which can be induced by numerous sclerogenic factors is the first pathological event in the arteriosclerosis.

4.   Lipidosis, calcinosis, cell necrosis, fibrinosis and thrombosis in the arterial wall are important but secondary events in the later stages of arteriosclerosis respectively atherosclerosis.

5.   Lipidosis, calcinosis, cell necrosis, fibrinosis and thrombosis in the arterial wall have correlations to the disturbed metabolism and pathological structure of the mesenchyme tissue in the arterial wall.

DR. WERTHESSEN: I do want to say that Dr. Friedman and Dr. Wissler, in their comments, have overlooked the critical significance of Dr. Lee's groups' findings. What a 0.3 dropout, 10 day regeneration time as compared to a normal of 0.5 dropout and 15 days regeneration time means when you observe a tissue is that (a) the tissue is metabolizing faster and (b) it is getting thicker or swelling. And so what Dr. Hauss has just said is significant. The nutrients from the plasma are going to have difficulty getting down through a swollen intima. So in Dr. Wissler's terms, sure it is a medial disease. But it's induced by the simple fact that the media now doesn't have what it needs coming through the intima. Let's leave that for Paris.

DR. CONSTANTINIDES: I would like to start by repeating the "Atherogenesis Equation" that appeared in my 1965 monograph "Experimental Atherosclerosis" and going on from there to see what progress we have made since that time. So we start off with a product relationship between lipemia and injury: A lot of lipemia can produce atherosclerosis (with little or no injury) and a little lipemia can do it - very little lipemia - in the presence of definite injury. How does injury increase atherosclerosis? Well, it could do it in three ways. First of all, let us assume as a working hypothesis that the normal arterial endothelium represents a barrier to very big molecules such as, the large lipoproteins and the particulate lipid - the chylomicrons. Let's think of the possibility that normally very few or no lipoproteins and certainly no chylomicrons cross the endothelium to get into the arterial wall. They would leave the arterial tree at the terminal bed through the perforated seeve-like sinusoids of the liver, intestine, endocrines and the spleen. Normally lipoproteins, as Dr. Werthessen would perhaps agree, are not utilizable directly by striated muscle, which derives most of its fuel from lipid in the form of fatty acid. Lipoproteins would have to split first into fatty acids and then the free fatty acids could be used as fuel by the skeletal muscle and could also cross the endothelium of arteries to get into the arterial wall. Injury will act on the arterial wall and break that endothelium barrier. It will open up doors, it

will make the endothelium of arteries perforated, like the endothelium in the liver sinusoids, and the subendothelial space might become like the space of Disse in the liver. Under the injured endothelium the subendothelial space might be inundated by big molecules
and chylomicrons, perhaps by everything that is in the plasma. That's
one mechanism through which injury could potentiate the deposition
of lipids. Secondly, injury never comes alone. If the injured tissue survives, it will immediately regenerate, produce new cells and
new extracellular material, new collagen, new elastic and new ground
substance, new sulfated mucopolysaccharides - which are all one package, which always come together in the regenerating arterial wall.
This is what Professor Hauss was so impressed with, the "mesenchymal
reaction," which certainly exists, it has been observed for half a
century and nobody quarrels with it. Thirdly, as a corollary of the
proliferation effect, the cells buried within the increasing matrix
of extracellular materials become more and more shut off from the
oxygen, become hypoxic and then gradually die off. But before they
do that, they will become less and less viable, less and less en-
zymatically active and less and less able to handle whatever lipid
gets into the wall. Thus both the cells within the thickening repair zone and the cells underneath the thickening repair zone would
suffer from the thickening. What factors can injure the arterial
wall? We know from animal experiments done a long time ago, that
calciferol can do it (the first experimental injury used in Russia
half a century ago). Now this has always been considered a terribly
artificial thing because nobody takes overdoses of calciferol, but,
in the face of what you have brought out, Dr. Werthessen, I think
there is a real possibility that altered cholesterol or derivatives
of heated cholesterol might have a calciferol-like action.

Vasoactive amines have been shown experimentally to injure the
arterial wall in concentrations of the order of a few gamma per cc.
Angiotensin certainly opened the door at one gamma per cc in the
endothelium of the femoral artery in my experiments, and Dr.
Robertson tells me he has used even a hundred times less than that
- ten nanograms per cc - and he gets evidence of gaps in the endothelium of the coronary capillaries by injecting angiotensin directly into the ventricles of rats. Next, antigen antibody complexes
can injure the arterial wall. They could come from two sources:
Either complexes arising from vascular or from nonvascular antigens. For example, whenever there is an antigen-antibody drama
somewhere else in the kidney for example, you get an immune nephritis.
But antigen-antibody complexes are not only limited to the kidney,
they circulate in the whole body and they attach to various parts of
the entire vascular tree - this has been clearly established by the
recent experiments of the La Jolla group and the Levy group. I was
very impressed at the Federation meeting one or two years ago when
Dr. Charles Cochrane showed us in animals in which he had produced
immune nephritis that within a few days the coronaries became severely injured, their internal elastic membrane was shattered to pieces,

their intima thickened greatly, there was a musculo-elastic hyperplasia with deposition of polysaccharides, and in the fragments of
the disintegrated internal elastica, as well as within the musculo-
elastic proliferated tissue of these injured coronaries, they could
show antigen-antibodies developing in the kidney and yet the coronaries
become injured by them too. So one may wonder how many times, when
we experience small episodes of apparently insignificant immune
disease, how many times this leaves its mark by burning up a little
of our endothelial barrier. In addition to the above there are other
injuring factors such as enzymes, radiation, variously induced hypoxia, kidney disease (acting through an as yet unknown factor) and
many others. Whatever is accomplished by the combination of lipemia
and injury, is further accentuated by an auxiliary hemodynamic factor.
As time goes on, we discover more and more faces of the hemodynamic
injury. At this meeting we have already focused on several. First
of all, the oldest one, the blood pressure. Secondly, blood turbulence, which produces little maelstroms that hit against the wall at
certain sites and may injure it in several different ways. Thirdly,
the systolic elongation that Dr. Fremont-Smith talked about. Fourth-
ly, although it is not strictly hemodynamic, the Gillman factor: A
remodeling of the artery due to growth which undoubtedly occurs both
in width and in length and seems to be similar to the remodeling
that accompanies growth in many of our tissues (including bone,
where we have to destroy old bone before we produce new bone). A
fifth hemodynamic factor could be something that has not yet been
studied very much, as I pointed out on Monday namely a reconstruction
and remodeling of the arterial wall that may very well result from
the rise in postnatal pressure right after birth. In the embryo,
the left side of the heart, the aorta and its branches are exposed
to much lower pressure than right after birth when the foramen ovale
closes and the blood pressure shoots up. This rise in pressure
might constitute a new hemodynamic stress that operates during the
first few postnatal months and contributes to the creation of musculo-elastic hyperplasia. Whatever these forces accomplish will increase with the passage of time. And since this system may operate
discontinuously, we may have a wave of lipemia or a wave of injury
lasting for a few days, weeks or months and then nothing, and each
wave will evidently add to the previous one, because advanced lesions
do not regress anymore than the calcified scar of an old tuberculosis
focus regresses. The successive episodes would show a summation or
accumulation effect leading to a gradual thickening of the lesion.
In addition to this lipemia-injury complex (you may call it the
"first complex" if you wish), we have a "second complex," and this
is thrombosis - mural thrombosis. Thrombosis undoubtedly occurs,
anybody who has looked at enough sections has been forced to accept
that. When I studied serial arterial sections for another purpose,
I was forced to see how often mural thrombi occurred one on top of
the other and became incorporated into the already atherosclerotic
wall and added to its thickness. We can have several waves, several
layers of fibrous thickening due to thrombosis, resulting in the

"multidecker" lesions which I showed at the beginning of this Conference. If we speak of the lipemia-injury complex as the A complex, and of thrombosis as the B complex, it is evident that as in all pluricausal phenomena one may have equal amounts of A and B, or a lot more A than B, or more B than A. I would say that the initial stages of atherosclerosis are almost always A, whereas the subsequent thickening in the coronaries is very much contributed to by B and so is, of course, the final occlusive episode, which can be lethal. I think we have, in the intervening five years, found out about several interactions among the above factors. First of all, there are increasing indications that lipemia itself may cause injury, and may so to speak, "open its own door" into the arterial wall.

Lipemic plasma in tissue cultures has been shown to injure cells. Furthermore, in experiments of the Albany group feeding cholesterol for only three days caused an increased endothelial DNA manufacture. Finally, I recently found that several lipids such as palmitic acid and phosphatidylethanolamine at only a few times their normal concentration, will injure or structurally alter the endothelium and open doors. If injury caused by too much fatty acid proves to be something real, it is interesting to speculate that whereas nature normally expects a release of free fatty acids to provide the fuel for intense muscular activity (for fighting), in our civilized society whenever we get emotionally excited or frustrated or angry, we do not have a muscular outlet and maybe this contributes to the episodic circulation of large amounts of fatty acids that injure our arteries. So we might have here a bridge between emotions and arterial injury. Finally, hemodynamic factors can cause injury and injury causes thrombosis, and there is the most recent possibility that thrombosis itself, (the platelet thrombi in Dr. Mustard's experiments that Dr. Wissler was impressed with) may also injure the endothelium by releasing serotonin or a phospholipid or something else.

DR. HAUST: What has been attempted here is to put the multitude of elements that have been discovered as being relevant to atherogenesis, into a dynamic process. There has been an emphasis on the role of the arterial wall which somehow hasn't been considered always. Now, we may "classify" the injurious element, no matter what its worth and intensity may be, as either belonging to the blood factors (Group I) (constituents and those in transit), hemodynamic factors (Group II) and, finally and very importantly, to factors as they relate to the makeup of the arterial wall itself (Group III). Now, suppose we say that an injurious factor, no matter where it may be derived from, i.e., either from Group I, Group II or Group III, affects the endothelium and results in an injury to endothelium alone; there may follow an altered permeability of the endothelium allowing for influx of whatever blood constituents may be at this given time in the blood stream, into the intima. Once in the intima, these blood factors will impair the mesenchymal components of the

intima, causing altered metabolism of the mesenchyme and further
changes. One can accommodate here Professor Hauss' concept of the
importance of vascular mesenchyme in atherogenesis. Alternatively,
the injury may be of a different nature and not altering the endothelium in any way, but instead, directly affecting the mesenchymal
components of the intima itself. That this is conceivable and possible was borne out of Dr. Bruce Taylor's experiments (Taylor, 1955)
many years ago; he showed that endothelium and other vascular components had a differential susceptibility to various injurious elements. Once these mesenchymal components are altered, so is their
metabolism, and this in turn may affect the endothelial lining with
resulting altered permeability and/or precipitation of mural thrombi.
This is the second possibility. And, finally, I should like to say
a few words on the third possibility and in keeping with the remarks
make today by Dr. Friedman. By its makeup and position the arterial
wall is in a milieu that is exposed to fluctuations dictated by many
factors whether they be hemodynamic, hormonal, blood, neurogenic,
etc. Thus, it may generate the injurious "stimulus" of abnormal
metabolism, so-to-say, in itself, in turn either altering the endothelial lining and allowing the influx of the blood constituents into
the vessel wall, or causing precipitation of mural thrombi. If there
is high lipid content in the blood, obviously this lipid will be also
deposited into the intima. The observations of, and the comments
made by, Dr. Scott today also refer to the factors of the arterial
wall and stress the importance of studying atherosclerosis of human
arteries in metabolic diseases.

DR. WOLF: Among other things we have learned in the past few
days, that the line between normal and abnormal is hazy. The initial
findings in atherosclerosis appear to indicate an accentuation of a
normal process. Some of what we have heard at this conference suggests that the early changes of arteriosclerosis may be adaptive and
that only the later changes are reparative. It may be very pertinent
to identify the trophic mechanisms that regulate the behavior of arterial tissue.* We have learned here that metabolic activity in the
arterial wall is enhanced by each one of a variety of experimental
ways of inducing atherosclerosis. Although the fuel requirement of
the vessel wall is doubtless enhanced, the associated accumulation
of lipids seems to far exceed the requirement. It is less clear that

---

*In an article published since the Lindau Conference (Austin and
Roberts et al., 1971) occular sympathectomy was found to result in
lipid deposition in the smooth muscle cells of the iris. In addition,
the authors reported that norepinephrine exerts a significant effect
on cholestérol ester breakdown and they found that cholesterol esterase activity was reduced to one-third of normal following sympathectomy.

oxygen is present in abundance. Indeed, a deficiency of oxygen may
contribute to the deterioration of muscle cells. At any rate when
the process of repair assumes dominance it is probable that only glucose and no longer lipids can serve the chemistry of healing. The
consequences of endothelial injury appear to include the opening up
of intercellular bridges and ultimately, with an actual rupture of
intima and exposure of collagen, the adherence of platelets and thrombosis. We have also heard that capillaries deep in the plaques may
rupture and that calcium may be deposited in the clot with further
damage to the wall. Underlying the many forces responsible for such
a chain of events a very important factor may be the rapidity of the
change and the intensity of the challenge to adaptation. The importance of dilatability of the coronary arteries to support effort was
emphasized and it was pointed out that this was related to sympathetic
activity. With age sympathetic activity in the artery appears to decrease and also, with age, there occurs a thickening of the intima
with longitudinal orientation of smooth muscle cells and increase
in lymphocytosis. Is there really a primary factor as there is in
infectious diseases for example, or is there necessarily a combination
of adequate factors in the algebra that produces atherosclerosis?

BIBLIOGRAPHY

Abdulla, Y.H., Adams, C.W.M. and Bayliss, O.B.: The Location of
    Lecithin: Cholesterol Transacylase Activity in the Athero-
    sclerotic Arterial Wall. J. Atheroscler. Res. 10: 229, 1969.

Abdulla, Y.H., Adams, C.W.M. and Morgan, R.S.: Connective-Tissue
    Reactions to Implantation of Purified Sterol, Sterol Esters,
    Phosphoglycerides, Glycerides and Free Fatty Acids. J. Path.
    Bact. 94(1):63, 1967.

Abt, A.F., von Schuching, S. and Roe, J.H.: I. Relation of Dietary
    and Tissue Levels of Ascorbic Acid to the Healing of Surgically-
    Induced Wounds in Guinea Pigs. Bull. Johns Hopkins Hosp. 104:
    163, 1959a.

Abt, A.F., von Schuching, S. and Roe, J.H.: II. The Effect of
    Vitamin C Deficiency on Healed Wounds. Bull. Johns Hopkins
    Hosp. 105: 67, 1959b.

Adams, C.W.M. and Bayliss, O.B.: The Relationship Between Diffuse
    Intimal Thickening, Medial Enzyme Failure and Intimal Lipid
    Deposition in Various Human Arteries. J. Atheroscler. Res.
    10: 327, 1969.

Adams, C.W.M., Morgan, R.S. and Bayliss, O.B.: The Differential
    Entry of (^{125}I) Albumin into Mildly and Severely Atheromatous
    Rabbit Aorta. J. Atheroscler. Res. 11: 119, 1970.

Alaupovic, P.: Recent Advances in Metabolism of Plasma Lipoproteins:
    Chemical Aspects. Progr. Biochem. Pharmacol. 4: 91, 1968.

Albrecht, W. and Schuler, W.: The Effect of Short-Term Cholesterol
    Feeding on the Development of Aortic Atheromatosis in the
    Rabbit. I. The Influence of Hypercholesterolaemia on Lipid
    Deposition in the Aorta, Liver and Adrenals. J. Atheroscler.
    Res. 5: 353, 1965.

Amenta, J.S.: A Rapid Chemical Method for Quantification of Lipids
    Separated by Thin-Layer Chromatography. J. Lipid Res. 5: 270,
    1964.

Anitschkow, N.: Ueber Experimentell Erzeugte Ablagerungen von
     Anisotropen Lipoidsubstanzen in der Milz und im Knochenmark.
     Beitr. Path. Anat. 57: 201, 1913.

Anliker, M., Histand, M.B. and Ogden, E.: Dispersion and Attenuation
     of Small Artificial Pressure Waves in the Canine Aorta. Cir-
     culat. Res. 23: 539, 1968.

Anliker, M. and Maxwell, J.A.: The Dispersion of Waves in Blood
     Vessels. Biomechanics Symposium, Proc. Amer. Soc. Mech. Engr.,
     New York, p. 47, 1966.

Anschutz, F.: Physical Activity and Aging. In: D. Brunner and E.
     Jokl (eds.), Medicine and Sport 4: 234, 1970. Basel and New
     York: S. Karger.

Ardlie, N.G. and Schwartz, C.J.: A Comparison of the Organization
     and Fate of Autologous Pulmonary Emboli and of Artificial Plasma
     Thrombi in the Anterior Chamber of the Eye in Normocholes-
     terolemic Rabbits. J. Path. Bact. 95: 1, 1968a.

Ardlie, N.G. and Schwartz, C.J.: The Organization and Fate of
     Autologous Pulmonary Emboli in Hypercholesterolemic Rabbits.
     J. Path. Bact. 95: 19, 1968b.

Armstrong, M.L., Warner, E.D. and Connor, W.E.: Regression of
     Coronary Atheromatosis in Rhesus Monkeys. Circulat. Res. 27:
     59, 1970.

Arndt, J.O.: Uber die Mechanik der Intakten A. Carotis Communis
     des Menschen unter Verschiedenen Kreislaufbedingungen. Archiv
     fur Kreislaufforschung 59: 153, 1969.

Ashford, T.P. and Freiman, D.G.: Platelet Aggregation at Sites of
     Minimal Endothelial Injury. Amer. J. Path. 53: 599, 1968.

Ashworth, L.A.E. and Green, C.: The Transfer of Lipids Between Human
     Alpha-Lipoprotein and Erythrocytes. Biochim. Biophys. Acta
     84: 182, 1964.

Asmussen, E. and Knudsen, E.O.E.: Studies in Acute but Moderate
     CO-Poisoning. Acta Physiol. Scand. 6: 67, 1943.

Astrup, P., Kjeldsen, K. and Wanstrup, J.: Enhancing Influence of
     Carbon Monoxide on the Development of Atheromatosis in Cho-
     lesterol-Fed Rabbits. J. Atheroscler. Res. 7: 343, 1967.

Austin, J., Roberts, W., Neville, H. and Armstrong, D.: The Role
     of the Sympathetic Nervous System in Lipid Deposition. I.

Increased Lipid Deposits in the Iris of the Sympathectomized
Eye in Rabbits Fed an Atherogenic Diet. Stroke 2(1): 23, 1971.

Baker, D.W. and Watkins, D.W.: A Phase Coherent Pulse Doppler System
for Cardiovascular Measurements. Proc. Ann. Conf. Engineering
in Med. and Biol. 9: 27, 1967.

Beaumont, J.L.: Autoimmune Hyperlipidemia. In: R.J. Jones (ed.),
Atherosclerosis: Proceedings of the Second International
Symposium, p. 166. New York, Heidelberg, Berlin: Springer-
Verlag, 1970.

Becker, C.G. and Murphy, G.E.: Demonstration of Contractile Protein
in Endothelium and Cells of the Heart Valves, Endocardium,
Intima, Arteriosclerotic Plaques and Aschoff Bodies of Rheu-
matic Heart Disease. Amer. J. Path. 55: 1, 1969.

Begent, N.A. and Born, G.V.R.: Growth Rate In Vivo of Platelet
Thrombi, Produced by Iontophoresis of ADP, as a Function of
Mean Blood Flow Velocity. Nature 227: 926, 1970.

Benkö, A. and Laki, K.: Studies on the Clot Stabilizing Enzyme in
Aorta of Rabbits under Normal Conditions and after Cholesterol
Feeding. Biochem. Biophys. Res. Commun. 31: 231, 1968.

Bennett, H.S.: Morphological Aspects of Extracellular Polysaccharides. J. Histochem. Cytochem. 11: 14, 1963.

Berne, R.M.: Cardiac Nucleotides in Hypoxia: Possible Role in
Regulation of Coronary Blood Flow. Amer. J. Physiol. 204:
317, 1963.

Bieber, C.P., Stinson, E.B., Shumway, N.E., Payne, R. and Kosek, J.:
Cardiac Transplantation in Man, VII Cardiac Allograft Pathology.
Circulation 41: 753, 1970.

Björkerud, S.: Reaction of the Aortic Wall of the Rabbit after
Superficial Longitudinal, Mechanical Trauma. Virchows Arch.
Path. Anat. 347, 197, 1969.

Blomstrand, R.J., Gurtler, J. and Werner, B.: Fatty Acid Esterification in Man during Fat Absorption. Acta Chem. Scand.
18(4): 1019, 1964.

Böttcher, C.J.F. and van Gent, C.M.: Changes in the Composition
of Phospholipids and of Phospholipid Fatty Acids Associated
with Atherosclerosis in the Human Aortic Wall. J. Atheroscler.
Res. 1: 36, 1961.

Böttcher, C.J.F. and Woodford, F.P.: Lipid and Fatty-Acid Composition of Plasma Lipoproteins in Cases of Aortic Atherosclerosis. J. Atheroscler. Res. 1: 434, 1961.

Böttcher, C.J.F., Woodford, F.P., Romeny-Wachter, C.T.H., Boelsma-van Houte, E. and van Gent, C.M.: Fatty-Acid Distribution in Lipids of the Aortic Wall. Lancet 1: 1378, 1960.

Bowyer, D.E., Howard, A.N. and Gresham, G.A.: Lipid Synthesis in Perfused Normal and Atherosclerotic Rabbit Aortas. Biochem. J. 103: 54P, 1967.

Bowyer, D.E., Howard, A.N., Gresham, G.A., Bates, D. and Palmer, B.V.: Aortic Perfusion in Experimental Animals Lipid Synthesis and Accumulation. Progr. Biochem. Pharmacol. 4: 235, 1968.

Bray, B.A. and Laki, K.: Glycopeptides from Fibrinogen and Fibrin. Biochemistry 7: 3119, 1968.

Buck, R.C. and Rossiter, R.J.: Lipids of Normal and Atherosclerotic Aortas; Chemical Study. Arch. Path. 51: 224, 1951.

Byers, S.A. and Friedman, M.: Effect of Infusions of Phosphatides upon the Atherosclerotic Aorta In Situ and as an Ocular Implant. J. Lipid Res. 1: 343, 1960.

Campbell, E.A.: The Serum Lipoproteins of the Domestic Animals. Res. Vet. Sci. 4: 56, 1963.

Campbell, J.A.: Tissue Oxygen Tension and Carbon Monoxide Poisoning. J. Physiol. 68: 81, 1929.

Caro, C.G., Fitz-Gerald, J.M. and Schroter, R.C.: Arterial Wall Shear and Distribution of Early Atheroma in Man. Nature 223: 1159, 1969.

Casley-Smith, J.R., Ardlie, N.G. and Schwartz, C.J.: Electron-Microscopical Observations on the Organization of Artificial Thrombi in the Rabbit Pulmonary Artery. Brit. J. Exp. Path. 48: 501, 1967.

Castelli, W.P., Nickerson, R.J., Newell, J.M. and Rutstein, D.D.: Serum NEFA Following Fat, Carbohydrate and Protein Ingestion, and During Fasting as Related to Intracellular Lipid Deposition. J. Atheroscler. Res. 6: 328, 1966.

Cavallero, C., Turolla, E. and Ricevuti, G.: Lesions Arterielles par Choi Orthostatique Chez le Lapin. Arch. Mal. Coeur. 62: suppl. 1: 10, 1969.

Chapman, I.: Morphogenesis of Occluding Coronary Artery Thrombosis.
    Arch. Path. 80: 256, 1965.

Chen, R. and Doolittle, R.F.: Isolation, Characterization and
    Location of a Donor-Acceptor Unit from Cross-Linked Fibrin.
    Proc. Natl. Acad. Sci. 66: 472, 1970.

Chobanian, A.V. and Hollander, W.: Phospholipid Synthesis in Human
    Blood Vessels. Clin. Res. 12: 178, 1964.

Choi, B.H., Florentin, R.A. and Thomas, W.A.: Effect of Various
    Concentrations of Hypercholesterolemic (HC) Serum on Mitotic
    Indices of Primary Aortic Cultures. Fed. Proc. 28(2): 682,
    1969.

Constantinides, P.: Plaque Fissures in Human Coronary Thrombosis.
    Fed. Proc. 23: 443, 1964a.

Constantinides, P.: Coronary Thrombosis Linked to Fissure in Athero-
    sclerotic Vessel Wall. JAMA 188: suppl.: 35, May 11, 1964b.

Constantinides, P.: Experimental Atherosclerosis, p. 40, 43.
    Amsterdam, London and New York: Elsevier Publishing Co., 1965.

Constantinides, P.: Plaque Fissures in Human Coronary Thrombosis.
    J. Atheroscler. Res. 6: 1, 1966.

Constantinides, P.: Pathogenesis of Cerebral Artery Thrombosis in
    Man. Arch. Path. 83: 422, 1967.

Constantinides, P.: Lipid Deposition in Injured Arteries. Electron
    Microscopic Study. Arch. Path. 85: 280, 1968.

Constantinides, P. and Robinson, M.: Ultrastructural Injury of
    Arterial Endothelium. 1. Effects of pH, Osmolarity, Anoxia
    and Temperature. Arch. Path. 88: 99, 1969a.

Constantinides, P. and Robinson, M.: Ultrastructural Injury of
    Arterial Endothelium. 2. Effects of Vasoactive Amines. Arch.
    Path. 88: 106, 1969b.

Constantinides, P. and Robinson, M.: Ultrastructural Injury of
    Arterial Endothelium. 3. Effects of Enzymes and Surfactants.
    Arch. Path. 88: 113, 1969c.

Cox, R.W. and Grant, R.A.: Native and Cross-Linked Collagen Fibrils
    and Ionizing Radiation with Electrons. J. Physiol. 200: 36P,
    1968.

Day, A.J.: Incorporation of ^{14}C-Labeled Acetate into Lipid by
Isolated Foam Cells and by Atherosclerotic Arterial Intima.
Circulat. Res. 21: 593, 1967.

Day, A.J., Newman, H.A. and Zilversmit, D.B.: Synthesis of Phospholipid by Foam Cells Isolated from Rabbit Atherosclerotic
Lesions. Circulat. Res. 19: 122, 1966.

Day, A.J. and Tume, R.K.: In Vitro Incorporation of ^{14}C-Labeled
Oleic Acid into Combined Lipid by Foam Cells Isolated from
Rabbit Atheromatous Lesions. J. Atheroscler. Res. 9: 141,
1969.

Day, A.J. and Tume, R.K.: Incorporation of ^{14}C-Labeled Oleic Acid
into Lipid by Foam Cells and by Other Fractions Separated from
Rabbit Atherosclerotic Lesions. Atherosclerosis 11: 291, 1970.

Day, A.J., and Wahlqvist, M.L.: Uptake and Metabolism of ^{14}C-Label-
ed Oleic Acid by Atherosclerotic Lesions in Rabbit Aorta. Circulat. Res. 23: 779, 1968.

Day, A.J. and Wahlqvist, M.L.: Localization by Autoradiography of
Phospholipid Synthesis in Rabbit Atherosclerotic Aorta. Exp.
Molec. Path. 11: 263, 1969.

Day, A.J., Wahlqvist, M. and Campbell, D.J.: Differential Uptake
of Cholesterol and of Different Cholesterol Esters by Atherosclerotic Intima In Vivo and In Vitro. Atherosclerosis 11:
301, 1970a.

Day, A.J., Wahlqvist, M. and Tume, R.K.: Incorporation of Different Fatty Acids into Combined Lipids in Rabbit Atherosclerotic
Lesions. Atherosclerosis 12: 253, 1970b.

Day, A.J. and Wilkinson, G.K.: Incorporation of ^{14}C-Labeled Acetate
into Lipid by Isolated Foam Cells and by Atherosclerotic Arterial Intima. Circulat. Res. 21: 593, 1967.

Dayton, S. and Hashimoto, S.: Movement of Labeled Cholesterol
Between Plasma Lipoprotein and Normal Arterial Wall Across
the Intimal Surface. Circulat. Res. 19: 1041, 1966.

Dayton, S. and Hashimoto, S.: Origin of Fatty Acids in Lipids of
Experimental Rabbit Atheroma. J. Atheroscler. Res. 8: 555,
1968.

Deppe, B.: Uber Hemodynamik des Arteriellen Systems. Z. Biol.
100: 427, 1940.

Dietrich, K.: Beitrage zur Pathologie der Arterien des Menschen.
     I. Mitteilung: Die Allgemeine Pathologie der groBen Muskulosen
     Arterien. Virchows Arch. Path. Anat. 274: 452, 1930.

Dieudonne, J.M.: Influence of Calcium on Acute Serotonin Toxicity
     in the Rat. Lab. Invest. 13: 222, 1964.

Dixon, F.J.: Personal Communication.

Drinker, C.K.: Pulmonary Oedema and Inflammation. Cambridge and
     Harvard: University Press, 1959.

Duckert, F., Jung, E. and Shmerling, D.H.: A Hitherto Undescribed
     Congenital Hemorrhagic Diathesis Probably due to Fibrin Sta-
     bilizing Factor Deficiency. Thromb. Diath. Haemorrh. 5: 179,
     1961.

Duling, B.R. and Berne, R.M.: Longitudinal Gradients in Peri-
     arteriolar Oxygen Tension in the Hamster Cheek Pouch.
     Fed. Proc. 29: 321, 1970.

Duling, B.R., Berne, R.M. and Born, G.V.R.: Microiontophoretic
     Application of Vasoactive Agents to the Microcirculation of
     the Hamster Cheek Pouch. Microvascular Res. 1: 158, 1968.

Duncan, L.E., Jr. and Buck, K.: Comparison of Rates at Which
     Albumin Enters Walls of Small and Large Aortas. Amer. J.
     Physiol. 203: 1167, 1962.

Dzoga, K., Jones, R., Vesselinovitch, D. and Wissler, R.W.:
     Use of Enzyme Labeled Antibodies to Identify Smooth Muscle
     Cells in Tissue Culture. Fed. Proc. 29: 1123, 1970.

Eisenberg, S., Rachmilewitz, D., Stein, O. and Stein, Y.: Biochim.
     Biophys. Acta, in press, 1970.

Eisenberg, S., Stein, Y. and Stein, O.: Phospholipases in Arterial
     Tissue. IV. The Role of Phosphatide Acylhydrolase, Lysophos-
     phatide Acyl-hydrolase, and Sphingomyelin Choline Phosphohydro-
     lase in the Regulation of Phospholipid Composition in the
     Normal Human Aorta with Age. J. Clin. Invest. 48: 2320, 1969a.

Eisenberg, S., Stein, Y. and Stein, O.: Phospholipases in Arterial
     Tissue. III. Phosphatide Acyl-hydrolase, Choline Phospho-
     hydrolase in Rat and Rabbit Aorta in Different Age Groups.
     Biochim. Biophys. Acta 176: 557, 1969b.

Erdos, E.G. (ed.): Bradykinin, Kallidin and Kallikrein. Hand-
     buck der Experimentellen Pharmakologie, pp. 1-850. Heidelberg:
     Springer-Verlag, 1970.

Evans, C.L.: The Velocity Factor in Cardiac Work. J. Physiol.
      52: 6, 1918.

Evans, C.L. and Matsuoka, L.: The Effects of Various Mechanical
      Conditions on the Gaseous Metabolism and Efficiency of the
      Mammalian Heart. J. Physiol. 49: 378, 1915.

Fahr, G.: Work of the Left Ventricle in Normal Hypertension and
      Arteriosclerosis. Proc. Soc. Exp. Biol. Med. 24: 405, 1927.

Farrell, J. and Laki, K.: Clotting of Bovine Fibrinogen by Liver
      Transamidase. Blood 35: 804, 1970.

Fleisch, J.H., Maling, H.M. and Brodie, B.B.: Beta-Receptor
      Activity in Aorta. Circulat. Res. 26: 151, 1970.

Florentin, R.A., Choi, B.H., Lee, K.T. and Thomas, W.A.: Stimula-
      tion of DNA Synthesis and Cell Division In Vitro by Serum
      From Cholesterol-Fed Swine. J. Cell Biol. 41: 641, 1969.

Florentin, R.A. and Nam, S.C.: Dietary Induced Atherosclerosis in
      Miniature Pigs. Exp. Molec. Path. 8: 263, 1968.

Florentin, R.A., Nam, S.C., Lee, K.T., Lee, K.J. and Thomas, W.A.:
      Increased Mitotic Activity in Aortas of Swine After Three Days
      of Cholesterol Feeding. Arch. Path. 88: 463, 1969b.

Florentin, R.A., Nam, S.C. and Thomas, W.A.: High Cell Division
      Rates in Aortic Cushion Region of Cholesterol-Fed Swine.
      Fed. Proc. 28(2): 682, 1969a.

Frank, O.: Die Elastizitat der Blutgefasse. Z. Biol. 37: 483, 1928.

Fredrickson, D.S. and Gordon, R.S., Jr.: Transport of Fatty Acids.
      Physiol. Rev. 38: 585, 1958.

Fredrickson, D.S., Levy, R.I. and Lees, R.S.: Fat Transport in
      Lipoproteins - An Integrated Approach to Mechanisms and Dis-
      orders. New Engl. J. Med. 276: 34, 94, 148, 215 and 273, 1967.

Fremont-Smith, F.: The Role of Elongation and Contraction of the
      Inferior Vena Cava, Coincident with Respiration, in the Return
      of Blood to the Heart: Report of an Observation on Man.
      J. Mount Sinai Hosp. 9: #4, Nov.-Dec., 1942.

Fremont-Smith, F.: Arterial Elongation During Systole. Modern
      Neurology. Boston: Little Brown & Co., 1969.

Friedman, M.: The Pathogenesis of Coronary Artery Disease. New
      York: McGraw-Hill Inc., 1969.

Friedman, M. and Byers, S.O.: Aortic Atherosclerosis Intensification
     in Rabbits by Prior Endothelial Denudation. Arch. Path. 79:
     345, 1965.

Friedman, M., Byers, S.O. and Elek, S.R.: The Induction of Neuro-
     genic Hypercholesterolemia. Proc. Soc. Exp. Biol. Med. 131:
     759, 1969.

Friedman, M., Byers, S.O. and St. George, S.: Site of Origin of the
     Luminal Foam Cells of Atherosclerosis. Amer. J. Clin. Path.
     45: 238, 1966.

Friedman, M. and VanDen Bovenkamp, G.I.: The Pathogenesis of a
     Coronary Thrombus. Amer. J. Path. 48: 19, 1966.

Fry, D.L.: Acute Vascular Endothelial Changes. Associated with
     Increased Blood Velocity Gradients. Circulat. Res. 22: 165,
     1968.

Fyfe, F.W., Gillman, T. and Oneson, I.B.: A Combined Quantitative
     Chemical, Light, and Electron Microscope Study of Aortic
     Development in Normal and Nitrile-treated Mice. Ann. N.Y.
     Acad. Sci. 149: Art. 2: 591, 1968.

Geer, J.C. and Malcolm, G.T.: Cholesterol Ester Fatty Acid
     Composition of Human Aorta Fatty Streak and Normal Intima.
     Exp. Molec. Path. 4: 400, 1965.

Geer, J.C., McGill, H.C., Jr. and Strong, J.P.: The Fine Struc-
     ture of Human Atherosclerotic Lesions. Amer. J. Path. 38: 263,
     1961.

Gillman, T.: Reduplication, Remodeling, Regeneration, Repair, and
     Degeneration of Arterial Elastic Membranes. Arch. Path. 67:
     624, 1959.

Gillman, T.: A Plea for Arterial Biology as a Basis for Under-
     standing Arterial Disease. In: D.G. Chalmers and G.A. Gresham
     (eds.), Biological Aspects of Occlusive Vascular Disease, pp.
     3-23. Cambridge: University Press, 1964.

Gillman, T.: Possible Significance of Arterial Hyperplasia or
     Growth Followed by Involution in the Genesis of Arterial De-
     generatory Diseases. In: Scebat, L. (ed.), Le Role de la Paroi
     Arterielle dans l'atherogenese. Centre National de la Recherche
     Scientifique, 1967.

Gillman, T.: On the Possible Roles of Arterial Growth, Remodeling,
     Repair, and Involution in the Genesis of Arterial Degeneration.
     Ann. N.Y. Acad. Sci. 149: Art. 2: 731, 1968.

Gillman, T., Grant, R.A. and Hathorn, M.: Histochemical and Chemical
    Studies of Calciferol-Induced Vascular Injuries. Exp. Path.
    41: 1, 1960.

Gillman, T. and Hathorn, M.: Rates of Growth and of Remodeling as
    Factors in the Genesis of Vascular and Osseous Lesions of
    Odoralism in Rats. J. Embryol. Exp. Morphol. 6: 270, 1958.

Gillman, T. and Hathorn, M.: Post-Natal Vascular Growth and Remodel-
    ing in the Pathogenesis of Arterial Lesions. Schweiz. Z. Path.
    Bakt. 22: 62, 1959.

Gillman, T., Hathorn, M. and Penn, J.: Microanatomy and Reactions
    to Injury of Vascular Elastic Membranes and Associated Poly-
    saccharides, p. 128. In: R.E. Tunbridge (ed.), Connective
    Tissue, A Symposium. Oxford: Blackwell, 1957.

Gillman, T., Penn, J., Bronks, D., and Roux, M.: Abnormal Elastic
    Fibers, Appearance in Cutaneous Carcinoma, Irradiation Injuries,
    and Arterial and Other Degenerative Connective Tissue Lesions
    in Man. Arch. Path. 59: 733, 1955.

Gladner, J.A., Murtaugh, P.A., Folk, J.E. and Laki, K.: Nature of
    Peptides Released by Fibrinogen. Ann. N.Y. Acad. Sci. 104:
    47, 1963.

Gofman, J.W. and Young, W.: The Filtration Concept of Athero-
    sclerosis and Serum Lipids in the Diagnosis of Atherosclerosis,
    p. 197. In: M. Sandler and G.H. Bourne (eds.), Atherosclerosis
    and Its Origin. New York: Academic Press, 1963.

Goodall, McC: Weightlessness. In: Encyclopedia of Science and
    Technology. New York: McGraw-Hill, in press, 1971.

Goodman, D.S. and Shiratori, T.: Fatty Acid Composition of Human
    Plasma Lipoprotein Fractions. J. Lipid Res. 5: 307, 1964.

Goth, A.: Mechanisms of Histamine Release by Polymeric Compounds
    of Biogenic Amines, pp. 371-378. Symposium on Biogenic Amines,
    Wenner Grene, Karolinska Institute. New York: Pergamon Press,
    1966.

Goth, A.: Effect of Drugs on Mast Cells, pp. 47-78. In: Advances
    in Pharmacology and Chemotherapy vol. 5. New York: Academic
    Press, 1967.

Goth, A., Nash, W.L., Nagler, M. and Holman, R.L.: Inhibition of
    Histamine Release in Experimental Diabetes. Amer. J. Physiol.
    191: 25, 1957.

Gould, R.G., Wissler, R.W. and Jones, R.J.: p. 205. In: R.J.
    Jones (ed.), The Evolution of the Atherosclerotic Plaque.
    Chicago: University of Chicago Press, 1963.

Graham, J.M. and Green, C.: The Binding of Sterols in Cellular
    Membranes. Biochem. J. 103: 16c, 1967.

Grant, R.A.: Preparation of Elastin-Like Material from Collagen
    by Cross-Linking Followed by Heat Treatment. Biochem. J.
    97: 5c, 1965.

Grant, R.A.: Content and Distribution of Aortic Collagen, Elastin
    and Carbohydrate in Different Species. J. Atheroscler. Res.
    7: 463, 1967.

Grant, R.A., Beale and Kent, C.M.: Personal Communication.

Grant, R.A., Cox, R.W. and Kent, C.M.: The Effects of Irradiation
    with High Energy Electrons on the Structure and Reactivity of
    Native and Cross-Linked Collagen Fibers. J. Cell Sci. 7:
    387, 1970.

Grant, R.A., Gillman, T. and Hathorn, M.: Prolonged Chemical and
    Histochemical Changes Associated with Widespread Calcification
    of Soft Tissues Following Brief Acute Calciferol Intoxication.
    Exp. Path. 44: 220, 1963.

Gresham, G.A., Howard, A.N., McGueen, J. and Bowyer, D.E.: Athero-
    sclerosis in Primates. Brit. J. Exp. Path. 46: 94, 1965.

Gunn, C.G., Friedman, M. and Byers, S.O.: Effects of Chronic Hypo-
    thalamic Stimulation upon Cholesterol Induced Atherosclerosis
    in the Rabbit. J. Clin. Invest. 39: 1963, 1960.

Gunn, C.G., Stout, L.C., Stout, W., Stamatis, J. and Williams, G.R.:
    The Influence of Arterial Denervation on Arterial Wall Lipid
    Storage and Synthesis, in preparation.

Gutstein, W.H., LaTaillade, J.N. and Lewis, L.: Role of Vasocon-
    striction in Experimental Arteriosclerosis. Circulat. Res.
    10: 925, 1962.

Gutstein, W.H., Robertson, A.L. and LaTaillade, J.N.: The Role of
    Local Arterial Irritability in the Development of Arterio-
    Atherosclerosis. Amer. J. Path. 42(1): 61, 1963.

Gutstein, W.H., Schneck, D.J. and Appleton, H.: Mechanism of Plasma
    Lipid Increases Following Brain Stimulation. Metabolism 18:
    300, 1969.

Guyton, A.C., Ross, J.M., Carrier, O., Jr. and Walker, J.R.: Evidence for Tissue Oxygen Demand as the Major Factor Causing Autoregulation. Circulat. Res. 15: 1, 1964.

Hagerman, J.S. and Gould, R.G.: The In Vitro Interchange of Cholesterol Between Plasma and Red Cells. Proc. Soc. Exp. Biol. Med. 78: 329, 1951.

Hand, R.A. and Chandler, A.B.: Atherosclerotic Metamorphosis of Autologous Pulmonary Thromboemboli in the Rabbit. Amer. J. Path. 40: 469, 1962.

Harland, W.A.: Pathogenesis of Myocardial Infarct and Coronary Thrombosis, p. 126. In: S. Sherry, K.M. Brinkhous, E. Genton and J.M. Stengle (eds.), Thrombosis. Washington, D.C.: Natl. Acad. Sci., 1969.

Harrison, C.V.: Experimental Pulmonary Arteriosclerosis. J. Path. Bact. 60: 289, 1948.

Hashimoto, S. and Dayton, S.: Transfer of Cholesterol and Cholesteryl Esters into Wall of Rat Aorta In Vitro. J. Atheroscler. Res. 6: 580, 1966.

Hass, G.M., Landerholm, W. and Hemmens, A.: Production of Calcific Athero-Arteriosclerosis and Thromboarteritis with Nicotine, Vitamin D and Dietary Cholesterol. Amer. J. Path. 49: 739, 1966.

Hass, G.M., Truehart, R.E. and Hemmens, A.: Experimental Arteriosclerosis Due to Hypervitaminosis D. Amer. J. Path. 37: 521, 1960.

Hauss, W.H.: Kreislauf und Emotion. Muskel u. Psyche, Symp. Wien 1963, pp. 155-166. Basel and New York: S. Karger, 1964.

Hauss, W.H.: The Role of the Mesenchymal Cells in Arteriosclerosis. Human Pathology, Framingham, in press, 1971.

Haust, M.D.: The Fibrils of Extracellular Space (Microfibrils). Their Structure and Role in Connective Tissue Organization. Amer. J. Path. 47: 1113, 1965.

Haust, M.D. and More, R.H.: Mechanism of Fibrosis in White Atherosclerotic Plaques of Human Aorta. An Electron Microscopic Study. Circulation 34: 14, 1966.

Haust, M.D. and More, R.H.: Electron Microscopy of Connective Tissues and Elastogenesis, pp. 352-376. In: D. Smith and B.

Wagner (eds.), Connective Tissues; Monograph #7, International Academy of Pathology. Baltimore: Williams and Wilkins Co., 1967.

Haust, M.D., More, R.H., Bencosme, S.A. and Balis, J.U.: Elastogenesis in Human Aorta; An Electron Microscopic Study. Exp. Molec. Path. 4: 508, 1965.

Haust, M.D., More, R.H. and Movat, H.Z.: The Mechanism of Fibrosis in Arteriosclerosis. Amer. J. Path. 35: 265, 1959.

Haust, M.D., More, R.H. and Movat, H.Z.: The Role of Smooth Muscle Cells in the Fibrogenesis of Arteriosclerosis. Amer. J. Path. 37: 377, 1960.

Hirsch, R.L. and Kellner, A.: New York Blood Center, New York, Unpublished Observations.

Histand, M.B.: An Experimental Study of the Transmission Characteristics of Pressure Waves in the Aorta. Ph.D. Dissertation, Stanford University, 1969.

Holman, R.L.: Atherosclerosis—A Pediatric Nutrition Problem? Amer. J. Clin. Nutr. 9: 565, 1961.

Honig, C.R.: Control of Smooth Muscle Actomysin by Phosphate and 5'AMP: Possible Role in Metabolic Autoregulation. Microvascular Res. 1: 133, 1968.

Howard, A.N.: Experimental Models for Atherosclerosis and the Study of Arterial Metabolism, p. 171. In: G. Cowgill, D.L. Estrich, and P.D. Wood (eds.), Proceedings of the 1968 Deuel Conference on 'The Turnover of Lipids and Lipoproteins'. Washington, D.C.: U.S. Department of Health, Education and Welfare, 1968.

Howard, A.N., Patelski, J., Bowyer, D.E. and Gresham, G.A.: Induction of Aortic Atherosclerosis in Hypercholesterolaemic Baboons by Immunological Injury, and the Effect of Modification of Aortic Cholesterol Esterase Activity. Circulation, in press, 1970.

Hurley, P.J. and Scott, P.J.: Plasma Turnover of S_f0-9 Low Density Lipoprotein in Normal Men and Women. Atherosclerosis 11: 51, 1970.

Imai, H., Lee, K.J., Lee, S.K., Lee, K.T., O'Neal, R.M. and Thomas, W.A.: Ultrastructural Features of Aortic Cells in Mitosis in Control and Cholesterol-Fed Swine. Lab. Invest. 23(4): 401, 1970.

Imai, H., Lee, K.T., Pastori, S., Ponlilio, E., Florentin, R. and
     Thomas, W.A.: Atherosclerosis in Rabbits. J. Exp. Molec.
     Path. 5: 273, 1966.

Kao, V. and Wissler, R.W.: A Study of the Immunohistochemical
     Localization of Serum Lipoproteins and Other Plasma Proteins
     in Human Atherosclerotic Lesions. J. Exp. Molec. Path. 4:
     465, 1965.

Kao, V.C.Y., Wissler, R.W. and Dzoga, K.: The Influence of Hyper-
     lipemic Serum on the Growth of Medial Smooth Muscle Cells of
     Rhesus Monkey Aorta In Vitro. Circulation 38: 4, 1968.

Karrer, H.E.: An Electron Microscope Study of Developing Chick
     Embryo Aorta. J. Ultrastructure Res. 4: 420, 1960.

Kayden, H.J., Franklin, E.C. and Rosenberg, B.: Interaction of
     Myeloma Gamma-Globulin with Human Beta-Lipoprotein. Circulation
     26: 659, 1962.

Kent, S.P., Vawter, G.F., Dowden, R.M. and Benson, R.E.: Hyper-
     vitaminosis D in Monkeys: A Clinical and Pathologic Study.
     Amer. J. Path. 34: 37, 1958.

Khouri, E.M., Gregg, D.E. and Howensohn, H.S.: Flow Measurements
     in the Major Branches of the Left Coronary Artery During Ex-
     perimental Coronary Insufficiency in the Unanesthetized Dog.
     Circulat. Res. 23: 99, 1968.

Kim, H.S., Suzuki, M. and O'Neal, R.: Leukocyte Lipids of Human
     Blood. Amer. J. Clin. Path. 48: 314, 1967.

Klausen, K., Rasmussen, B., Gjellerod, H., Madsen, H. and Petersen,
     E.: Circulation, Metabolism and Ventilation During Prolonged
     Exposure to Carbon Monoxide and to High Altitude. Scand. J.
     Clin. Lab. Invest. 22: suppl. 103: 26, 1968.

Klip, W., van Loon, P. and Klip, D.A.: Formulas for Phase Velocity
     and Damping of Longitudinal Waves in Thick-Walled Viscoelastic
     Tubes. J. Appl. Physics 38: 3745, 1967.

Klynstra, F.B., Bottcher, C.J.F., Van Melsen, J.A. and Van der Laan,
     E.J.: Distribution and Composition of Acid Mucopolysaccharides
     in Normal and Atherosclerotic Human Aorta. J. Atheroscler. Res.
     7: 301, 1967.

Knieriem, H.J., Kao, V.C.Y. and Wissler, R.W.: Actomysin and Myosin
     and the Deposition of Lipids and Serum Lipoproteins. Arch.
     Path. 84: 118, 1967.

Knieriem, H.J., Kao, V.C.Y. and Wissler, R.W.: Demonstration of
    Smooth Muscle Cells in Bovine Arteriosclerosis: An Immuno-
    histochemical Study. J. Atheroscler. Res. 8: 125, 1968.

Kosek, J. and Bieber, C.P.: Atheroma in a Transplanted Heart.
    Lancet 1: 563, 1970.

Kumar, V., Berenson, G.S., Ruiz, H., Dalferes, E.R. and Strong, J.P.:
    Acid Mucopolysaccharides of Human Aorta. 2. Variations with
    Atherosclerotic Involvement. J. Atheroscler. Res. 7: 583, 1967.

Lagunoff, D. and Benditt, E.P.: Mast Cell Degranulation and
    Histamine Release Observed in a New In Vitro System. J. Exp.
    Med. 112: 571, 1960.

Laki, K.: Enzymatic Effects of Thrombin. Fed. Proc. 24: 794, 1965.

Laki, K.: Fibrinogen. New York: Marcel Dekker, Inc., 1968.

Laki, K. and Lorand, L.: On the Solubility of Fibrin Clots.
    Science 108: 280, 1948.

Lang, P.D. and Insull, W., Jr.: Lipid Droplets in Atherosclerotic
    Fatty Streaks of Human Aorta. J. Clin. Invest. 49: 1479, 1970.

Langer, T., Strober, W. and Levy, R.L.: Familial Type II Hyper-
    lipoproteinaemia: Defect of Beta-Lipoprotein Apoprotein
    Catabolism? J. Clin. Invest. 48: 49a, 1969.

Lee, D. and Alaupovic, P.: Studies of the Composition and Structure
    of Plasma Lipoproteins. Isolation, Composition and Immuno-
    chemical Characterization of Low Density Lipoprotein Sub-
    fractions of Human Plasma. Biochemistry 9: 2244, 1970.

Lee, V.A.: Individual Trends in the Total Serum Cholesterol of
    Children and Adolescents over a Ten-Year Period. Amer. J.
    Clin. Nutr. 20: 5, 1967.

Levy, L.: A Form of Immunological Atherosclerosis, p. 426. In:
    N.R.D. Luzio and R. Paoletti (eds.), Advances in Experimental
    Medicine and Biology, vol. 1. New York: Plenum Press, 1967.

Levy, R.S. and Day, C.E.: Low Density Lipoprotein Structure and
    its Relation to Atherogenesis, pp. 186-189. In: R.J. Jones
    (ed.), Atherosclerosis: Proceedings of the Second International
    Symposium. New York, Heidelberg, Berlin: Springer-Verlag,
    1970.

Lewis, Thomas: Observations upon Reactions of Vessels of Human
    Skin to Cold. Heart 15: 177, 1930.

Liu, L.B. and Taylor, C.B.: Defect of Nicotine and Vitamin D on
     the Genesis of Dietary Hypercholesterolemia and Experimental
     Arteriosclerosis in Rhesus Monkeys. Fed. Proc. 29(2): abs. 796,
     March-April, 1970.

Lofland, H.B. and Clarkson, T.B.: The Bi-Directional Transfer of
     Cholesterol in Normal Aorta, Fatty Streaks, and Atheromatous
     Plaques. Proc. Soc. Exp. Biol. Med. 133: 1, 1970.

Lopez, A., Krehl, W.A. and Hodges, R.E.: Relationship Between Total
     Cholesterol and Cholesteryl Esters with Age in Human Blood
     Plasma. Amer. J. Clin. Nutr. 20: 808, 1967.

Lorand, J., Urayama, T. and Lorand, L.: Transglutaminase as a Blood
     Clotting Enzyme. Biochem. Biophys. Res. Commun. 23: 838, 1966.

Malmros, H. and Sternby, N.H.: Induction of Atherosclerosis in Dogs
     by a Thiouracil-Free Semisynthetic Diet Containing Cholesterol
     and Hydrogenated Coconut Oil. Progr. Biochem. Pharmacol. 4:
     482, 1968.

Mariniscu, V., Pausescu, E., Pavelescu, I. and Fagarasanu, D.:
     Functional and Structural Changes of the Artery Wall after
     Sympathectomy. J. Cardiovasc. Surg. (Turino) 9: 54, 1968.

Matacic, S. and Loewy, A.G.: The Identification of Isopeptide Cross-
     Links in Insoluble Fibrin. Biochem. Biophys. Res. Commun. 30:
     356, 1968.

Matthews, C.M.E.: The Theory of Tracer Experiments with ^{131}I-Labeled
     Plasma Proteins. Phys. in Med. Biol. 2: 36, 1957.

McCandless, E.L. and Zilversmit, D.B.: The Effect of Cholesterol on
     the Turnover of Lecithin, Cephalin and Sphingomyelin in the
     Rabbit. Arch. Biochem. Biophys. 62: 402, 1956.

McGill, H.C., Strong, J.P., Holman, R.L. and Werthessen, N.T.:
     Arterial Lesions in the Kenya Baboon. Circulat. Res. 8: 670,
     1960.

McLeod, F.D.: Calibration of CW and Pulse Doppler Flowmeters. Proc.
     Ann. Conf. Engineering in Med. and Biol. 12: 271, 1970.

Meyer, W.W.: Monatsschr. Kenderheilk, in press, 1971.

Meyer, W.W. and Stelzig, H.H.: Verkalkundgs Formen Der Inneren
     Elastischen Membran der Beinarterien und ihre Bedeutung fur
     die Mediaverkalkung. Virchows Arch. Path. Anat. 342: 361, 1967.

Minick, C.R.:   The Induction of Athero-Arteriosclerosis in Rabbits
     by Repeated Injections of Foreign Serum and Diets Rich in Lipids.
     Bull. N.Y. Acad. Med. 42: 159, 1966.

Minick, C.R., Murphy, G.E. and Campbell, W.G., Jr.:   Experimental
     Induction of Athero-Arteriosclerosis by the Synergy of Allergic
     Injury to Arteries and Lipid-Rich Diet.   J. Exp. Med. 124:
     635, 1966.

Mitchell, J.R.A., Schwartz, C.J. and Zinger, A.:   Relationship
     Between Aortic Plaques and Age, Sex and Blood Pressure.
     Brit. Med. J. 5377: 205, 1964.

Moore, S. and Lough, J.:   Lipid Accumulation in Renal Arterioles
     Due to Platelet Aggregate Embolism.   Amer. J. Path. 58(2):
     283, 1970.

Moritz, W.E.:   Transmission Characteristics of Distension Torsion
     and Axial Waves in Arteries.   Ph.D. Dissertation, Stanford
     University, 1969.

Movat, H.Z., Haust, M.D. and More, R.H.:   The Morphologic Elements
     in the Early Lesions of Arteriosclerosis.   Amer. J. Path. 35:
     93, 1959.

Murphy, T.O., Haglin, J.J. and Felder, D.A.:   The Progression of
     Experimental Atherosclerosis after Lumbar Sympathectomy.   Surg.
     Forum 7: 332, 1957.

Mustard, J.F.:   Recent Advances in Molecular Pathology.   A Review.
     Platelet Aggregation, Vascular Injury and Atherosclerosis.
     Exp. Molec. Path. 7: 366, 1967.

Mustard, J.F., Murphy, E.A., Rowsell, H.C. and Downie, H.G.:
     Platelets and Atherosclerosis.   J. Atheroscler. Res. 4: 1, 1964.

Nam, S.C., Florentin, R.A., Reiner, J.M., Lee, K.T. and Thomas, W.A.:
     Hyperlipemic Diets and Kinetic Parameters of Swine Aortic Cells.
     I. Fundamental Theory and Initial Evaluation for Smooth Muscle
     Cells, in preparation.

Nestel, P.J., Hirsch, E.Z. and Couzens, E.A.:   The Effect of Chloro-
     phenoxyisobutyric Acid and Ethinyl Estradiol on Cholesterol
     Turnover.   J. Clin. Invest. 44: 891, 1965.

Newman, H.A., Day, A.J. and Zilversmit, D.B.:   In Vitro Phospho-
     lipid Synthesis in Normal and Atheromatous Rabbit Aortas.
     Circulat. Res. 19: 132, 1966.

Newman, H.A., McCandless, E.L. and Zilversmit, D.B.: The Synthesis
    of C^{14} -Lipids in Rabbit Atheromatous Lesions. J. Biol. Chem.
    236: 1264, 1961.

Newman, H.A. and Zilversmit, D.B.: Quantitative Aspects of Choles-
    terol Flux in Rabbit Atheromatous Lesions. J. Biol. Chem. 237:
    2078, 1962.

Newman, H.A. and Zilversmit, D.B.: Uptake and Release of Choles-
    terol by Rabbit Atheromatous Lesions. Circulat. Res. 18: 293,
    1966.

Okishio, T.: Studies on the Transfer of I^{131}-Labeled Serum Lipopro-
    teins into the Aorta of Rabbits with Experimental Atheroscle-
    rosis. Med. J. Osaka Univ. 11: 367, 1961.

Olsson, R.A.: Changes in Content of Purine Nucleoside in Canine
    Myocardium During Coronary Occlusion. Circulat. Res. 26:
    301, 1970.

Packham, W.A., Rowsell, H.C., Jorgensen, L. and Mustard, J.F.:
    Localization Protein Accumulation in the Wall of the Aorta.
    Exp. Molec. Path. 7: 214, 1967.

Page, I.H.: Atherosclerosis: An Introduction. Circulation 10:
    1, 1954.

Partridge, S.M., Elsden, D.F. and Thomas, J.: Constitution of the
    Cross-Linkages in Elastin. Nature (London) 197: 1297, 1963.

Patelski, J., Bowyer, D.E., Howard, A.N. and Gresham, G.A.:
    Changes in Phospholipase A, Lipase and Cholesterol Esterase
    Activity in the Aorta in Experimental Atherosclerosis in the
    Rabbit and Rat. J. Atheroscler. Res. 8: 221, 1968.

Patelski, J., Bowyer, D.E., Howard, A.N., Jennings, I.W., Thorne,
    C.J.R. and Gresham, G.A.: Modification of Enzyme Activities
    in Experimental Atherosclerosis in the Rabbit. Atherosclerosis
    12: 41, 1970.

Patterson, J.C.: Capillary Rupture with Intimal Hemorrhage as
    Causative Factor in Coronary Thrombosis. Arch. Path. 25:
    474, 1938.

Peronneau, P.A. and Leger, F.: Doppler Ultrasonic Pulsed Blood
    Flowmeter. Proc. 8th International Conf. on Medical and
    Biological Engineering, Chicago, Ill., p. 10, 1969.

Peterson, L., Lessen, M. and Shepard, R.: Some Current Problems
    in Circulatory Physiology. C.R. II. Intl. Congr. Angiol.
    Fribourg, p. 11. Basel: Schwabe, 1956.

Pirani, C.L. and Levenson, S.M.: Effect of Vitamin C Deficiency on
    Healed Wounds. Proc. Soc. Exp. Biol. Med. 82: 95, 1953.

Pisano, J.J., Finlayson, J.S. and Peyton, M.P.: Cross-Link in Fibrin
    Polymerized by Factor XIII: ε-(γ-glutamyl) Lysine. Science
    160: 892, 1968.

Poole, J.C., Sanders, A.G. and Florey, H.W.: The Regeneration of
    Aortic Endothelium. J. Path. Bact. 75: 133, 1958.

Pyorala, K., Punsar, S., Seppala, F. and Carlsson, K.: Mucopoly-
    saccharides of the Aorta and Epiphyseal Cartilage in Lathyritic
    Growing Rats and Rat Fetuses. Acta Path. Microbiol. Scand. 41:
    497, 1957.

Rein, H.: Untersuchungen am Herzlungenpraparat mit Verschiedener
    Windkesselgrosse. Ges. Naturwissenschaft Gottingen Klasse
    VI(3): 270, 1937-40.

Remington, J.W.: Volume Quantitation of the Aortic Pressure Pulse.
    Fed. Proc. 11: 750, 1952.

Reynolds, S.M.R., Light, F.W., Jr., Ardran, G.M. and Prichard, M.M.L.:
    The Qualitative Nature of Pulsatile Flow in Umbilical Blood
    Vessels, with Observations on Flow in the Aorta. Bull. Johns
    Hopkins Hosp. 91: 83, 1952.

Rindfleisch, E.: A Manual of Pathological Histology, vol. I.
    London: New Sydenham Society, 1872.

Robertson, A.L.: Metabolism and Ultrastructure of the Arterial
    Wall in Atherosclerosis. Cleveland Clinic Quart. 32(3): 99,
    1965a.

Robertson, A.L.: Intracellular Incorporation of Plasma Lipoproteins
    by Arterial Intima in Relation to Early Stages of Intravascular
    Thrombosis, pp. 267-274. In: P.N. Sawyer (ed.), Biophysical
    Mechanisms in Vascular Homeostasis and Intravascular Thrombosis.
    New York: Appleton-Century-Crofts, 1965b.

Robertson, A.L.: Transport of Plasma Lipoproteins and Ultrastructure
    of Human Arterial Intimacytes in Culture. Wistar Institute
    Symposium "Lipid Metabolism in Tissue Culture Cells" Monograph
    6: 115, 1967.

Robertson, A.L.: Oxygen Requirements of Arterial Intima in Athero-
      genesis. International Symposium on Recent Advances in Athero-
      sclerosis. Progr. Biochem. Pharmacol. 4: 305, 1968.

Robertson, A.L. and Insull, W.: Dissection of Normal and Athero-
      sclerotic Human Artery with Proteolytic Enzymes In Vitro.
      Nature 214: 821, 1967.

Rutstein, D.D. Castelli, W.P. and Nickerson, R.J.: Effect of Carbo-
      hydrate Ingestion in Humans on Intracellular Lipid Deposition
      in Tissue Culture. Amer. J. Clin. Nutr. 20: 98, 1967.

Rutstein, D.D., Castelli, W.P. and Nickerson, R.J.: Heparin and
      Human Lipid Metabolism. Lancet 1: 1003, May 17, 1969.

Rutstein, D.D., Castelli, W.P., Sullivan, J.C. Newell, J.M. and
      Nickerson, R.J.: Effects of Fat and Carbohydrate Ingestion in
      Human Beings on Serum Lipids and Intracellular Lipid Deposition
      in Tissue Culture. New Engl. J. Med. 271: 1, 1964.

Sanwald, R., Ritz, E. and Hug, B.: Untersuchungen zum Stoffwechsel
      der Sauren Mucopolysaccharide in Normalen und Arteriosklerotisch
      Veranderten Frischen Menschlichen Arterien. J. Atheroscler.
      Res. 8: 433, 1968.

Schatz, J.D. and Williams, R.H.: The Effect of Acute Insulin
      Deficiency in the Rat on Adipose Tissue Lipolytic Activity
      and Plasma Lipids. Diabetes 12: 174, 1963.

Schmidtmann, M.: Vigantolversuche. Verhandl. Dtsch. Path. Ges.
      24: 75, 1929.

Schmitt, G., Knoche, H., Junge-Hulsing, G., Koch, R. and Hauss.,
      W.H.: Uber die Reduplikation von Aortenwandzellen bei
      Arterielles Hypertonie. Z. Kreislaufforschg. 6: 481, 1970.

Schrade, W, Bohle, E. and Biegler, R.: The Fatty Acids and Blood
      Lipids in Health and in Atherosclerosis and Their Modifications
      by Exogenous Influences, p. 454. In: S. Garattini and R.
      Paoletti (eds.), Drugs Affecting Lipid Metabolism. Amsterdam:
      Elsevier, 1961.

Schwartz, C.J.: Personal Communication.

Schwartz, C.J., Ardlie, N.G., Carter, R.F. and Patterson, J.C.:
      Gross Aortic Sudanophilia and Hemosiderin Deposition. A
      Study on Infants, Children and Young Adults. Arch. Path.
      83: 325, 1967.

Schwartz, C.J. and Mitchell, J.R.A.: Observations on Localization
    of Arterial Plaques. Circulat. Res. 11: 63, 1962.

Schwartz, C.J., Nishizawa, E.E., Somer, J.B. and Mustard, J.F.:
    Focal ^{3}H and ^{14}C Cholesterol Accumulation in the Pig Aorta.
    Circulation 38: suppl. 6: 22, 1968.

Schwartz, C.J. Stenhouse, N.S., Taylor, A.E. and White, T.A.:
    Coronary Disease Severity at Necropsy. Brit. Heart J. 28: 731,
    1965.

Scott, P.J. and Hurley, P.J.: The Distribution of Radio-Iodinated
    Serum Albumin and Low Density Lipoprotein in Tissues and the
    Arterial Wall. J. Atheroscler. Res. 11: 77, 1970.

Scott, P.J., White, B.M., Winterbourn, C.C. and Hurley, P.J.: Low
    Density Lipoprotein Peptide Metabolism in Nephrotic Syndrome;
    A Comparison with Patterns Observed in Other Syndromes Char-
    acterized by Hyperlipoproteinaemia. Aust. Ann. Med. 1: 1, 1970.

Scott, P.J. and Winterbourn, C.C.: Low Density Lipoprotein Ac-
    cumulation in Actively Growing Xanthomas. J. Atheroscler.
    Res. 7: 207, 1967.

Scott, R.F., Jarmolych, J., Fritz, K.E., Imai, H., Kim, D.N. and
    Morrison, E.S.: Reactions of Endothelial and Smooth Muscle
    Cells in the Atherosclerotic Lesions, p. 50. In: R.J. Jones
    (ed.), Atherosclerosis: Proceedings of the Second Internation-
    al Symposium. New York, Heidelberg, Berlin: Springer-Verlag,
    1970.

Seelig, M.S.: Vitamin D. and Cardiovascular, Renal, and Brain Damage
    in Infancy and Childhood. Ann. N.Y. Acad. Sci. 147: 537, 1969.

Serafini-Fracassini, A.: Electron Microscope and X-Ray Crystal
    Analysis of the Calciferol Elastic Tissue. J. Atheroscler.
    Res. 3: 178, 1963.

Shimamoto, T.: Damages to Silicone-Like Property of Vascular Endo-
    thelial Cells and Prevention of Monoamine Oxidase Inhibitor,
    Nialamide. Asian Med. J. 3: 479, 1960.

Siggaard-Andersen, J.P., Bonde, F., Hansen, T.I. and Mellemgaard, K:
    Plasma Volume and Vascular Permeability During Hypoxia and
    Carbon Monoxide Exposure. Scand. J. Clin. Lab. Invest. 22:
    suppl. 103: 39, 1968.

Simon, R.C., Still, W.J. and O'Neal, R.M.: The Circulating Lipo-
    phage and Experimental Atherosclerosis. J. Atheroscler. Res.
    1: 395, 1961.

Sinapius, D.: Uber Wandveranderungen bei Coronarthrombose.
    Bemerkungen zur Haufigkeit, Entstehung und Bedeutung. Klin.
    Wschr. 43: 875, 1965.

Singh, I., Khanna, P.K., Srivastava, M.C., Lal, M., Roy, S.B. and
    Subramanyam, C.S.V.: Acute Mountain Sickness. New Engl. J.
    Med. 280: 175, 1969.

Smith, E.B.: The Influence of Age and Atherosclerosis on the
    Chemistry of Aortic Intima. I. The Lipid. J. Atheroscler.
    Res. 5: 224, 1965a.

Smith, E.B.: The Influence of Age and Atherosclerosis on the
    Chemistry of Aortic Intima. II. Collagen and Mucopolysac-
    charides. J. Atheroscler. Res. 5: 241, 1965b.

Smith, E.B.: Quantitative and Qualitative Comparison of the Lipids
    in Platelets, Aortic Intima and Mural Thrombi. Cardiovascular
    Res. 1: 111, 1967.

Smith, E.B., Evans, P.H. and Downham, M.D.: Lipid in the Aortic
    Intima. The Correlation of Morphological and Chemical Char-
    acteristics. J. Atheroscler. Res. 7: 171, 1967.

Smith, E.B. and Slater, R.S.: The Chemical and Immunological Assay
    of Low Density Lipoproteins Extracted from Human Aortic Intima.
    Atherosclerosis 11: 417, 1970a.

Smith, E.B. and Slater, R.S.: The Lipoproteins of the Lesions, p. 42.
    In: R.J. Jones (ed.), Atherosclerosis: Proceedings of the
    Second International Symposium. New York, Heidelberg, Berlin:
    Springer-Verlag, 1970b.

Smith, E.B. and Slater, R.S.: Manuscript in Preparation.

Smith, E.B., Slater, R.S. and Chu, P.K.: The Lipids in Raised Fatty
    and Fibrous Lesions in Human Aorta. A Comparison of the Changes
    at Different Stages of Development. J. Atheroscler. Res. 8:
    399, 1968.

Snyder, D.D. and Campbell, G.S.: Effect of Aortic Constriction on
    Experimental Atherosclerosis in Rabbits. Proc. Soc. Exp. Biol.
    Med. 99: 563, 1958.

Solowjew, A.: Uber Experimentell Hervorgerufene Elasticarisse der
    Arterien und deren Bedeutung fur die Lipoidablagerung. Virchows
    Arch. Path. Anat. 283: 213, 1932.

Somoza, C.: Serum Cholesterol Levels and Aortic Medical Calcifi-
    cations in Rabbits with Lesions in the Brain. Amer. J. Path.
    47: 271, 1965.

Spraragen, S.C., Bond, V.F. and Dahl, L.K.: Role of Hyperplasia in
    Vascular Lesions of Cholesterol-Fed Rabbits Studied with Thy-
    midine-^{3}H Autoradiography.. Circulat. Res. 11: 329, 1962.

St. Clair, R.W., Lofland, H.B., Jr. and Clarkson, T.B.: Composition
    and Synthesis of Fatty Acids in Atherosclerotic Aortas of the
    Pigeon. J. Atheroscler. Res. 9: 739, 1968.

St. Clair, R.W., Lofland, H.B., Jr. and Clarkson, T.B.: Influence
    of Atherosclerosis on the Composition, Synthesis, and Esterifi-
    cation of Lipids in Aorta of Squirrel Monkeys (Saimiri Sciureus).
    J. Atheroscler. Res. 10: 193, 1969.

St. Clair, R.W., Lofland, H.B., Jr. and Clarkson, T.B.: Influence
    of Duration of Cholesterol Feeding on Esterification of Fatty
    Acids by Cell-Free Preparation and Pigeon Aorta. Studies on
    the Mechanism of Cholesterol Esterification. Circulat. Res.
    27: 213, 1970.

Stary, H.C.: Cell Proliferation in the Experimental Atheroma as
    Revealed by Radioautography After Injection of Thymidine-^{3}H.
    Circulation 36: suppl 2: 11, 1967.

Stary, H.C. and McMillan, G.C.: Kinetics of Cell Proliferation in
    Experimental Atherosclerosis. Arch. Path. 89: 173, 1970.

Stein, O., Eisenberg, S. and Stein, Y.: Aging of Aortic Smooth
    Muscle Cells in Rats and Rabbits. A Morphologic and Biochemical
    Study. Lab. Invest. 21: 386, 1969.

Stein, O., Rachmilewitz, D., Eisenberg, S. and Stein, Y.: Aortic
    Phospholipids. Localization in Normal Adult Aorta. Israel
    J. Med. Sci. 6: 53, 1970.

Stein, O., Selinger, Z., Stein, Y.: Incorporation of (1-^{14}C)-
    Linoleic Acid into Lipids of Human Umbilical Arteries. J.
    Atheroscler. Res. 3: 189, 1963.

Stein, O. and Stein, Y.: Lipid Synthesis and Transport in the Nor-
    mal and Atherosclerotic Aorta. An Autoradiographic Study of
    Rat and Rabbit Aortae Incubated and Perfused with Choline-H^3
    and Oleic Acid-H^3. Lab. Invest. 23: 556, 1970.

Stein, Y. and Stein, O.: Incorporation of Fatty Acids into Lipids
    of Aortic Slices of Rabbits, Dogs, Rats and Baboons. J. Athero-
    scler. Res. 2: 400, 1962.

Stein, Y., Stein, O. and Shapiro, B.: Enzymic Pathways of Glyceride
    and Phospholipid Synthesis in Aortic Homogenates. Biochim.
    Biophys. Acta. 70: 33, 1963.

Sternby, N.H.: Atherosclerosis in a Defined Population. An Autopsy
     Survey in Malmo, Sweden. Acta Path. Microbiol. Scand., Suppl.
     194: 5+, 1968.

Stetten, M.R.: Some Aspects of Metabolism of Hydroxyproline, Studied
     with Aid of Isotopic Nitrogen. J. Biol. Chem. 181: 31, 1949.

Still, W.J.S.: An Electron Microscopic Study of the Organization
     of Experimental Thrombo-Emboli in the Rabbit. Lab. Invest. 15:
     1492, 1966.

Stoltzner, G.: Electron Microscopic Studies Concerning the Presence
     of Platelet Specific Antigen in Atheromas. Thesis presented for
     M.S. degree, University of Chicago, 1968.

Strong, J.P. and McGill, H.C., Jr.: The Natural History of Coronary
     Atherosclerosis. Amer. J. Path. 40: 37, 1962.

Strong, J.P., Richard, M.L., McGill, H.C., Jr., Eggen, D.A. and
     McMurry, M.T.: On the Association of Cigarette Smoking with
     Coronary and Aortic Atherosclerosis. J. Atheroscler. Res. 10:
     303, 1969.

Suzuki, M. and O'Neal, R.: Circulating Lipophages, Serum Lipids,
     and Atherosclerosis in Rats. Arch. Path. 83: 169, 1967.

Tanner, J.M. and Whitehouse, R.H.: Standards for Subcutaneous Fat
     in British Children. Percentiles for Thickness of Skinfolds
     over Triceps and Below Scapula. Brit. Med. J. 5276: 446,
     Feb. 17, 1962.

Taylor, C.B.: The Reaction of Arteries to Injury by Physical Agents.
     With a Discussion of Arterial Repair and Its Relationship to
     Atherosclerosis, pp. 74-90. In: Symposium on Atherosclerosis.
     National Academy of Sciences - National Research Council
     Publication 338, 1955.

Taylor, C.B., Cox, G.E., Hall-Taylor, B.J. and Nelson, L.G.: Athero-
     sclerosis in Areas of Vascular Injury in Monkeys with Mild
     Hypercholesterolemia. Circulation 10: 613, 1954.

Taylor, C.B., Cox, G.E., Manalo-Estrella, P., Southworth, J., Patton,
     D.E. and Cathcart, C.: Atherosclerosis in Rhesus Monkeys.
     II. Arterial Lesions Associated with Hypercholesterolemia
     Induced by Dietary Fat and Cholesterol. Arch. Path. 74: 16,
     1962.

Taylor, C.B., Trueheart, R.E. and Cox, G.E.: Atherosclerosis in
     Rhesus Monkeys: III. The Role of Increased Thickness of Ar-
     terial Walls in Atherogenesis. Arch. Path. 76: 14, 1963.

Texon, M.: A Hemodynamic Concept of Atherosclerosis, with Partic-
    ular Reference to Coronary Occlusion. Arch. Int. Med. 99: 418,
    1957.

Thienes, C.H.: Chronic Nicotine Poisoning. Ann. N.Y. Acad. Sci.
    90: 239, 1960.

Thomas, W.A., Florentin, R.A., Nam, S.C., Kim, D.N., Jones, R.M.
    and Lee, K.T.: Pre-Proliferative Phase of Atherosclerosis in
    Swine Fed Cholesterol. Arch. Path. 86: 621, 1968.

Thomson, J.G.: Production of Severe Atheroma in a Transplanted
    Human Heart. Lancet 2: 1088, Nov. 22, 1969.

Todd, A.S.: The Histological Localization of Fibrinolysin Activator.
    J. Path. Bact. 78: 281, 1959.

Tyler, H.M. and Laki, K.: Purification and Properties of a Fibrin
    Cross-Linking Transamindase from Rabbit Liver. Biochemistry
    6: 3259, 1967.

Ueda, H., Ebihara, A., Ishii, M., Taiceda, T. and Ikeda, T.: Effects
    of Chronic Electrical Stimulation of Diencephalon on Aortas
    in Rabbits. Jap. Heart J. 6: 325, 1965.

Unna, P.G.: The Histopathology of the Diseases of the Skin.
    Translated by N. Walker. Edinburgh: Wm. F. Clay, 1896.

Uvnas, B. and Thon, I.L.: Mechanisms of Release of Biogenic Amines,
    pp. 361-370, Symposium on Biogenic Amines, Wenner Grene,
    Karolinska Institute. New York: Pergamon Press, 1966.

Van Citters, R.L. and Watson, N.W.: Coronary Disease in Spawning
    Steelhead Trout Salmo Gairdnerii. Science 159: 105, 1968.

Van Winkle, M. and Levy, L.: Effect of Removal of Cholesterol Diet
    upon Serum Sickness-Cholesterol-Induced Atherosclerosis. J.
    Exptl. Med. 128: 497, 1968.

Vane, J.R.: The Release and Fate of Vaso-Active Hormones in the
    Circulation. Brit. J. Pharmacol. 35: 209, 1969.

Vihert, A.M., Zhdanov, V.S. and Matova, E.E.: Atherosclerosis of
    the Aorta and Coronary Vessels of the Heart in Cases of Various
    Diseases. J. Atheroscler. Res. 9: 179, 1969.

Vlodaver, Z., Kahn, H.A. and Neufeld, H.N.: The Coronary Arteries
    in Early Life in Three Different Ethnic Groups. Circulation
    39: 541, 1969.

Volwiler, J.W., Goldsworthy, P.D., MacMartin, M.P., Wood, P.A.,
    Mackay, I.R. and Fremont-Smith, K.: Biosynthetic Determination
    with Radioactive Sulfur of Turn-Over Rates of Various Plasma
    Proteins in Normal and Cirrhotic Man. J. Clin. Invest. 34:
    1126, 1955.

Vost, A.: Lipid Accretion in the Perfused Rabbit Aorta. J. Athero-
    scler. Res. 9: 221, 1969.

Wahlqvist, M.L. and Day, A.J.: Phospholipid Synthesis by Foam Cells
    in Human Atheroma. Exp. Molec. Path. 11: 275, 1969.

Wahlqvist, M.L., Day, A.J. and Tume, R.K.: Incorporation of Oleic
    Acid into Lipid by Foam Cells in Human Atherosclerotic Lesions.
    Circulat. Res. 24: 123, 1969.

Waisman, J., Carnes, W.H. and Weissman, N.: Some Properties of the
    Microfibrils of Vascular Elastic Membranes in Normal and Cooper-
    Deficient Swine. Amer. J. Path. 54: 107, 1969.

Walton, K.W., Scott, P.J., Dykes, P.W. and Davies, J.W.L.: The
    Significance of Alterations in Serum Lipids in Thyroid Dys-
    function. II. Alterations of the Metabolism and Turnover of
    ^{131}I-Low-Density-Lipoproteins in Hypothyroidism and Thyrotox-
    icosis. Clin. Sci. 29: 217, 1965.

Walton, K.W. and Williamson, N.: Histological and Immunofluorescent
    Studies on the Evolution of the Human Atheromatous Plaque.
    J. Atheroscler. Res. 8: 599, 1968.

Wanstrup, J., Kjeldsen, K. and Astrup, P.: Acceleration of Sponta-
    neous Intimal-Subintimal Changes in Rabbit Aorta by a Prolonged
    Moderate Carbon Monoxide Exposure. Acta Path. Microbiol. Scand.
    75: 353, 1969.

Warren, B.A.: Fibrinolytic Properties of Vascular Endothelium.
    Brit. J. Exp. Path. 44: 365, 1963.

Watts, H.F.: The Mechanism of Arterial Lipid Accumulation in Human
    Coronary Artery Atherosclerosis, pp. 98-113. In: W. Likoff
    and J.H. Moyer (eds.), Coronary Heart Disease. New York:
    Greene and Stratton, Inc., 1963a.

Watts, H.F.: Role of Lipoprotein in the Formation of Atherosclerotic
    Lesions, pp. 117-132. In: R.J. Jones (ed.), Evolution of the
    Atherosclerotic Plaque. Chicago: University of Chicago Press,
    1963b.

Weller, R.O.: Cytochemistry of Lipids in Atherosclerosis. J. Path.
    Bact. 94: 171, 1967.

Wenzel, D.G., Turner, J.A. and Kissil, D.: Effect of Nicotine on
     Cholesterol-Induced Atherosclerosis in the Rabbit. Circulat.
     Res. 7: 256, 1959.

Werthessen, N.T., Beall, J.R. and James, A.T.: Semiautomatic
     Chromatographic Determination of Neutral Lipids. J. Chromatog.
     46: 149, 1970.

Wiggers, C.J.: Physical and Physiological Aspects of Arterioscle-
     rosis and Hypertension. Ann. Int. Med. 6: 12, 1932.

Wilens, S.L. and McCluskey, R.T.: Permeability of Excised Arteries
     and Other Tissues to Serum Lipid. Circulat. Res. 2: 175, 1954.

Wissler, R.W.: How Does "Spontaneous" Atherosclerosis in Animals
     Compare to that in Man? p. 342. In: J.C. Roberts, Jr. and R.
     Straus (eds.), Comparative Atherosclerosis. New York:
     Hoeber, Inc., 1965.

Wissler, R.W.: Discussion Following Papers by Dr. R. Foster Scott
     and Dr. L. Robert, p. 72. In: R.J. Jones (ed.), Atheroscle-
     rosis: Proceedings of the Second International Symposium.
     New York, Heidelberg, Berlin: Springer-Verlag, 1970a.

Wissler, R.W.: Introduction: Pathogenesis of Atherosclerosis, p. 3.
     In: R.J. Jones (ed.), Atherosclerosis: Proceedings of the
     Second International Symposium. New York, Heidelberg, Berlin:
     Springer-Verlag, 1970b.

Wissler, R.W. and Kao, V.: Immunohistochemical Studies of the
     Human Aorta. Fed. Proc. 21: 95, 1962.

Wissler, R.W., Moskowitz, M.S., Hughes, R.H. and Petrie, L.: A
     Study of the Histogenesis of Atherosclerosis in Man. Circu-
     lation 18: 497, 1958.

Wissler, R.W. and Vesselinovitch, D.: Experimental Models of Human
     Atherosclerosis. Ann. N.Y. Acad. Sci. 149(2): 907, 1968.

Wojcik, J.D., D.L. Van Horn, A.J. Webber, and S.A. Johnson: Mech-
     anism Whereby Platelets Support the Endothelium. Transfusion
     9: 324, 1969.

Wolinsky, H. and Glagov, S.: Structural Basis for the Static
     Mechanical Properties of the Aortic Media. Circulat. Res.
     14: 400, 1964.

Wolinsky, H. and Glagov, S.: Comparison of Abdominal and Thoracic
     Aortic Medical Structure in Mammals: Deviation of Man from the
     Usual Pattern. Circulat. Res. 25(6): 677, 1969.

Wright, H.P.: Thromb. Diath. Haemorrh., in press, 1971.

Wyllie, J. and Haust, M.D.: Demonstration of Fibrin in Early Fatty
    Lesions of Human Arteriosclerosis by Fluorescent Antibody
    Method. Fed. Proc. 22: 251, 1963.

Yang, H.Y.T., Erdos, E.G., Jenssen, T.A. and Levin, Y.: Character-
    ization of an Angiotensin I Converting Enzyme. Fed. Proc. 29:
    281, 1970a.

Yang, H.Y.T., Erdos, E.G. and Levin, Y.: A Dipeptidyl Carboxy-
    peptidase that Converts Angiotensin II and Inactivates Brady-
    kinin. Biochim. Biophys. Acta 214: 374, 1970b.

Yang, H.Y.T., Erdos, E.G. and Levin, Y.: J. Pharmacol. Exp. Therapy,
    in press, 1971.

Yates, W.G.: Experimental Studies of the Variations in the Mechan-
    ical Properties of the Canine Abdominal Vena Cava. Ph.D.
    Dissertation, Stanford University, 1969.

Yu, S.Y. and Blumenthal, H.T.: The Calcification of Elastic Fibers.
    I. Biochemical Studies. J. Geront. 18: 127, 1963.

ADDENDUM

A prominent topic for discussion at the Conference was the
connective tissue proliferation characteristic of arteriosclerosis.
Following the Conference the following highly relevant publications
appeared:
    Rodbard, S.: Negative Feedback Mechanisms in the Architecture
        and Function of the Connective and Cardiovascular Tissues.
        Perspectives in Biol. Med. 13, #4: 507, Summer, 1970.

Dr. Robert was unable to attend the Conference, but his work,
and that of his collaborators, concerning enzymes of human platelets,
was referred to by several of the speakers, two of the references
are as follows:
    Robert, B., Szigeti, M., Robert, L., Legrand, Y., Pignaud, G.
        and Caen, J.: Release of Elastolytic Activity from
        Blood Platelets. Nature 227, #5264: 1248, Sept. 19, 1970.

    Legrand, Y., Robert, B., Szigeti, M., Pignaud, G., Caen, J.
        and Robert, L.: Etudes Sur Une Protease Elastinolytique
        des Plaquettes Sanguines Humaines. Atherosclerosis 12:
        451, 1970.

MIX
Papier aus verantwortungsvollen Quellen
Paper from responsible sources
FSC® C105338

If you have any concerns about our products,
you can contact us on
ProductSafety@springernature.com

In case Publisher is established outside the EU,
the EU authorized representative is:
Springer Nature Customer Service Center GmbH
Europaplatz 3, 69115 Heidelberg, Germany

Printed by Libri Plureos GmbH
in Hamburg, Germany